Asthma and Infections

LUNG BIOLOGY IN HEALTH AND DISEASE

Executive Editor

Claude Lenfant

Former Director, National Heart, Lung, and Blood Institute
National Institutes of Health
Bethesda, Maryland

For information on volumes 25–188 in the *Lung Biology in Health and Disease* series, please visit www.informahealthcare.com

The opinions expressed in these volumes do not necessarily represent the views of the National Institutes of Health.

Asthma and Infections

edited by

Richard J. Martin
National Jewish Health
University of Colorado Denver
Denver, Colorado, USA

E. Rand Sutherland
National Jewish Health
University of Colorado Denver
Denver, Colorado, USA

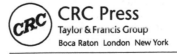

CRC Press
Taylor & Francis Group
Boca Raton London New York

CRC Press is an imprint of the
Taylor & Francis Group, an **Informa** business

First published 2010 by Informa Healthcare, Inc.

Published 2019 by CRC Press
Taylor & Francis Group
6000 Broken Sound Parkway NW, Suite 300
Boca Raton, FL 33487-2742

First issued in paperback 2019

No claim to original U.S. Government works

ISBN 13: 978-0-367-44601-7 (pbk)
ISBN 13: 978-1-4200-9299-8 (hbk)

Visit the Taylor & Francis Web site at
http://www.taylorandfrancis.com

and the CRC Press Web site at
http://www.crcpress.com

Library of Congress Cataloging-in-Publication Data

Asthma and infections / edited by Richard J. Martin, E. Rand Sutherland.
    p. ; cm. – (Lung biology in health and disease ; v. 238)
    Includes bibliographical references and index.
    ISBN-13: 978-1-4200-9299-8 (hb : alk. paper)
    ISBN-10: 1-4200-9299-5 (hb : alk. paper) 1. Respiratory infections.
2. Asthma. I. Martin, Richard J. (Richard Jay), 1946- II. Sutherland, E. Rand. III. Series: Lung biology in health and disease ; v. 238.
    [DNLM: 1. Respiratory Tract Infections–diagnosis. 2. Asthma–microbiology.
3. Hypersensitivity–immunology. W1 LU62 v.238 2009 / WF 553 A85472 2009]
    RC740.A88 2009
    616.2'38–dc22

                                                    2009031091

To Elana Rose Schaffer, my granddaughter who adds so much to life
Richard Martin

To my wife and children, Julie, Sam, Emma, and Eliza with love and appreciation
E. Rand Sutherland

Introduction

For many years, the clinical community, especially pediatricians, have suspected an association of pulmonary infection with asthma. The object of this matter has been primarily focused on the possible link between asthma and respiratory syncytial virus (RSV), but questions have been raised about the role of bacterial organisms as well.

The main point of attention has been whether viral infections are a determinant risk factor for asthma exacerbations, but the question has also been raised about whether RSV infection may be the cause of asthma. An editorial by C. K. Kuehni and E. M. Silverman titled "Causal Links Between RSV Infection and Asthma: No Clear Answers to an Old Question" (1) identifies the problems and admits that research has not clearly answered the questions but has raised many new ones.

Bacterial infections, including atypical ones such as *Clamydia pneumoniae* and more common ones such as *Streptococcus pneumoniae*, have also been linked to asthma mostly as exacerbating factors. However, while the questions about bacteria-asthma associations are of dominant importance, they have received less attention than the virus-asthma association.

This volume, edited by Richard J. Martin and E. Rand Sutherland and titled *Asthma and Infections* opens the door on the entire "landscape" of the important question of the relationship between asthma and infection. Not only does it present the facts but raises questions that will stimulate the clinical and research communities to explore new avenues that may provide "clear answers to old questions!" The editors and contributors are internationally recognized in the field of asthma research and clinical care, and thus, the series of monographs Lung Biology in Health and Disease is very grateful to them for the opportunity to present this volume to its readership.

Claude Lenfant, MD
Vancouver, Washington, U.S.A.

Reference

1. Kuehni CK, Silverman EM. Causal links between RSV infection and asthma: no clear answers to an old question. Am J Respir Crit Care Med 2009; 179:1079–1080.

Preface

The area of how infection alters asthma has been speculated on for centuries. More recently, newer techniques have been developed to increase accuracy in determining if bacteria or viruses populate the airways of patients. This has led to renewed scientific investigation about the interaction between infection and the acute exacerbation of asthma, as well as the propagation of asthma on a chronic basis. This publication will assist the reader to understand the role of microbes in acute and chronic asthma, learn how infection alters innate and adaptive immunity, and understand how antibiotic and anti-inflammatory agents affect bacteria and asthma. Knowledge will be gained with respect to the interaction between allergen and infection and how this interaction propagates chronic asthma. Furthermore, the text will help the reader to determine the best techniques to diagnose respiratory infection.

Both the clinician and the researcher will derive benefit from this text. In the clinical setting, this volume will be invaluable to pulmonologists, allergists/clinical immunologists, and infectious disease specialists with information about presentation, diagnosis, and therapy. For a basic, translational, and clinical researcher investigating asthma with relationship to bacterial and viral infection, inflammation, and allergic responses, this text will bring up-to-date information to help guide ideas and suggest potential future investigation that is needed.

Richard J. Martin
E. Rand Sutherland

Contributors

Hong W. Chu   National Jewish Health, Denver, Colorado, U.S.A.

Fabienne Gally   National Jewish Health, Denver, Colorado, U.S.A.

James E. Gern   University of Wisconsin Medical School, Madison, Wisconsin, U.S.A.

Ronald J. Harbeck   Advanced Diagnostic Laboratories, National Jewish Health, Denver, Colorado, U.S.A.

Druhan Howell   Duke University Medical Center, Durham, North Carolina, U.S.A.

Sebastian L. Johnston   National Heart and Lung Institute, Imperial College London, London, U.K.

Monica Kraft   Duke University Medical Center, Durham, North Carolina, U.S.A.

Andrew H. Liu   National Jewish Health and University of Colorado Denver School of Medicine, Denver, Colorado, U.S.A.

Jonathan D. R. Macintyre   National Heart and Lung Institute, Imperial College London, London, U.K.

Richard J. Martin   National Jewish Health, Denver, Colorado, U.S.A.

Fernando D. Martinez   Arizona Respiratory Center, The University of Arizona, Tucson, Arizona, U.S.A.

Dawn C. Newcomb   Vanderbilt University Medical School, Nashville, Tennessee, U.S.A.

Mari Numata   National Jewish Health, Denver, Colorado, U.S.A.

R. Stokes Peebles, Jr.   Vanderbilt University Medical School, Nashville, Tennessee, U.S.A.

Kaharu Sumino   Washington University School of Medicine, St. Louis, Missouri, U.S.A.

E. Rand Sutherland   National Jewish Health and University of Colorado Health Sciences Center, Denver, Colorado, U.S.A.

Annemarie Sykes   National Heart and Lung Institute, Imperial College London, London, U.K.

Dennis R. Voelker   National Jewish Health, Denver, Colorado, U.S.A.

Michael J. Walter   Washington University School of Medicine, St. Louis, Missouri, U.S.A.

Contents

1

Overview of the Infection, Allergy, and Asthma Relationship

DAWN C. NEWCOMB and R. STOKES PEEBLES, JR.
Vanderbilt University Medical School, Nashville, Tennessee, U.S.A.

I. Introduction

Infections and asthma are intricately interwoven disease processes. Infections have been associated with acute exacerbations of asthma, the maintenance of a chronic asthma phenotype, as well as asthma inception. New evidence suggests that the innate immune response of persons with asthma is unique compared with that of nonasthmatics, leading to the profound differences in severity of illness between these two populations. In this chapter, we will focus on the relationship between bacteria and asthma; namely, first, whether bacterial infections cause asthma symptoms; second, whether asthmatics are more susceptible to bacterial infections; and last, recent data suggesting that bacterial infections may be involved in asthma inception. Next, we will review the relationship between viral infections and asthma; first, examining the overwhelming data that viral infections are causative for asthma exacerbations; second, exploring whether asthmatics experience more severe consequences to viral infection; and last, new data proposing that early-life viral infections may be a major determinant of the development of asthma in childhood.

II. Bacterial Infections and Asthma Exacerbations

Infections have long been recognized as a cause of asthma exacerbations. Sir William Osler wrote in his 1892 initial edition of *Principles and Practice of Medicine*, which is considered to be the first textbook of modern medicine, that paroxysms of asthma could be elicited by local climate conditions, breathing the air of certain rooms, emanations of animals, diet, and "every fresh cold" (1).

During Osler's time, viruses had not yet been identified, and in the first few decades of the 20th century, many physicians who took care of asthma patients believed that bacteria, presumed to cause upper respiratory tract infections, were responsible for worsening of asthma, although this premise was not universally held (2). For those who were advocates of "bacterial asthma," the prevailing concept was that subjects who experienced asthma exacerbations with bacterial infections had immediate-type hypersensitivity to bacterial antigens and the allergic reaction to these antigens triggered the exacerbation (2). Data in support of bacterial hypersensitivity causing asthma flares largely came from uncontrolled trials of autogenous vaccine preparations used for the diagnosis of bacterial allergy and prevention of exacerbations. In a 1924 report from

Thomas and Touart, the vaccines used in their study consisted of cultures from a subject's own sputum, excised tonsils, nares, pharynx, or tonsils in situ (2). However, in this report, when vaccines did not provide positive skin tests, they were made from bacterial cultures of stool. Such vaccines were administered at an initial dose of 100 million killed organisms with two to three days intervals between injections. The dose was then escalated to 400 million organisms per injection, with intervals between injections increased to every five to seven days. Once symptoms improved, the interval between injections was increased from once per week to once per month to prevent relapses of asthma exacerbations. These authors reported that in 62 asthmatic patients who had positive skin tests to the vaccine material prepared from that specific patient's body fluid or tissues, 87.1% had either "complete relief or material improvement" of their asthma when treated with the vaccine (2).

By 1933, the controversy over the use of bacterial vaccines in asthma treatment was increasing. Wilmer and Cobe wrote that "the actual status of vaccine therapy in general ranges today from utter condemnation by one class of internists to complete dependence by another class" (3). While Wilmer and Cobe wrote that bacterial vaccines were "'gunshot' methods of diagnosis and treatment" and that such indiscriminate use of vaccines should be condemned, they also noted that "allergists will protest loudly that vaccines are impractical and unscientific and continue to use them as blindly as when they were first put on the market." However, after their investigation of 150 asthmatic subjects who were treated with either "stock" bacterial vaccines prepared by commercial biologic laboratories or autogenous vaccines, these authors concluded that "bacterial allergy is a definite pathologic entity which responds to bacterin therapy, either through desensitization, increased phagocytosis, or stimulated antibody formation. Selective vaccines based on skin reactions give the best results and appear to be on a more scientific basis than other types of vaccines." These conclusions were based on the authors' observations that 63.6% of 66 asthma cases were either cured or improved with autogenous vaccine therapy in an uncontrolled trial (3). Detractors of the bacterial allergy theory pointed out that while extracts of environmental allergens such as pollens or animal dander could produce positive immediate skin test results in sensitive subjects, bacterial extracts did not provoke such hypersensitivity reactions and instead caused local erythematous reactions (4).

The era of "bacterial allergy" as an etiology of asthma exacerbations and the use of autogenous bacterial vaccines in the treatment of asthma came to an end in the late 1950s and early 1960s. Large placebo-controlled trials revealed that vaccines consisting primarily of *Streptococcus viridans*, *Hemophilus influenzae*, pneumococcus (mixed types), *Staphylococcus* (mixed types), *Moraxella catarrhalis*, and *Klebsiella pneumoniae* improved asthma symptoms in approximately 50% to 65% of patients; however, this response rate was the same as that in case of placebo injections (4–6). The conclusion of these studies was that "ordinary palliative measures, combined with the psychologic support supplied by a weekly visit to and injection by the patient's own doctor, are capable of giving prolonged benefit to half the patients" (6).

Although the belief that bacteria caused asthma exacerbations though they induced immediate hypersensitivity reactions fell out of favor by the 1960s, the concept that bacterial infections might be involved in exacerbation pathogenesis continued to be investigated in the 1970s and 1980s. In separate studies, McIntosh and Hudgel sought to determine if bacteria could be isolated more frequently in the respiratory tract secretions of subjects who were experiencing asthma exacerbations compared with times when the same subjects were asymptomatic (7,8). McIntosh and colleagues reported that the identification rate of *pneumococcus, H. influenzae,* and *Staphylococcus* was as frequent when subjects were in exacerbation as when they were without wheezing, suggesting that bacterial infections were not etiologic for worsening symptoms (8). Hudgel also found that bacterial cultures were positive at the same rate when subjects experienced asthma flares as when they were well (7). These studies suggested that bacterial infections may not be responsible for asthma exacerbations.

To more definitively determine whether bacterial infections might impact disease pathogenesis and disease course, intervention studies were necessary. Shapiro and colleagues noted that in the early 1970s, antibiotics were often recommended in the management of severe asthma exacerbations, despite a lack of conclusive clinical evidence that bacterial infections were present in disease flares (9). Therefore, these investigators performed a randomized, double-blind, placebo-controlled trial comparing treatment with hetacillin, the active form of which was ampicillin, in children hospitalized with status asthmaticus. They found that hetacillin had no impact on hospital length of stay, hospital course, complications, or pulmonary function and concluded that the use of broad-spectrum antibiotics in children with severe asthma exacerbations was of no clinical benefit in the absence of clear bacterial disease (9). Similarly, Graham and colleagues reported in 1982 that in a randomized, placebo-controlled trial of 60 adult subjects admitted to the hospital with asthma exacerbations, amoxicillin had no impact on hospital length of stay, the time necessary for a 50% improvement in symptoms, symptom scores, and pulmonary function either during the hospital course or at the time of discharge (10). These authors also concluded that antibiotic therapy should not routinely be administered to patients admitted with acute asthma exacerbations.

The studies in the 1970s and 1980s examining the impact of bacterial infections on asthma exacerbations focused predominantly on the organisms that cause the majority of respiratory tract infections, primarily encapsulated organisms such as *Streptococcus pneumoniae, H. influenzae,* and *M. catarrhalis,* and the antibiotics chosen in the intervention studies were active against these pathogens; however, atypical bacteria such as *Mycoplasma pneumoniae* and *Chlamydia pneumoniae* were not investigated. The possibility that these pathogens might be an important cause of asthma exacerbations was proposed by Kraft and Martin who found that *M. pneumoniae* was detected in the respiratory tract secretions by polymerase chain reaction (PCR) in 10 of 18 (55%) subjects with chronic stable asthma and only 1 of 11 (9%) nonasthmatic control subjects (11). The importance of PCR for detection of *Mycoplasma* was critical as cultures, enzyme-linked immunoassay, and serology were all negative for this organism (11). In contrast, PCR and cultures were negative for *C. pneumoniae* in the subjects with chronic stable asthma; however, 9 of the 18 (50%) of these subjects had positive serology for *M. pneumoniae,* while only 1 of 11 (9%) nonasthmatic control subjects had positive serology (11). A larger follow-up study by this same group revealed that 25 of 55 (45%) chronic stable asthma subjects had either bronchoalveolar lavage fluid or lung biopsy specimens that were PCR positive for *M. pneumoniae,* while 6 of 55 (11%) subjects had detectable *C. pneumoniae* by PCR on these same specimens (12). Lieberman and colleagues also found an increased prevalence of *M. pneumoniae* in the respiratory tract secretions of Israeli adults with acute asthma exacerbations compared with control subjects (13). While there was no difference in the detection rate of

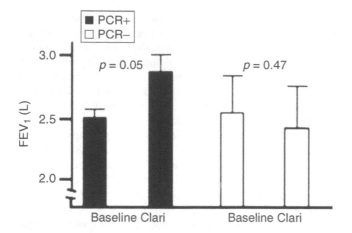

Figure 1 FEV$_1$ before and after treatment in the clarithromycin (Clari) groups with positive PCR findings (PCR$^+$) and negative PCR findings (PCR$^-$). *Abbreviations*: FEV$_1$, forced expiratory volume in 1 second; PCR, polymerase chain reaction. *Source*: From Ref. 14.

S. pneumoniae, *Legionella* species, or *C. pneumoniae* between asthmatic subjects in exacerbation and controls, *M. pneumoniae* was detected in 18% of adults with asthma exacerbations and in only 3% of controls (13).

To further explore the possible contribution of atypical bacteria such as *M. pneumoniae* and *C. pneumoniae* to asthma pathogenesis, Kraft and Martin performed an intervention study in which they treated subjects with chronic stable asthma with clarithromycin, an antibiotic that has activity against both these pathogens (14). Subjects who had *Mycoplasma pneumoniae* and *Chlamydia pneumoniae* detectable by PCR in airway biopsies or bronchoalveolar lavage fluid (BAL) fluid had a significant improvement in forced expiratory volume in 1 second (FEV$_1$) following clarithromycin treatment (Fig. 1), while there was no such improvement in the pulmonary function of those subjects that were PCR negative for these organisms (14). Clarithromycin also reduced proinflammatory cytokine mRNA expression in the airways of both the subjects that were PCR positive for *M. pneumoniae* and *C. pneumoniae* (decreased in TNF, IL-5, and IL-12 mRNA in BAL and TNF mRNA in airway tissue) and those that were PCR negative for these atypical bacterial (reduction in TNF and IL-12 mRNA in BAL and TNF-α mRNA in airway tissue) (14).

Another invention study using macrolide antibiotics was performed in subjects with an acute exacerbation of asthma by Johnston and colleagues (15). In a double-blind, randomized, placebo-controlled study of 278 subjects who were enrolled within 24 hours of an acute exacerbation, telithromycin or placebo was initiated in addition to usual asthma care. In this study, subjects who received telithromycin had a statistically significant greater reduction in asthma symptoms compared with the placebo-treated group; however, there was no relationship in symptom improvement based on *M. pneumoniae* and *C. pneumoniae*, nor did treatment have an impact on morning peak flow rates (15).

It is important to note that there are important differences in the patient populations between the Kraft and Martin study and the one performed by Johnston and colleagues; most notably, that one examined chronic stable asthmatics, while the other was in adults with acute exacerbations, and these population differences may be a critical factor in the outcomes witnessed (14,15). To further define the role of atypical bacterial and macrolide treatment in asthma care, the Asthma Clinical Research Network (ACRN) trial has a currently ongoing trial called Macrolides in Asthma (MIA) in which 144 subjects are proposed to be enrolled who will be treated with 16 weeks of clarithromycin 500 mg twice daily plus an inhaled steroid (fluticasone propionate 88 mcg twice daily) or the same dose of inhaled steroid alone (ClinicalTrials.gov identifier NCT00318708). The primary end point is asthma control as determined by standardized questionnaire, with secondary end points including symptoms, rescue medication use, pulmonary function, methacholine reactivity, and exhaled nitric oxide levels. Completion of this study is scheduled for August 2009 and will hopefully clarify the importance of *Mycoplasma* and *Chlamydia*, and focused treatment for these organisms on the course of asthmatic symptoms.

III. Asthma and Severity of Bacterial Infections

S. pneumoniae is an important cause of morbidity and mortality in the United States. The 23-valent pneumococcal vaccine is currently recommended by the Center for Disease Control and Prevention (CDC) for persons with chronic obstructive lung diseases such as emphysema and chronic bronchitis, but these recommendations specifically exclude asthma as a cause for vaccination (16). Talbot and colleagues performed a nested case control study of persons aged 2 to 49 years enrolled in the Tennessee Medicaid from 1995 to 1999 to determine if persons with asthma were at greater risk for invasive pneumococcal disease than nonasthmatics (17). Invasive pneumococcal disease was defined as the isolation of *S. pneumoniae* from a site that is normally sterile, such as blood, cerebrospinal fluid, pleural fluid, peritoneal fluid, pericardial fluid, surgical aspirate, bone, or joint fluid. Among subjects without coexisting conditions that increased the risk for invasive pneumococcal disease, persons with high-risk asthma (defined as having had an asthma-related hospitalization or emergency department visit in the last year, an oral corticosteroid course, or three or more β-agonist prescriptions in the last year) had an annual incidence of invasive pneumococcal disease that was 4.2 episodes per 10,000 persons, while the incidence was 2.3 episodes in persons with low-risk asthma (outpatient visits for asthma and prescription of medications specific for asthma), and 1.2 episodes in persons without asthma (17). These results suggested that asthma was an independent risk factor for invasive pneumococcal disease in that the risk was at least double for asthmatics than that for controls. These results were supported by Juhn and colleagues who performed a retrospective case control study of residents of Rochester, Minnesota from 1964 to 1983 (18). In this analysis, they reported that severe pneumococcal disease (invasive pneumococcal disease, pneumococcal pneumonia, or both) was associated with asthma, with a significantly increased odds ratio of 6.7 in adults, controlling for high-risk conditions for invasive pneumococcal disease and smoking exposure (18). These two studies, in very different patient populations over two different time periods, suggest that asthma is a high-risk condition for serious pneumococcal disease.

The possibility that asthma might be a risk factor not only for invasive pneumococcal disease but also for community-acquired pneumonia was strengthened by Almirall and colleagues who performed a population-based, case control study of 859,033 persons who lived on the eastern coast of Spain in 1999 to 2000 (19). These investigators found in multivariate analysis that, in addition to cigarette smoking, usual contact with children, inhalational therapy, oxygen therapy, and chronic bronchitis, asthma was a significant independent risk factor for community-acquired pneumonia (19).

These three epidemiologic studies could have a profound impact on routine asthma care, vaccination practices, and health utilization costs. The Advisory Committee of Immunization Practices for the Department of Health and Human Services and the CDC recently unanimously voted that asthma be included among the chronic obstructive pulmonary diseases for which the 23-valent pneumococcal polysaccharide vaccine be recommended (20). It is currently estimated that 20 million persons have asthma (21). The private-sector cost of the 23-valent pneumococcal polysaccharide vaccine is $32.99 (22), therefore, the cost of vaccinating all asthmatics in the United States would be approximately $660,000,000. In addition, the treatment guidelines for asthma would need to be changed as they do not currently include the 23-valent pneumococcal polysaccharide vaccine as a recommendation (23).

These epidemiologic studies only reveal that there is an increased risk for invasive pneumococcal disease and community-acquired pneumonia in asthmatic subjects but do not inform as to the mechanisms by which this increased risk occurs. Possible contributing factors might include the disrupted airway epithelial barrier that is noted in bronchial biopsy specimens from asthmatics, augmented mucus production, defective innate and/or adaptive immunity, and possible genetic factors linked to asthma that may alter the immune response to infectious organisms (24). The possibility that the airway epithelium of asthmatic subjects is different from that of non-asthmatic persons is supported by Kraft and colleagues who found that *M. pneumoniae* induced the major airway mucin (MUC)5AC mRNA and protein expression in airway epithelial cells isolated from asthmatic subjects but not from similarly cultured epithelial cells from control subjects (25). More work will need to be performed to determine the actual mechanisms by which asthmatics are at greater risk for more severe pneumococcal disease.

IV. Bacterial Infection and Inception of Asthma

There are few studies examining the relationship between bacterial infection in early life and the subsequent development of asthma. In examining this issue, it is difficult to know if an increased presence of certain bacteria in the airway of children who later develop asthma predispose to the development of asthma or whether the immune response that is a consequence of factors specific to asthma is responsible for a certain bacterial colonization pattern. In the latter case, the underlying immune response that is responsible for asthma defines the bacteria present in the airway, and the bacteria themselves have no impact on asthma development. Bisgaard and colleagues recently examined the association between bacterial colonization in the hypopharynx of neonates and the subsequent phenotype of wheeze, asthma, and allergy at age 5 (26). The subjects were offsprings of mothers who had asthma and were enrolled in the Copenhagen Prospective Study on Asthma in Childhood birth cohort. In this study population, 21% of infants who had hypopharyngeal colonization at one month of age with *S. pneumoniae*, *M. catarrhalis*, *H. influenzae*, or a combination of these organisms had a significantly increased hazard ratio of having persistent wheeze, acute severe exacerbation of wheeze, and hospitalization for wheeze. In addition, children colonized with the above organisms at one month of age also had significantly increased blood eosinophilia and total, but not antigen-specific, IgE. Colonization at 12 months had no impact on the wheezing phenotypes mentioned above (26). The mechanism by which the bacterial colonization pattern seen in this study may impact asthma development is unclear. Bacterial activation of certain toll-like receptors, or perhaps lack of activation of others, may predispose to the development of asthma (27). On the other hand, perhaps the presence of the bacteria found by Bisgaard in subjects who later had wheezing is solely a consequence of a defective innate immune response related to asthma (27). Further studies will be necessary to fully define the relationship between early-life bacterial infections and asthma.

A. Viral Infections and Asthma Exacerbations

As Osler noted, every fresh cold was a predisposing factor for asthma exacerbations (1). One of the reasons it took almost a century to prove Osler right is that the detection methods for viral infections were relatively insensitive and, up until the advent of PCR, led to false negative results. Similar to studies performed in the 1970s to determine if upper respiratory bacterial infections were more common in asthmatic subjects when they were wheezing compared with when they were asymptomatic (which, as mentioned earlier, was not the case), investigators also sought to determine if the viruses could be detected more frequently when asthmatics were wheezing than when they felt well. Studies using the relatively insensitive viral detection techniques such as culture, immunofluorescence, and serology revealed that viruses were present from two to five times more frequently when asthmatic subjects were in exacerbation compared with when they were without symptoms (7,28–30).

By the mid-1990s, PCR technology was being used in clinical research studies and revealed that viruses could be detected in the respiratory tract secretions far more frequently during asthma exacerbations than previously considered (Table 1).

In a landmark report, Johnston and colleagues found in a community-based 13-month longitudinal study of British children 9 to 11 years old that viruses could be detected in the respiratory tract secretions in 80% of reported episodes of reduced peak expiratory flow, 80% of reported episodes of wheeze, and 85% of reported episodes of upper respiratory symptoms, cough, wheeze, and a fall in peak expiratory flow (31). Atmar and colleagues also found that viruses were detected at a high rate in adults who experienced asthma exacerbations in Houston, Texas (35). In a longitudinal cohort study of asthmatic adults who were recruited from the pulmonary clinic of an urban county hospital, 44% of asthma exacerbations were associated with a respiratory tract viral infection (35). In asthmatic adults presenting to the emergency department with acute symptoms, 55% of asthma exacerbations were associated with a respiratory tract viral infection. Fifty percent of the asthmatic subjects admitted from the emergency department with an asthma exacerbation had detectable virus in the respiratory tract secretions. It is important to note that 60% of the picornavirus infections and 71% of the 31 coronavirus infections were identified using only reverse transcriptase (RT)-PCR, thus emphasizing the importance of a sensitive method in detecting the presence of viral infections (35). In both the studies of British school children and adults in Houston, rhinoviruses, members of the picornavirus family, were by far the most common type of

Table 1 Pathogens Detected from Patients with Asthma Exacerbations

Pathogen	Nucleic acid of pathogen	Subtypes	Diseases	Percentage detected in exacerbations (12,13,31–34)
Adenovirus	Nonenveloped dsRNA	1–49	Pneumonia, acute respiratory distress	<1
Coronavirus	Enveloped (+) ssRNA	229E, OC43, SARS	Common cold (229E and OC43), SARS	26–40
Human metapneumovirus	Enveloped (−) ssRNA	A–D	Cold-like symptoms (URI), bronchiolitis, pneumonia (LRI)	7
Influenza	Enveloped (−) ssRNA	A–C	Pneumonia	2–9
Parainfluenza	Enveloped (−) ssRNA	1–4	Croup, common cold,	3–9
Respiratory syncytial virus	Enveloped (−) ssRNA	A–B	Cold-like symptoms (URI), bronchiolitis, pneumonia (LRI)	1–12
Rhinovirus	Nonenveloped (+) ssRNA	A–C (100+ serotypes)	Common cold	34–75
Mycoplasma pneumoniae Atypical bacteria	DNA/RNA	–	URI, pneumonia, pleural effusions	18–46
Chlamydia pneumoniae Atypical bacteria	DNA/RNA	–	Pneumonia bronchiolitis	2–12

Abbreviations: SARS, severe acute respiratory syndrome; dsRNA, double-stranded RNA; ssRNA, single-stranded RNA; URI, upper respiratory infection; LRI, lower respiratory infection.

virus detected in the respiratory tract secretions of asthmatic subjects. Since rhinoviruses are an important cause of asthma exacerbations, one might expect to see an increase in asthma exacerbations during the peak of the rhinovirus season, and this is indeed the case. Sears and Johnston noted that hospital admissions, emergency department visits, and outpatient physician visits for childhood asthma predictably increase each September in many Northern Hemisphere countries, which is the peak of rhinovirus detection in these countries (36). Such asthma epidemics have been reported in the United States, the United Kingdom, Mexico, Israel, Finland, Trinidad, and Canada, where one-fifth to one quarter of all childhood asthma exacerbations requiring hospitalization occur in September (36).

B. Asthma and Severity of Viral Infection

There have been few studies performed examining the difference in severity of illness between asthmatics and nonasthmatics who are infected with viral respiratory infections. Corne and colleagues investigated 76 cohabiting couples in which one person in each of the couple had aeroallergen sensitivity by skin testing and asthma and the other member of the couple was not allergic and did not have asthma (37). They followed these couples over a four-month period, and every two weeks nasal aspirates were obtained and examined for rhinovirus by PCR. There was no significant difference between the rhinovirus detection rate for the allergic asthmatic subjects and nonasthmatic controls (10.1% vs. 8.5%, respectively) (37). After adjusting for confounding factors, asthma did not significantly increase the risk of rhinovirus infection. However, the first rhinovirus infection was associated more frequently with lower respiratory tract symptoms (wheeze, cough, shortness of breath, or chest tightness) in persons with asthma than in the nonasthmatics. In addition, the symptoms of lower respiratory tract infection were significantly more severe and longer lasting in subjects with asthma than in the nonasthmatics (37).

Other respiratory tract viruses also cause greater severity of illness in asthmatics compared with those without asthma. Pregnant women with asthma have a much greater morbidity associated with influenza infection than nonasthmatic women (38). Hartert and colleagues performed a matched cohort study utilizing an administrative database of pregnant women aged 15 to 44 years enrolled in the Tennessee Medicaid population to determine pregnancy outcomes associated with respiratory hospitalizations during influenza season (38). Pregnant women hospitalized during influenza seasons 1985 to 1993 were matched by gestational age and presence of comorbidity with pregnant control subjects without a respiratory hospitalization. These investigators found that during the study period, women with singleton pregnancies had respiratory disease hospitalizations at a rate of 5.1:1000. However, women with asthma had a log increase in rate of such hospitalization at 59.7:1000. Despite the greater hospitalization rate among the asthmatic women with respiratory-related hospitalization, there was no difference between asthmatic and nonasthmatic women in mode of delivery, delivery length of stay, episodes of preterm labor, prevalence of prematurity, and low infant birth weight (38).

As with bacterial infections, the mechanisms by which asthmatics have more severe symptoms with viral infection are unknown; however, defective innate immunity may be a common thread. Wark and colleagues found that primary bronchial epithelial cells from asthmatic subjects had decreased interferon (IFN)-β production compared with primary epithelial cells obtained from healthy control subjects (39). Additionally, the bronchial epithelial cells from asthmatic subjects had delayed virus-induced cell lysis, decreased caspase activity and apoptosis, and a 50-fold increase in viral RNA expression compared with the control bronchial epithelial cells (39). Similarly, Contoli and colleagues found that primary bronchial epithelial cells from asthmatic subjects produced significantly lower levels of IFN-λ compared with control bronchial epithelial cells and that there was a significant correlation between severity of rhinovirus-induced asthma exacerbations and virus load (40). Thus, there is evidence that airway epithelial cells are functionally different between asthmatics and nonasthmatics, even in vitro, after the other factors associated with the asthmatic milieu are no longer present.

V.   Viral Infection and Inception of Asthma

In contrast to the few studies examining the relationship between early-life bacterial infection and the subsequent asthma phenotype, there are many studies examining the relationship between early viral bronchiolitis and the later diagnosis of asthma. Most of these studies have focused on respiratory syncytial virus (RSV) as this is the predominant virus associated with infant hospitalization for wheezing (41). Two long-term longitudinal studies have followed children who experienced lower respiratory tract infections with RSV during infancy and examined the subsequent rate of asthma diagnosis. Sigurs and colleagues enrolled 47 infants who had severe RSV bronchiolitis to the degree that they were hospitalized in the winter of 1989 to 1990 (42). They matched these infants with 93 controls who were admitted to the hospital for other diagnoses, and have then followed them at regular intervals up to age 13. The children with severe RSV bronchiolitis during infancy consistently had significantly higher rates of physician-diagnosed asthma at age 1, 3, 7½, and 13 compared with control subjects. In addition, the children who experienced severe infant RSV bronchiolitis also have had significantly greater allergic sensitization as diagnosed by both skin test reactivity and measurement of antigen-specific IgE (42). Stein and colleagues followed over 1200 children enrolled prospectively in the Tucson Children's Respiratory Study and found that children with lower respiratory tract infection with RSV before age 1 had a significant increase in the odds ratio of having both frequent and infrequent wheezes at ages 6 and 11 compared with children who did not experience a lower respiratory tract infection in infancy (43). However, there was no increased risk of wheezing at age 13 in the children with the RSV lower respiratory tract infection during infancy (43). A possible explanation for the differences seen in the Sigurs and Stein studies is that the subjects in the Sigurs study required hospitalization and may have experienced more severe bronchiolitis than the children who were outpatients in the Stein cohort.

The relationship between severity of illness during bronchiolitis and subsequent development of asthma later in childhood has been further explored by Wu and colleagues who found that birth timing in relationship to the peak of hospitalization for bronchiolitis determines the risk of severe bronchiolitis during infancy, as well as the risk of developing asthma (44). Their results suggest that severe bronchiolitis, or some factor closely associated with this phenotype, might cause asthma. In this investigation, a cohort of over 95,000 children enrolled in the Tennessee Medicaid program who were born between 1995 and 2000 were followed over their first five viral seasons until the age of 5½ years. This cohort includes approximately one quarter of the births each year in that state. First, the timing of infant birth in relationship to the winter virus peak, as defined as the first day of the week with the highest number of bronchiolitis hospitalizations for that winter season, predicted the likelihood of developing clinically significant bronchiolitis (Fig. 2) (44). Clinically significant bronchiolitis was defined as hospitalization, emergency department visit, or outpatient visit. After adjusting for other factors previously reported to be associated with severe bronchiolitis, infants 122 days (95% CI, 118–126 days) old at the winter virus peak had the greatest risk of developing clinically significant bronchiolitis. Second, the timing of infant birth in relationship to the winter virus peak predicted the likelihood of developing childhood asthma as defined ICD-9 code or medication use for asthma (Fig. 3). Children who were 121 days (95% CI, 108–131 days) old at the winter virus peak had the greatest risk of developing high-risk asthma when a comparison was made with children who were either older or younger at the peak of the winter virus season (44). Compared with children who were 365 days old at the winter virus peak, there was a 29% increase in odds of developing high-risk childhood asthma for children who were 121 days of age at the winter virus peak, the

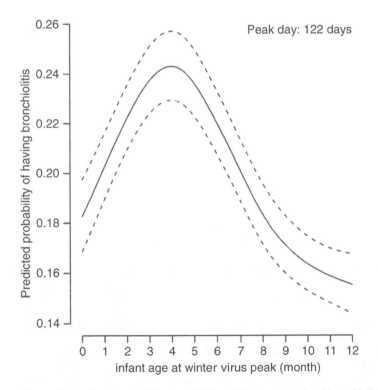

Figure 2 Predicted probability and 95% confidence intervals of bronchiolitis requiring a health care visit during infancy (hospitalization, emergency department visit, or outpatient visit) by infant age in months at the winter virus peak ($\chi_3^2 = 345.52$; $p < 0.001$). Results were obtained from a multivariable logistic regression model. Effect was adjusted for gender, infant race, birth weight, gestational age, number of living siblings, region of residence, maternal smoking, marital status, maternal education, and season. *Source*: From Ref. 44.

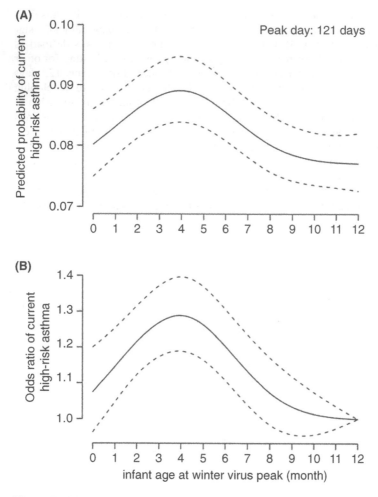

Figure 3 Differential risk of developing current high-risk childhood asthma in relationship to infant age at the winter virus peak. Results were obtained from a multivariable logistic regression model adjusted for gender, infant race, birth weight, gestational age, number of living siblings, region of residence, maternal smoking, marital status, maternal education, and season. (**A**) Predicted probability and 95% CI of developing current high-risk childhood asthma by infant age in months at the winter virus peak ($\chi_3^2 = 49.05$; $p < 0.001$). The area under the curve is equal to the asthma prevalence of the population. (**B**) Adjusted odds ratio and 95% CI of developing current high-risk childhood asthma relative to children who were 12 months of age at the winter virus peak. Infants who were one year of age at the winter virus peak served as the reference group. *Abbreviation*: CI, confidence interval. *Source*: From Ref. 44.

almost identical infant age at winter virus peak that conferred the greatest risk of bronchiolitis. High-risk asthma was defined as asthma-related hospitalization, emergency department treatment, or rescue corticosteroid prescription. Despite the fact that the winter virus peak shifted as much as six weeks over the five viral seasons studied for each child, this relationship of age at peak viral season with the subsequent development of asthma was not affected when subgroup analysis was conducted on children who encountered early or late winter virus peaks. Interestingly, maternal history of asthma had no effect on this analysis (44).

Wu and colleagues speculated that two possible explanations for the relationship between the timing of the peak of the viral season and the increased risk of developing both significant bronchiolitis and high-risk asthma might exist (44). The first is that a common genetic predisposition could result in both severe winter viral bronchiolitis and asthma, while another possibility is that an environmental exposure such as winter viral infection leads to asthma. The data presented does not exclude either or both of these possibilities. One of the most interesting aspects of this study is the risk of developing either bronchiolitis or asthma by timing of birth in relationship to the winter virus peak present for every year analyzed, despite the fact that the timing of the viral peak shifted from year to year. Thus, birth around four months of age (120 days) before the peak of the viral season led to a significantly increased risk of developing both bronchiolitis and subsequent asthma (44).

While most of the exploration of the relationship between early-life viral infection and asthma inception has centered on RSV, new data suggests that rhinovirus lower respiratory tract infection in infancy may be an important risk factor for later asthma development. Jackson and colleagues have found that rhinovirus infections that result in wheezing illness in the first three years of life predict asthma development in children who are deemed high risk because of a family history of allergy or asthma and that this risk surpasses that associated with early-life wheezing from RSV infection (45). In this study, 259 children enrolled in the University of Wisconsin Childhood Origins of Asthma (COAST) study were followed prospectively for six years and had met entry criteria because either one or both parents had a history of positive skin tests to aeroallergens or physician-diagnosed asthma (45). The presence of virus in respiratory tract secretions in early life was determined by PCR and standard viral detection techniques at scheduled monthly intervals during the first year of life and when subjects developed respiratory tract illnesses. The assays incorporated potential detection for rhinovirus, RSV, parainfluenza virus types 1 to 4, influenza types A and B, adenovirus, enterovirus, coronavirus, and metapneumovirus (45).

Analysis of respiratory tract secretions revealed that viruses were present in these fluids 90% of the time that wheezing illnesses occurred in the first three years of life. Rhinovirus was the virus most frequently detected (48%), followed by RSV (21%) and parainfluenza viruses (12%), with the other viruses being detected in less than 10% of the respiratory tract secretions (45). In approximately 10% of wheezing illnesses, more than one virus was detected in the respiratory tract secretions. In this high-risk population, 28% of the subjects met the criteria for asthma diagnosis at age 6 on the basis of National Asthma Education and Prevention program guidelines. When an analysis was performed to determine which viruses were most often detected in the respiratory tract secretions during wheezing illnesses before age 3 and associated with the diagnosis of asthma at age 6, rhinovirus was the most common virus identified. The odds ratio of having asthma at age 6 was 9.8 when rhinovirus was detected in the first three years of life during wheezing, and the odds ratio was 2.6 for RSV when the referent was neither virus being detected in the nasal secretions. When both rhinovirus and RSV were detected, the odds ratio of having asthma at age 6 was 10. Wheezing illness with any of the other viruses included in the viral detection assays was not associated with asthma diagnosis at age 6 (45).

This study strongly suggests that rhinovirus infection in early life may be causative for the subsequent development of asthma and that future studies examining the relationship between infant infections and asthma needs to include assays for the detection of rhinovirus and the inclusion of this virus in the data analysis.

VI. Conclusion

As can be seen, there is a complex relationship between infections and asthma. Infections are known to cause exacerbations of asthma, and underlying asthma can lead to more severe infections. In addition, there is increasing evidence that severe viral infections in early life are associated with the development of asthma later in childhood. Although the relationship between infection and asthma has been investigated for over 100 years, additional work is necessary to completely dissect the interactions between these two disease processes and more fully understand how interventions to prevent either infection or asthma will affect the other.

Acknowledgment

Sources of support:
F32 HL091653-01 (DCN)
R01 AI 070672, R01 AI 054660, R01 HL 069449, 5P50GM015431 (RSP)

References

1. Osler W. Diseases of the respiratory system. In: Osler W, ed. The Principles and Practice of Medicine. New York: D. Appleton and Company, 1892:474–556.
2. Thomas WS, Tuoart MD. Treatment of asthma with autogenous vaccines. Arch Int Med 1924; 34:79–84.
3. Wilmer HB, Cobe HM. Vaccine therapy: the uses and misuses. J Allergy 1933; 4:414–425.
4. Helander E. Bacterial vaccines in the treatment of bronchial asthma. Acta Allergologica 1959; 13:47–66.
5. Aas K, Berdal P, Henriksen SD, et al. "Bacterial allergy" in childhood asthma and the effect of vaccine treatment. Acta Paediatr 1963; 52:338–344.
6. Frankland AW, Hughes WH, Gorland RH. Autogenous bacterial vaccines in treatment of asthma. BMJ 1955; 2:941–944.
7. Hudgel DW, Langston L, Jr., Selner JC, et al. Viral and bacterial infections in adults with chronic asthma. Am Rev Respir Dis 1979; 120(2):393–397.
8. McIntosh K, Ellis EF, Hoffman LS, et al. The association of viral and bacterial respiratory infections with exacerbations of wheezing in young asthmatic children. J Pediatr 1973; 82(4):578–590.
9. Shapiro GG, Eggleston PA, Pierson WE, et al. Double-blind study of the effectiveness of a broad spectrum antibiotic in status asthmaticus. Pediatrics 1974; 53(6):867–872.
10. Graham VA, Milton AF, Knowles GK, et al. Routine antibiotics in hospital management of acute asthma. Lancet 1982; 1(8269):418–420.

11. Kraft M, Cassell GH, Henson JE, et al. Detection of Mycoplasma pneumoniae in the airways of adults with chronic asthma. Am J Respir Crit Care Med 1998; 158(3):998–1001.
12. Martin RJ, Kraft M, Chu HW, et al. A link between chronic asthma and chronic infection. J Allergy Clin Immunol 2001; 107(4):595–601.
13. Lieberman D, Lieberman D, Printz S, et al. Atypical pathogen infection in adults with acute exacerbation of bronchial asthma. Am J Respir Crit Care Med 2003; 167(3):406–410.
14. Kraft M, Cassell GH, Pak J, et al. Mycoplasma pneumoniae and Chlamydia pneumoniae in asthma: effect of clarithromycin. Chest 2002; 121(6):1782–1788.
15. Johnston SL, Blasi F, Black PN, et al. The effect of telithromycin in acute exacerbations of asthma. N Engl J Med 2006; 354(15):1589–1600.
16. Prevention of pneumococcal disease: recommendations of the Advisory Committee on Immunization Practices (ACIP). MMWR Recomm Rep 1997; 46(RR-8):1–24.
17. Talbot TR, Hartert TV, Mitchel E, et al. Asthma as a risk factor for invasive pneumococcal disease. N Engl J Med 2005; 352(20):2082–2090.
18. Juhn YJ, Kita H, Yawn BP, et al. Increased risk of serious pneumococcal disease in patients with asthma. J Allergy Clin Immunol 2008; 122(4):719–723.
19. Almirall J, Bolibar I, Serra-Prat M, et al. New evidence of risk factors for community-acquired pneumonia: a population-based study. Eur Respir J 2008; 31(6):1274–1284.
20. Centers for Disease Control and Prevention. Available at: http://www.cdc.gov/mmwr/PDF/wk/mm5753.pdf.
21. Centers for Disease Control and Prevention. Available at: http://www.cdc.gov/asthma/asthmadata.htm.
22. Centers for Disease Control and Prevention. Available at: http://www.cdc.gov/vaccines/programs/vfc/cdc-vac-price-list.htm.
23. National Heart Lung and Blood Institute. Available at: http://www.nhlbi.nih.gov/guidelines/asthma/index.htm.
24. Hartert TV. Are persons with asthma at increased risk of pneumococcal infections, and can we prevent them? J Allergy Clin Immunol 2008; 122(4):724–725.
25. Kraft M, Adler KB, Ingram JL, et al. Mycoplasma pneumoniae induces airway epithelial cell expression of MUC5AC in asthma. Eur Respir J 2008; 31(1):43–46.
26. Bisgaard H, Hermansen MN, Buchvald F, et al. Childhood asthma after bacterial colonization of the airway in neonates. N Engl J Med 2007; 357(15):1487–1495.
27. von Mutius E. Of attraction and rejection—asthma and the microbial world. N Engl J Med 2007; 357(15):1545–1547.
28. Horn ME, Reed SE, Taylor P. Role of viruses and bacteria in acute wheezy bronchitis in childhood: a study of sputum. Arch Dis Child 1979; 54(8):587–592.
29. Jennings LC, Barns G, Dawson KP. The association of viruses with acute asthma. N Z Med J 1987; 100(829):488–490.
30. Mitchell I, Inglis JM, Simpson H. Viral infection as a precipitant of wheeze in children. Combined home and hospital study. Arch Dis Child 1978; 53(2):106–111.
31. Johnston SL, Pattemore PK, Sanderson G, et al. Community study of role of viral infections in exacerbations of asthma in 9–11 year old children [see comments]. BMJ 1995; 310(6989):1225–1229.
32. Nicholson KG, Kent J, Ireland DC. Respiratory viruses and exacerbations of asthma in adults. BMJ 1993; 307(6910):982–986.
33. Wark PA, Johnston SL, Moric I, et al. Neutrophil degranulation and cell lysis is associated with clinical severity in virus-induced asthma. Eur Respir J 2002; 19(1):68–75.
34. Williams JV, Crowe JE, Jr., Enriquez R, et al. Human metapneumovirus infection plays an etiologic role in acute asthma exacerbations requiring hospitalization in adults. J Infect Dis 2005; 192(7):1149–1153.

35. Atmar RL, Guy E, Guntupalli KK, et al. Respiratory tract viral infections in inner-city asthmatic adults. Arch Intern Med 1998; 158(22):2453–2459.
36. Sears MR, Johnston NW. Understanding the September asthma epidemic. J Allergy Clin Immunol 2007; 120(3):526–529.
37. Corne JM, Marshall C, Smith S, et al. Frequency, severity, and duration of rhinovirus infections in asthmatic and non-asthmatic individuals: a longitudinal cohort study. Lancet 2002; 359(9309):831–834.
38. Hartert TV, Neuzil KM, Shintani AK, et al. Maternal morbidity and perinatal outcomes among pregnant women with respiratory hospitalizations during influenza season. Am J Obstet Gynecol 2003; 189(6):1705–1712.
39. Wark PA, Johnston SL, Bucchieri F, et al. Asthmatic bronchial epithelial cells have a deficient innate immune response to infection with rhinovirus. J Exp Med 2005; 201(6):937–947.
40. Contoli M, Message SD, Laza-Stanca V, et al. Role of deficient type III interferon-lambda production in asthma exacerbations. Nat Med 2006; 12(9):1023–1026.
41. Heymann PW, Carper HT, Murphy DD, et al. Viral infections in relation to age, atopy, and season of admission among children hospitalized for wheezing. J Allergy Clin Immunol 2004; 114(2):239–247.
42. Sigurs N, Gustafsson PM, Bjarnason R, et al. Severe respiratory syncytial virus bronchiolitis in infancy and asthma and allergy at age 13. Am J Respir Crit Care Med 2005; 171(2):137–141.
43. Stein RT, Sherrill D, Morgan WJ, et al. Respiratory syncytial virus in early life and risk of wheeze and allergy by age 13 years [see comments]. Lancet 1999; 354(9178):541–545.
44. Wu P, Dupont WD, Griffin MR, et al. Evidence of a causal role of winter virus infection during infancy in early childhood asthma. Am J Respir Crit Care Med 2008; 178(11):1123–1129.
45. Jackson DJ, Gangnon RE, Evans MD, et al. Wheezing rhinovirus illnesses in early life predict asthma development in high-risk children. Am J Respir Crit Care Med 2008; 178(7):667–672.

2

Laboratory Diagnosis of Respiratory Infections

RONALD J. HARBECK
Advanced Diagnostic Laboratories, National Jewish Health, Denver, Colorado, U.S.A.

I. Introduction

Respiratory tract infections are among the most common type of infections in children and adults and are one of the most common reasons for prescribing antibiotics. A majority of antibiotic prescriptions in children are due to acute respiratory tract infections, although in most cases without clear evidence of a bacterial infection. Determining the agent responsible for the infection can often be a challenge to the clinical microbiology laboratory. The process of identification of the specific organism that is involved is complicated by the presence of a number of different organisms that can lead to infections in the upper and lower respiratory tracts including bacteria, viruses, fungi, protozoa, and helminthes. The emergence of new pathogens also provides additional challenges.

The status of early detection of infectious agents by point-of-care (POC) testing may be useful for reducing prescriptions of unnecessary antibiotics and lead to appropriate infection control measures. POC tests for the early diagnosis of lower respiratory tract infections have been recently reviewed (1).

The presence of abundant normal microbial flora within the oral cavity poses difficulties for obtaining uncontaminated specimens. The question then becomes: are the organisms isolated and identified by the laboratory a cause of the infectious process or are they merely colonizing the oropharynx? However, the presence of some microorganisms such as *Legionella pneumophila*, *Mycobacterium tuberculosis*, *Pneumocystis carinii*, most viruses, and pathogenic dimorphic fungi is often considered proof that these are the etiological agents of an ongoing disease. Other potentially pathogenic organisms such as *Streptococcus pneumoniae*, *Haemophilus influenzae*, *Moraxella catarrhalis*, *Staphylococcus aureus*, and gram-negative rods, the latter two being especially common in hospitalized patients, may, in fact, be colonizing the oropharynx. *Mycoplasma pneumoniae* and *Chlamydia pneumoniae* can also be found in throat samples without evidence of ongoing disease.

Because of the diversity of potentially pathogenic microorganisms present in the respiratory tract, the selection of the appropriate testing strategy is of extreme importance. In general, there are several means where a laboratory diagnosis of respiratory tract infections may be made and include identification of the causative microorganism itself by culture and biochemical tests, determination of the presence of an antigenic cellular or subcellular product of the microorganism, by the detection of specific nucleic acid sequences, and/or determination of a specific antibody response in the host to the agent.

Thus, considering these variables, it is important to consider the source and how the specimen is obtained to make an informed decision regarding the role of the organism in making the diagnosis. In light of this, the interpretation of very sensitive methods such as the polymerase chain reaction (PCR) must be made cautiously. Uncontaminated material obtained from aseptic aspiration of pleural, paranasal sinus, or middle ear effusions, and percutaneous fine-needle aspiration of a pneumonic process offers the best proof that the isolated organism is the etiological agent. In certain respiratory tract infections such as severe cases of pneumonia, sinusitis, and epiglottitis, a blood culture will often establish the etiological agent.

This review will primarily stress the means of identification of bacteria and viruses associated with upper and lower respiratory infections. For a complete description of the identification of fungi and parasitic infections, the reader should refer to more recent texts (2).

II. Bacteria
A. Specimen Collection and Transport

One of the most important considerations in diagnosing a lower or upper respiratory tract infection is to obtain an appropriate specimen (3). When swabbing the throat for subsequent culture, one must swab the tonsils, arches, and uvula to avoid false-negative results. Specimens for lower respiratory tract infections are submitted to determine if an individual has an airway disease such as tracheitis and bronchitis, pneumonia, lung abscess, and empyema. Specimens that are usually obtained from the lower respiratory tract include expectorated sputum, induced sputum, endotracheal tube aspirations, bronchial brushings, washes, or alveolar lavage fluid and pleural fluid. It is critical that the specimens be delivered to the laboratory as soon as possible after collection and processed by the laboratory within one hour. The specimen should be refrigerated if it is not possible to deliver in a timely manner.

One of the ways in which the quality of sputum is assessed is by counting the number of squamous epithelial cells per $10\times$ objective microscopic field (3). Epithelial cells greater than 10 per field indicate contamination from the oropharyngeal areas. Many laboratories have instituted policies that will reject specimens that contain greater than 10 epithelial cells per $10\times$ microscopic field. However, for the detection of *M. pneumoniae*, *Legionella* spp., dimorphic fungi, and *M. tuberculosis*, there is no need to access the quality of the sputum prior to culture (3).

Gram-stained smears should be prepared from sputum specimens and examined for potential pathogens. Bacteria not present in sufficient quantity or not having morphology resembling a pathogen could be reported preliminarily as normal flora. Cultures of respiratory tract specimens should include plating on sheep blood agar, a selective gram-negative medium, such as MacConkey's agar, and chocolate agar, for the detection of *Haemophilus* spp. Culture plates should be incubated at 35°C in 3% to 5% CO_2 for two days and only reported out as negative after 48 hours. Cultures are examined for numbers and types of bacteria that grow on the culture plates. Interpretative guidelines have been established for bacterial lower respiratory tract culture results (4). Bacteria isolated from sputum, either coughed or induced, and from endotracheal tube aspirates are most likely to be the cause of the infection if it is the predominant potential pathogen in gram stain and culture and there is an abundance of neutrophils. It is not likely to be significant if the growth of the organism is modest on culture and not present on a Gram stain and the neutrophils are not abundant on the gram stain. For bronchoalveolar lavage (BAL) fluid, the potential pathogen should be seen by Gram stain in every $100\times$ field and quantitative culture should detect $>10^5$ CFU/mL.

B. Detection of Bacterial Infections

For lower respiratory tract infections where quantitative cultures of respiratory secretions when the risk of contamination is minimized and quantitative studies are performed, a number of studies have indicated that when at least 10^5 colony-forming units (CFU)/mL of respiratory tract secretions are obtained, then the specificity that this is the causative agent is increased (5). Transtracheal aspirations, percutaneous lung puncture, bronchoscopic protected specimen brushes, and BAL are included in these types of specimens. Adequate induction and sampling of sputum are critical since it is much more difficult to obtain with sputum specimens since the number of bacteria colonizing the oropharynx can exceed 10^6 CFU/mL. The combination of a Gram stain and quantitative culture makes the results of sputum analysis much more reliable especially if the patient is able to produce a purulent specimen. Regardless of the specimen, the sensitivity of culture is seriously compromised if it is obtained after the start of antibiotic therapy.

C. Diagnosis of Bacterial Upper Respiratory Tract Infections
Antigen Detection Methods

Several antigen detection methods using immunoassays have been developed to diagnose bacterial respiratory infections (6). Any antigen can be measured if the appropriate, specific antibody to that antigen can be developed. There are three general immunoassay methods that have been developed: label free, reagent excess, and reagent limited. Label-free assays depend on the ability of the antigen and antibody to interact and form a visible agglutination or precipitin. Tests of this nature include precipitin tests to measure antibodies to fungal antigen, for example, *Coccidioides*, *Aspergillus*, and *Histoplasma*. The reagent excess methods require an excess of labeled antigen or antibody and use immunoblotting and solid-phase enzyme-linked immunoabsorbent assay. These are the most commonly employed tests for antigen detection by clinical microbiology laboratories today. The reagent-limited assays are competitive-based tests and employ a limited amount of either antigen or antibody. Classical enzyme-linked immunoassays (EIA) or radioimmunoassay (RIA) fall within this category.

There are several rapid immunological tests available in the marketplace for the detection of bacterial antigens or bacterial cell components from throat swabs especially for the diagnosis of group A streptococci. These tests can be performed as POC tests in a doctor's office, a clinic, or a standard clinical microbiology laboratory. While the specificity of these commercially available tests approaches 100%, their sensitivity can be variable depending on the test kit and quality of specimen collected (6,7); thus, a positive test can be considered diagnostic, while a negative test does not exclude a streptococcal etiology. It is recommended that a culture be performed for the definitive diagnosis (6,7). In addition, cultures can detect other agents of pharyngitis including group C and G streptococcus, a relatively common cause of pharyngitis, as well as *Arcanobacterium haemolyticum*.

For the more unusual cases of bacterial pharyngitis such as those caused by
Corynebacterium diphtheriae, A. haemolyticum, and *Neisseria gonorrhea,* special media
is required. If these organisms are suspected on clinical grounds, then this information
should be communicated to the clinical microbiology laboratory so that the appropriate
cultures can be performed.

A number of different bacteria as well as fungi and viruses have been associated
with sinusitis. These include *S. pneumoniae* and *H. influenzae* in about half of all the
cases. To a lesser extent, *M. catarrhalis, Streptococcus pyogenes, S. aureus,* and gram-
negative rods have been detected. It is likely that these bacteria originate from the nose
and nasopharynx and their presence is often a diagnostic dilemma in the interpretation of
the significance of the culture results. Specimens obtained by sinus puncture should be
the method of choice for determining the etiological agent on the basis of culture. The
aspirated material should be transported to the laboratory promptly after collection and
should be kept in an oxygen-free environment so that anaerobe viability is not significantly compromised.

D. Bacterial Diagnosis of Infections of the Lower Respiratory Tract

For the diagnosis of community-acquired pneumonia, the examination of sputum by
Gram stain or culture has been questioned since many of the elderly or severely ill
patients fail to produce any sputum or produce only nonpurulent specimens. In
addition, many patients are on antibiotic therapy prior to sampling (8). *M. pneumoniae,*
C. pneumoniae, and *Legionella* species are the most important causes of "atypical"
bacterial pneumonia. As discussed in chapter 9 of this book, there is growing evidence to
suggest the presence of *M. pneumoniae* and *C. pneumoniae* with wheezing and asthma
(9,10). *M. pneumoniae* belongs to the Mollicutes class and are unique among bacteria.
They are smaller in cellular and genome size than conventional bacteria, making them
the smallest free-living organisms known. In addition, they also lack a cell wall and are
contained by a trilayered cell membrane. The lack of a cell wall makes these organisms
resistant to β-lactam antimicrobials, prevents them from being gram stained, and is
responsible for their pleomorphic forms.

Mycoplasmas are extremely sensitive to drying and heat. For collection of
specimens for mycoplasma isolation, it is recommended that the samples be immediately
placed in appropriate transport or culture media (9). Because mycoplasmas lack a cell
wall, they cannot be visualized by routine microscopic examination after Gram staining.
Similarly culture of mycoplasma organisms can be challenging because of their slow
growth and requirement for specific growth factors in the culture media. There is no
standard culture media that will allow for the growth of all mycoplasma since different
species require different pHs and substrates. The colonies are microscopic and, once
detected, cannot be easily identified in most clinical microbiology laboratories.

Since culture is slow and insensitive, laboratory diagnosis has relied on serology
until recently when nucleic acid amplification methods have been successfully applied
(9,11–16). In one study, PCR was found to be superior to serology for diagnosis of
M. pneumoniae infection during the early phases of infection (17). Persistent, sometimes
long-term, carriage of *M. pneumoniae* in the throat was common following acute
infection and was not affected by antibiotic therapy.

C. pneumoniae are nonmotile, obligate intracellular prokaryotic organisms characterized by a unique biphasic developmental cycle. Each cycle differs in morphology

and function. The so-called elementary bodies (EBs) of *Chlamydia* infect eukaryotic cells and can survive for only a limited amount of time outside of the host cell. Once they have infected the host cell, they differentiate into a metabolically active reticulate body (RB), which multiply by binary fission within vacuoles. At the end of the developmental cycle, RBs convert back to EBs, which are released from the host cell to continue the infectious process.*C. pneumoniae* can cause both upper and lower respiratory tract infections such as sinusitis, pharyngitis, bronchitis, and pneumonia (18).

C. pneumoniae is rapidly inactivated at room temperature, so specimens collected for identification should be kept at 4°C to 8°C in *Chlamydia* transport media (19). The method of choice for detection of *C. pneumoniae* is nucleic acid amplification techniques. Recently, several techniques have been described (13,20).

III. Procalcitonin as an Agent to Distinguish Bacterial from Viral Infections

Procalcitonin (PCT), a prohormone of calcitonin, is elevated in bacterial infections but is low in viral infections (21). As a precursor to calcitonin, procalcitonin is inhibited by endotoxin and cytokines that are released during bacterial infections. Thus, in individuals with bacterial, not viral, infections, the levels of PCT are increased by a factor of several tens of thousands during sepsis (22,23). Because PCT is downregulated in viral infections, PCT may help in defining the need for antibiotic therapy among patients with radiographic evidence of pneumonia. PCT guidance has been shown to substantially reduce antibiotic use in patients with lower respiratory infections without compromising outcomes (23,24). Studies using PCT levels can lead to the safe withholding of antibiotics among patients with low PCT levels (<0.25 μg/L), with no clinical signs of severe illness (25). Serial measurements of PCT have been reported to correlate with clinical response to therapy and may be able to guide short durations of therapy. In a recent review addressing the usefulness of serum markers in community-acquired pneumonia and ventilator-associated pneumonia, it was indicated that serum markers such as PCT and C-reactive protein (CRP) should be used to support a clinical approach and guide culture sampling and empirical antibiotic prescription (26). They are also useful in monitoring the clinical course, adjusting antibiotic therapy, and identifying nonresponders to apply a more aggressive approach to therapy to prevent clinical deterioration (21,26). In a retrospective analysis, serum levels of PCT values below 0.1 ng/mL might be a marker to identify children with acute respiratory tract infections in whom antibiotic treatment could however be withheld; the authors caution that only a prospective interventional trial will prove the general safety of such an approach (21). PCT can be detected in the BAL; however, the utility of its measurement in the BAL is no better than detection in serum from patients with ventilator-associated pneumonia (27).

IV. Detection of Viral Infections

A. Specimen Collection and Transport: Viruses

There are three general diagnostic methods for the detection of viruses; cell culture, viral antigen detection, and molecular techniques. As with all microbiological detection methods, proper collections, transport, and processing are required for a successful and accurate diagnosis.

For respiratory specimens, the viruses that are most frequently detected are influenza, parainfluenza, respiratory syncytial virus (RSV), adenoviruses, and rhinoviruses. Many of these viruses infect the ciliated epithelium of the nasopharynx. Studies comparing nasopharyngeal swabs and aspirates for immunoassay detection of viruses indicate that nasopharyngeal swabs are generally collected from older children and adults, while nasopharyngeal aspirates are the method of choice for infants and young children (28,29). In general, nasal washes are not obtained because of the low yield of virus-infected cells. For lower respiratory tract infections, the specimens of choice are BAL and bronchial specimens, both which are less invasive to open lung biopsy.

Nasopharyngeal swabs are collected by inserting a fine-shafted, flexible, sterile swab into the nares, past the point of resistance, and gently rubbing or rotating the swab in the posterior pharynx and nasal turbinates. The swab should immediately be placed in an appropriate viral transport media (VTM) (30). For the collection of aspirates, a small tube or a catheter is placed in the nasal passage and the aspirate material is withdrawn with a syringe or some other mechanical suction device and placed in VTM (31). Nasal washes are obtained by instilling several milliliters of saline into the nasal passage with the patient's head tilted back slightly. The patient's head is then brought forward and the instilled saline is allowed to flow into a collection cup. BAL and bronchial specimens are obtained using a fiber-optic bronchoscope into the involved area of the lung, instilling sterile saline and removing the saline by suction.

Once the respiratory specimen(s) has been collected, it should be transported to the laboratory as quickly as possible especially if culture methods are being used for its identification (32). The specimens should be transported in VTM and on ice if the transport time is greater than one hour. One should avoid freezing of the specimens especially since the recovery of RSV, CMV, and VZV may be seriously compromised (33). However, if there is a delay of beyond 24 hours in getting the sample to the laboratory, one should freeze the samples on dry ice. If in doubt as how best to transport the specimen, the virology laboratory should be contacted before beginning any procedure.

Acute respiratory disease accounts for an estimated 75% of all acute morbidities in developed countries, and upward of 80% these infections are viral. Technologies are constantly being developed to diagnose viral infections including respiratory viral infections. In the past 20 years, virus isolation and serology have been the most common means of diagnosing respiratory virus infections. Infectivity of cell lines and the use of embryonated hen eggs for influenza virus have been the means to isolate viruses. The serological tests used have included hemagglutination inhibition tests, complement fixation, and enzyme immunoassays.

B.   Methods for Detection of Viral Infections

Over several years, an increasing number of new assay systems have been available commercially. These vary in methodology, efficiency, sensitivity, specificity, accuracy, and cost. Laboratories are continually faced with decisions on the best method to employ and the best system for patient care. In addition to molecular-based methods for viral detection, there are a number of other procedures that have been used. These include electron microscopy, rapid antigen testing, immunofluorescence antibody staining, conventional cell culture, and rapid cell cultures. For each of the viral infections, a table of the usefulness of the various detection methods has been described (34). The "gold standard" method has always been cell culture; however, this too has its potential drawbacks including a long incubation period with results not often available during the initial stages of the patient's infection. In practice, electron microscopy is rarely used in the diagnosis of respiratory infections, but it may be useful for epidemiological studies or for the diagnosis of unusual conditions. Thus, it will not be discussed further in this chapter.

Rapid Antigen Detection

The most common nonmolecular rapid antigen tests for viruses are based on an immunoassay format. In general, they require approximately 10^5 to 10^6 viral particles to yield a positive result, while cell culture and molecular methods require as few as 10 viral particles (35). The tests are easy to perform with time to results from 15 to 30 minutes. Many are considered waived tests by the Clinical Laboratory Improvement Act (CLIA) (36) and can be performed outside of the clinical laboratory, for example, in physician offices, emergency departments, and clinics. During the respiratory infection season, the specificity for RSV and influenza antigen tests is high; however, when outside the season, the specificity and positive predictive value is lower (37). The sensitivities of the various detection systems vary widely from 44% to 95% for influenza virus and 59% to 89% for RSV (35,37). It is recommended that if a positive result is obtained outside of the infectious season, then it should be confirmed preferably by culture.

Rapid Antigen Immunofluorescence-Based Tests

Many laboratories perform immunofluorescence detection of virus directly on cell preparations obtained from the respiratory sample. With the use of fluorescent-labeled viral-specific antibody and the location of the virus within the cell, one can identify the viral agent. A mixture of two dual-labeled antibodies can assist in the identification of two or more viruses in the specimen. Immunofluorescence provides for a relatively rapid turnaround time, and results can be obtained within 30 to 90 minutes. Additional advantages offered by this testing are better sensitivity than cell culture for RSV and the detection of nonviable virus. The disadvantages are that these tests are less sensitive than cell culture, especially for adenovirus, and the level of expertise required for reading the results. Reagents and kits are available to detect influenza A and B, RSV, parainfluenza 1, 2, and 3, adenovirus, and metapneumovirus.

Conventional Cell Culture

Details of the use of cell cultures for the detection of respiratory viruses have been recently reviewed (35,38). The 1970s saw the accelerated growth in the number of diagnostic virology laboratories due, in large part, to the availability of susceptible cell lines and reagents. Cell cultures of primary, diploid, and heteroploid cells are used in various combinations to support the growth of common respiratory viruses. Most laboratories can now purchase cell lines that will support the growth of the viruses that may be of interest. Cell culture is the method by which all other methods have been compared, including molecular diagnostic methods. The advantages of cell culture is the broad range of viruses that can be detected, increased sensitivity over the rapid antigen methods, and the ability to isolate the virus for further study if needed. The disadvantages are the long detection time for some of the viruses, less sensitivity than the antigen detection methods for RSV, the level of expertise that is required to read the cultures for cytopathic effects (CPE), and, while the culture reagents and supplies are relatively low in cost, the technical labor time is increased.

Rapid Cell Culture Formats

The use of centrifugation of a respiratory specimen onto a cell monolayer grown in microwell plates or on cover slips in shell vials has improved significantly the time to identification of viruses (38,39). After incubation for 24 to 72 hours, the cells are examined for CPE and generally stained with antibodies specific to the virus. The advantages of the rapid cell cultures are the shorter time for detection of a virus compared with the conventional cell culture method (40), the detection of viruses that replicate poorly in cell culture, and the need for less expertise in reading the cultures for CPE. Among the disadvantages of the rapid cell culture method are the decreased sensitivity for RSV and adenovirus detection and the increased amount of time for reading and staining of the cells.

C. Detection of Respiratory Pathogens by Molecular Methods

In recent years, there have been major advances in the diagnosis of respiratory infections (11). This is a dynamic area of pathogen diagnosis with ever increasing gains made in new technologies including polymerase chain. Nucleic acid amplification techniques are commonly used in clinical microbiology laboratories to diagnose infectious diseases. Recent publications suggest that molecular testing for viral agents can be more sensitive and specific than viral culture and/or immunoassays (41–43). The commercialization of many kits and reagents in the past several years has facilitated the employment of these technologies in the clinical laboratory. The PCR has led this advancement; however, many other rapid and sensitive techniques have followed.

The application of molecular technology to the diagnosis of upper and lower respiratory infections has made tremendous gains in the past few years. The advantage of molecular detection is that results are available much more rapidly than in standard culture and with the capability of identifying fastidious organisms that may not be easily cultured for identification. Furthermore, increased sensitivity and specificity are obtained with the added advantage of organism quantitation.

Nonamplified Nucleic Acid Probes

Nucleic acid probes are segments of DNA or RNA labeled with radioisotopes, enzymes or chemiluminescent reporter molecules that can bind to complementary nucleic acid sequences. These probes can bind with a high degree of specificity. The probes can be designed to identify any microbe. There are a number of commercial kits that can be obtained to be used to directly identify a pathogen in a clinical specimen or one that has been isolated after culture. One of the more commonly used formats for identification of the organism is called the liquid-phase "probe hybridization protection assay" (Gen-Probe, Inc., San Diego, California, U.S.). In this assay, the process can be completed with a few hours. Nevertheless, nonamplified nucleic acid probe assays are relatively insensitive and are most useful when there are a high number of organisms in the clinical sample, for example, with group A streptococcal pharyngitis or genital tract infections with *N. gonorrhoeae and C. trachomatis* (44). In addition, these techniques can be used to confirm the culture identification of mycobacteria and systemic dimorphic fungi.

A unique characteristic of viruses is that they contain either DNA or RNA, and never both, as in other infectious agents. Some viruses are able to be grown in cell culture lines, but the speed of detection by these methods has been a drawback. Early antigen detection, for example, by immunofluorescence using virus-specific antibodies, can often shorten the time to one to two days. With the application of the PCR, a widely used technique in molecular biology, the identification can take less than 24 hours.

Target Amplification Techniques

Target amplification techniques have several features in common (44). They all use enzyme-medicated processes in which the enzyme(s) synthesize copies of the target nucleic acid. In addition, the amplification product is detected by oligonucleotide primers that bind to complementary sequences on opposite strands of double-stranded targets. The final outcome of the amplification product is millions of copies of the target sequence in hours.

The development of the PCR in 1988 was the start of molecular diagnostics (45). PCR derives its name from the fact that a key enzyme, that is, DNA polymerase, is used to amplify the DNA in vitro by enzymatic replication. As new DNA is generated, it serves as new templates for further replication, and thus, copies of the original DNA in the sample are exponentially produced. The DNA polymerase used in PCR reactions is a heat-stable enzyme, termed "Taq polymerase," which was originally isolated from the thermophilic bacteria *Thermus aquaticus*. The Taq polymerase assembles nucleotides by using a single-stranded DNA as a template along with DNA primers or a short strand that, generally around 20 nuclcotides in length of DNA, serves as a starting point for DNA replication. The majority of PCR reactions use thermal cycling, alternating heating to physically unwind the strands of the DNA double helix and cooling to allow for replication to occur on the two strands. With each cycle of denaturing, annealing, and synthesis, the specific DNA fragment is amplified exponentially. The specificity of the reaction is determined in the primers, which target the region of the DNA to be amplified. By this process, millions of copies of the DNA are synthesized after roughly 25 to 30 cycles.

When the virus is a RNA-containing virus, a process called reverse transcription polymerase chain reaction (RT-PCR) is employed. In this procedure, the RNA is first transcribed into its DNA complement (or cDNA) by a reverse transcriptase reaction followed by the amplification of the DNA by the standard PCR reaction.

Real-Time PCR

Real-time PCR, also known as quantitative real-time PCR (Q-PCR or qPCR), is a procedure that uses amplification with the simultaneous quantitation of a target DNA molecule. The PCR product is detected as it is produced by the intercalation of fluorescence dyes into the double-stranded DNA (ds-DNA). Dyes such as SYBR Green will bind to the ds-DNA products and fluorescence (20).

RT-PCR

RT-PCR should not be confused with Q-PCR. The Q-PCR is a laboratory technique that is based on the PCR; however, during the amplification steps, one can use fluorescent dyes that intercalate with the ds-DNA that are produced or modified DNA oligonucleotides probes that fluoresce when hybridized with the complementary DNA. Thus, as the PCR reaction progresses with the synthesis of more and more ds-DNA with each cycle of the thermocycler, more fluorescence is generated, which can be measured with a detector. Commercially available kits from Roche Diagnostics (Indianapolis, Indiana, U.S.) that use a single enzyme technology are available for certain viruses.

Real-time PCR has had a significant impact in research and the clinical microbiology laboratory where improvements in the time to diagnosis have been obtained. However, one must be cautious when using the PCR for diagnosis of respiratory infections because of its extreme sensitivity.

Nested PCR

Nested PCR offers the advantage of increased sensitivity and specificity (46). Two sets of primers are used in two successive PCR reactions. In the first reaction, one pair of primers is used to generate DNA products, which, besides the intended target, may still consist of nonspecifically amplified DNA fragments. The product(s) are then used in a second PCR reaction with a set of primers, or "nested" primers that are different from the first primer set but still within the intended DNA target. Nested PCR is often more useful than conventional PCR in amplifying long fragments of DNA; however, it requires more detailed information of the targeted sequences. Care must be taken since contamination can occur when the first-round product is transferred for the second round of PCR.

Multiplex PCR

One of the more encouraging areas of diagnostic procedures to be developed in recent years is the multiplexing assays for respiratory pathogens, especially viruses. Several of these assays have been developed in recent years, which allow the detection of multiple viral nucleic acid targets in a single specimen (47–58). Recently, a multiplex system was described to measure 17 viruses that commonly cause respiratory infections including influenza A and B, parainfluenza virus (PIV) 1, 2, 3, 4a, and 4b, RSV A and B, human rhinovirus (HRV), coronaviruses 229E/NL63 and OC43, adenovirus B, C, and E, and human metapneumovirus (59). The respiratory specimens came from throat and/or nasopharyngeal swabs. The investigators used a multiplex system developed by EraGen Biosciences, Inc. (Madison, Wisconsin, U.S.) and called MultiCode-PLx assay. In brief, in a single well of a 96-well plate, the viral cDNAs were amplified by PCR, target-specific extension of tagged primers, capture of the target-specific products to labeled microspheres, and readout of the fluorescent signal on each microsphere using a multiplex microbead reading system. The authors concluded that this assay showed an overall sensitivity of 99% and specificity of 87% compared with conventional identification techniques, that is, real-time PCR and routine viral culture.

Using the Luminex xTAG respiratory viral panel for the detection of 20 respiratory virus targets, it has been reported that it compared favorably with the real-time nucleic acid amplification tests for the individual viruses with the exception of lower sensitivity for detection of adenovirus (60).

Recently, a multiplex PCR assay (Seegene Inc., Seoul, Korea) has been described, which allows for the simultaneous detection and identification of nine respiratory viruses using RT-PCR assay (61), and in a subsequent paper, two primer mixes were used for detection of 12 respiratory viruses (62). The analytical sensitivity of the later assay was 10 to 100 copies for each virus with good correlation with detection by viral culture and immunofluorescence. In a publication, five separate multiplex nested PCR assays were used for the detection of 20 respiratory viruses and three atypical bacteria, that is, influenza A and B group specific, and subtypes H1, H3, H5, PIV type 1, 2, 3, and 4, RSV groups A and B, rhinovirus, enteroviruses, coronaviruses OC43, 229E, SARS-CoV, human metapneumovirus, and *M. pneumoniae*, *C. pneumoniae*, and *L. pneumophila* (63).

Signal Amplification Techniques

Although PCR is the most developed technique, other techniques have been developed, which have clinical utility. One of these is signal amplification. In this method, the measurement of the labeled molecules attached to the target nucleic acid is detected, which allows for greater sensitivity of the assay. Another assay in use is the branched DNA assay. In a signal amplification test, the presence of specific nucleic acids is measured by the signal-generated "branched," labeled (generally enzymatic) DNA probes. This test detects an amplified luminescent signal whose brightness depends on the amount of viral nucleic acid present (64).

Hybrid Capture Assays

The hybrid capture system, also called the hybridization antibody capture assay, uses chemiluminescence detection of the hybrid molecules. The target DNA in the specimen is denatured and then hybridized with a specific RNA probe. Next, the DNA-RNA hybrids are captured by antihybrid antibodies. The presence of the hybrids is detected with an enzyme-conjugated antihybrid antibody, which, with the addition of a substrate, produces either a color change or chemiluminescence; the intensity of which is proportional to the amount of target in the original sample (65).

Other Molecular Methods: 16S rRNA

The 16S rRNA gene sequences have been used to identify both culturable and non-culturable bacteria since it is present in most bacteria (66,67). Also, gene sequencing is a more objective method of identification compared with the classical methods of biochemical analysis and physical properties of the organisms. Gene sequencing is also not dependent on optimal growth or even on whether the organism(s) are viable. 16S rRNA (or 16S rDNA) is an approximately 1500–base pair gene that codes for a part of the 39S ribosome, and a partial sequence of about 500 base pairs has proven to be an accurate and faster method for identifying most aerobic and anaerobic bacteria including *M. tuberculosis* in the clinical laboratory (45,68,69). A disadvantage of 16S rDNA sequencing is that certain bacteria share similar sequences and cannot be separated reliably by their genomic DNA. This is likely due to the acquisition of virulence plasmids. For example, *Bacillus cereus* and *B. anthracis* have the identical 16S rDNA and genomic DNA sequences (67). To accurately classify a gene sequence to a specific, a bacteria requires an analysis with a reference library, for example, MicroSeq (Applied Biosystems, Foster City, California, U.S.), GenBank (70), Ribosomal Database Project (Center for Microbial Ecology, Michigan State University, East Lansing, Michigan, U.S.), Ribosomal Differentiation of Medical Microorganisms Database (RIDOM) (71), SILVA (72), and SmartGene (73).

References

1. Charles PG. Early diagnosis of lower respiratory tract infections (point-of-care tests). Curr Opin Pulm Med 2008; 14(3):176–182.
2. Manual of Clinical Microbiology. 9th ed. Washington, D.C.: ASM Press, 2007.
3. Thomson RB, Miller JM. Specimen collection, transport, and processing: bacteriology. In: Murray PR Baron EJ, Jorgensen JH, et al. eds. Manual of Clinical Microbiology. 8th ed. Washington, DC: ASM Press, 2003:286–330.
4. Thomson RB. Use of microbiology laboratory tests in the diagnosis of infectious disease. In: Tan J, ed. Expert Guide to Infectious Diseases. Philadelphia: American College of Physicians, 2002:1–41.
5. Kalin M, Petrini B. The laboratory diagnosis of respiratory infections. In: Michael Ellis, ed. Infectious Diseases of the Respiratory Tract. Cambridge, UK: Cambridge University Press, 1998:3–31.
6. Carpenter AB. Immunoassays for the diagnosis of infectious diseases. In: Murray PR, Baron EJ, Jorgensen JH, et al. eds. Manual of Clinical Microbiology. 8th ed. Washington, D.C.: ASM Press, 2007:257–270.
7. Leung AK, Newman R, Kumar A, et al. Rapid antigen detection testing in diagnosing group A beta-hemolytic streptococcal pharyngitis. Expert Rev Mol Diagn 2006; 6(5):761–766.
8. Bartlett JG. Diagnostic test for etiologic agents of community-acquired pneumonia. Infect Dis Clin North Am 2004; 18(4):809–827.
9. Waites KB, Taylor-Robinson D. Mycoplasma and Ureaplasma. In: Murray PR, Baron EJ, Jorgensen JH, et al. eds. Manual of Clinical Microbiology. 9th ed. Washington, D.C.: ASM Press, 2007:1004–1020.
10. Waites KB, Balish MF, Atkinson TP. New insights into the pathogenesis and detection of Mycoplasma pneumoniae infections. Future Microbiol 2008; 3:635–648.
11. Murdoch DR. Molecular genetic methods in the diagnosis of lower respiratory tract infections. Apmis 2004; 112(11–12):713–727.
12. Hamano-Hasegawa K, Morozumi M, Nakayama E, et al. Comprehensive detection of causative pathogens using real-time PCR to diagnose pediatric community-acquired pneumonia. J Infect Chemother 2008; 14(6):424–432.
13. Kumar S, Hammerschlag MR. Acute respiratory infection due to Chlamydia pneumoniae: current status of diagnostic methods. Clin Infect Dis 2007; 44(4):568–576.
14. Martinez MA, Ruiz M, Zunino E, et al. Detection of Mycoplasma pneumoniae in adult community-acquired pneumonia by PCR and serology. J Med Microbiol 2008; 57(pt 12): 1491–1495.
15. Dumke R, Jacobs E. Comparison of commercial and in-house real-time PCR assays to detect Mycoplasma pneumoniae. J Clin Microbiol 2009; 47(2):441–444.
16. Winchell JM, Thurman KA, Mitchell SL, et al. Evaluation of three real-time PCR assays for detection of Mycoplasma pneumoniae in an outbreak investigation. J Clin Microbiol 2008; 46(9):3116–3118.
17. Nilsson AC, Bjorkman P, Persson K. Polymerase chain reaction is superior to serology for the diagnosis of acute Mycoplasma pneumoniae infection and reveals a high rate of persistent infection. BMC Microbiol 2008; 8:93.
18. Kuo CC, Jackson LA, Campbell LA, et al. Chlamydia pneumoniae (TWAR). Clin Microbiol Rev 1995; 8(4):451–461.
19. Essig A. Chlamydia and Chlamydophila. In: Murray PR, Baron EJ, Jorgensen JH, et al. eds. Manual of Clinical Microbiology. 9th ed. Washington, D.C.: ASM Press, 2007:1021–1035.
20. Ieven M. Currently used nucleic acid amplification tests for the detection of viruses and atypicals in acute respiratory infections. J Clin Virol 2007; 40(4):259–276.
21. Schutzle H, Forster J, Superti-Furga A, et al. Is serum procalcitonin a reliable diagnostic marker in children with acute respiratory tract infections? A retrospective analysis. Eur J Pediatr 2008.

22. Christ-Crain M, Mulle B. Biomarkers in respiratory tract infections: diagnostic guides to antibiotic prescription, prognostic markers and mediators. Eur Respir J 2007; 30(3):556–573.

23. Christ-Crain M, Jaccard-Stolz D, Bingisser R, et al. Effect of procalcitonin-guided treatment on antibiotic use and outcome in lower respiratory tract infections: cluster-randomised, single-blinded intervention trial. Lancet 2004; 363(9409):600–607.

24. Briel M, Schuetz P, Mueller B, et al. Procalcitonin-guided antibiotic use vs a standard approach for acute respiratory tract infections in primary care. Arch Intern Med 2008; 168(18):2000–2007.

25. Niederman MS. Biological markers to determine eligibility in trails for community-acquired pneumonia: a focus on procalcitonin. Clin Infect Dis 2008; 47:S127–S132.

26. Povoa P. Serum markers in community-acquired pneumonia and ventilator-associated pneumonia. Curr Opin Infect Dis 2008; 21(2):157–162.

27. Linssen CF, Bekers O, Drent M, et al. C-reactive protein and procalitonin concentration in bronchoalveolar lavage fluid as a predictor of ventilator-associated pneumonia. Ann Clin Biochem 2008; 45(3):293–298.

28. Ahluwalia G, Embree J, McNicol P, et al. Comparison of nasopharyngeal aspirate and nasopharyngeal swab specimens for respiratory syncytial virus diagnosis by cell culture, indirect immunofluorescence assay, and enzyme-linked immunosorbent assay. J Clin Microbiol 1987; 25(5):763–767.

29. Landry ML, Cohen S, Ferguson D. Impact of sample type on rapid detection of influenza virus A by cytospin-enhanced immunofluorescence and membrane enzyme-linked immunosorbent assay. J Clin Microbiol 2000; 38(1):429–430.

30. Chapin K. Reagents, stains, media, and cell lines: virology. In: Murray PR, Baron EJ, Jorgensen JH, et al. eds. Manual of Clinical Microbiology. 9th ed. Washington, D.C.: ASM Press, 2007:1297–1303.

31. Miller JM, Krisher K, Holmes HT. General principles of specimen collection and handling. In: Murray PR, Baron EJ, Jorgensen JH, et al. eds. Manual of Clinical Microbiology. 9th ed. Washington, D.C.: ASM Press, 2007:43–54.

32. Wilson ML. General principles of specimen collection and transport. Clin Infect Dis 1996; 22(5):766–777.

33. Forman MS, Valsamakis A, eds. Specimen Collection, Transport, and Processing: Virology. 9th ed. Washington, D.C.: ASM Press, 2007.

34. Landry AL, Caliendo AM, Tang Y-W, et al. Algorithms for detection and identification of viruses. In: Murray PR, Baron EJ, Jorgensen JH, et al. eds. Manual of Clinical Microbiology. 9th ed. Washington, D.C.: ASM Press, 2007:1304–1307.

35. Ginocchio CC. Detection of respiratory viruses using non-molecular based methods. J Clin Virol 2007; 40(suppl 1):S11–S14.

36. Administration HCF. Medicare, Medicaid, and CLIA programs. Regulations implementing the Clinical Laboratory Improvement Amendments of 1988 (CLIA). Eur J Pediatr 2009; 168(9): 1117–1124.

37. Leland DS, Ginocchio CC. Role of cell culture for virus detection in the age of technology. Clin Microbiol Rev 2007; 20(1):49–78.

38. Hughes JH. Physical and chemical methods for enhancing rapid detection of viruses and other agents. Clin Microbiol Rev 1993; 6(2):150–175.

39. Fong CK, Lee MK, Griffith BP. Evaluation of R-Mix FreshCells in shell vials for detection of respiratory viruses. J Clin Microbiol 2000; 38(12):4660–4662.

40. Barenfanger J, Drake C, Mueller T, et al. R-Mix cells are faster, at least as sensitive and marginally more costly than conventional cell lines for the detection of respiratory viruses. J Clin Virol 2001; 22(1):101–110.

41. Frisbie B, Tang YW, Griffin M, et al. Surveillance of childhood influenza virus infection: what is the best diagnostic method to use for archival samples? J Clin Microbiol 2004; 42(3):1181–1184.

42. Grondahl B, Puppe W, Weigl J, et al. Comparison of the BD Directigen Flu A+B Kit and the Abbott TestPack RSV with a multiplex RT-PCR ELISA for rapid detection of influenza viruses and respiratory syncytial virus. Clin Microbiol Infect 2005; 11(10):848–850.

43. Smith AB, Mock V, Melear R, et al. Rapid detection of influenza A and B viruses in clinical specimens by Light Cycler real time RT-PCR. J Clin Virol 2003; 28(1):51–58.

44. Nolte FS, Caliendo AM. Molecular detection and identification of microoganisms. In: Murrany PR, Baron EJ, Jorgensen JH, et al. eds. Manual of Clinical Microbiology. Washington, D.C.: ASM Press, 2007:218–244.

45. Saiki RK, Gelfand DH, Stoffel S, et al. Primer-directed enzymatic amplification of DNA with a thermostable DNA polymerase. Science 1988; 239(4839):487–491.

46. Haqqi TM, Sarkar G, David CS, et al. Specific amplification with PCR of a refractory segment of genomic DNA. Nucleic Acids Res 1988; 16(24):11844.

47. Boivin G, Cote S, Dery P, et al. Multiplex real-time PCR assay for detection of influenza and human respiratory syncytial viruses. J Clin Microbiol 2004; 42(1):45–51.

48. Brunstein J, Thomas E. Direct screening of clinical specimens for multiple respiratory pathogens using the Genaco Respiratory Panels 1 and 2. Diagn Mol Pathol 2006; 15(3):169–173.

49. Coiras MT, Aguilar JC, Garcia ML, et al. Simultaneous detection of fourteen respiratory viruses in clinical specimens by two multiplex reverse transcription nested-PCR assays. J Med Virol 2004; 72(3):484–495.

50. Coiras MT, Lopez-Huertas MR, Lopez-Campos G, et al. Oligonucleotide array for simultaneous detection of respiratory viruses using a reverse-line blot hybridization assay. J Med Virol 2005; 76(2):256–264.

51. Kehl SC, Henrickson KJ, Hua W, et al. Evaluation of the Hexaplex assay for detection of respiratory viruses in children. J Clin Microbiol 2001; 39(5):1696–1701.

52. Kessler N, Ferraris O, Palmer K, et al. Use of the DNA flow-thru chip, a three-dimensional biochip, for typing and subtyping of influenza viruses. J Clin Microbiol 2004; 42(5):2173–2185.

53. Mahony J, Chong S, Merante F, et al. Development of a respiratory virus panel test for detection of twenty human respiratory viruses by use of multiplex PCR and a fluid microbead-based assay. J Clin Microbiol 2007; 45(9):2965–2970.

54. Puppe W, Weigl JA, Aron G, et al. Evaluation of a multiplex reverse transcriptase PCR ELISA for the detection of nine respiratory tract pathogens. J Clin Virol 2004; 30(2):165–174.

55. Stockton J, Ellis JS, Saville M, et al. Multiplex PCR for typing and subtyping influenza and respiratory syncytial viruses. J Clin Microbiol 1998; 36(10):2990–2995.

56. Syrmis MW, Whiley DM, Thomas M, et al. A sensitive, specific, and cost-effective multiplex reverse transcriptase-PCR assay for the detection of seven common respiratory viruses in respiratory samples. J Mol Diagn 2004; 6(2):125–131.

57. Templeton KE, Scheltinga SA, Beersma MF, et al. Rapid and sensitive method using multiplex real-time PCR for diagnosis of infections by influenza a and influenza B viruses, respiratory syncytial virus, and parainfluenza viruses 1, 2, 3, and 4. J Clin Microbiol 2004; 42(4):1564–1569.

58. Wang D, Coscoy L, Zylberberg M, et al. Microarray-based detection and genotyping of viral pathogens. Proc Natl Acad Sci U S A 2002; 99(24):15687–15692.

59. Marshall DJ, Reisdorf E, Harms G, et al. Evaluation of a multiplexed PCR assay for detection of respiratory viral pathogens in a public health laboratory setting. J Clin Microbiol 2007; 45(12):3875–3882.

60. Pabbaraju K, Tokaryk KL, Wong S, et al. Comparison of the Luminex xTAG respiratory viral panel with in-house nucleic acid amplification tests for diagnosis of respiratory virus infections. J Clin Microbiol 2008; 46(9):3056–3062.

61. Roh KH, Kim J, Nam MH, et al. Comparison of the Seeplex reverse transcription PCR assay with the R-mix viral culture and immunofluorescence techniques for detection of eight respiratory viruses. Ann Clin Lab Sci 2008; 38(1):41–46.
62. Kim SR, Ki CS, Lee NY. Rapid detection and identification of 12 respiratory viruses using a dual priming oligonucleotide system-based multiplex PCR assay. J Virol Methods 2009; 156:111–116.
63. Sung RYT, Chan PKS, Tsen T, et al. Identification of viral and atypical bacterial pathogen in children hospitalized with acute respiratory infections in Hong Kong by multiplex PCR assays. J Med Virol 2009; 81:153–159.
64. Chernoff DN. The significance of HIV viral load assay precision: a review of the package insert specifications of two commercial kits. J Int Assoc Physicians AIDS Care (Chic Ill) 2002; 1(4):134–140.
65. Hodinka RL. The clinical utility of viral quantitation using molecular methods. Clin Diagn Virol 1998; 10(1):25–47.
66. Janda JM, Abbott SL. 16S rRNA gene sequencing for bacterial identification in the diagnostic laboratory: pluses, perils, and pitfalls. J Clin Microbiol 2007; 45(9):2761–2764.
67. Petti CA. Detection and identification of microorganisms by gene amplification and sequencing. Clin Infect Dis 2007; 44(8):1108–1114.
68. Tang YW, Ellis NM, Hopkins MK, et al. Comparison of phenotypic and genotypic techniques for identification of unusual aerobic pathogenic gram-negative bacilli. J Clin Microbiol 1998; 36(12):3674–3679.
69. Hall L, Doerr KA, Wohlfiel SL, et al. Evaluation of the MicroSeq system for identification of mycobacteria by 16S ribosomal DNA sequencing and its integration into a routine clinical mycobacteriology laboratory. J Clin Microbiol 2003; 41(4):1447–1453.
70. National Center for Biotechnology Information. What does NCBI do? Available at: www.ncbi.nlm.nih.gov.
71. Harmsen D, Rothganger J, Frosch M, et al. RIDOM: ribosomal differentiation of medical micro-organisms database. Nucleic Acids Res 2002; 30(1):416–417.
72. Pruesse E, Quast C, Knittel K, et al. SILVA: a comprehensive online resource for quality checked and aligned ribosomal RNA sequence data compatible with ARB. Nucleic Acids Res 2007; 35(21):7188–7196.
73. Simmon KE, Croft AC, Petti CA. Application of SmartGene IDNS software to partial 16S rRNA gene sequences for a diverse group of bacteria in a clinical laboratory. J Clin Microbiol 2006; 44(12):4400–4406.

3
Hygiene Hypothesis for Allergy and Asthma

ANDREW H. LIU
National Jewish Health and University of Colorado Denver School of Medicine, Denver, Colorado, U.S.A.

I. Introduction

The hygiene hypothesis proposes that naturally occurring microbial exposures in early-life steer immune development away from the allergic march of childhood (Fig. 1). Consequently, secular reductions in infections and microbial exposures have contributed to the global rise in allergic diseases and asthma in the past century. This can seem counterintuitive since any benefit from microbial exposures must be reconciled with the harm of infections. A contemporary paradigm is that microbial exposures can promote immune and respiratory health, without causing severe or chronic illness. This is dependent on certain conditions of exposure: (*i*) early persistent timing, prior to disease onset, (*ii*) moderate, nontoxic dosage, (*iii*) little to no pathogenicity, (*iv*) diverse microbial burden of exposure, and (*v*) favorable genetics. The clinical, translational, and epidemiologic evidence for these key determinants of healthful outcomes from microbial exposures will be presented in this chapter. The hygiene hypothesis may be more than theory, but health benefits from this knowledge have not yet been realized.

II. Historical and Epidemiologic Trends Initiating the Hygiene Hypothesis

Two current epidemiologic trends might be explained, in part, by the hygiene hypothesis: (*i*) the global rise in allergy and asthma prevalence and (*ii*) the broad variation in allergy and asthma prevalence in different locales. To understand the hygiene hypothesis, one should begin with a historical perspective on the secular changes in public and personal hygiene of the past century.

A. A Historical Perspective on Hygiene

The foundation of public and personal hygiene is the germ theory of disease, which came into wide acceptance in the late 1800s (1). Before the discovery and widespread use of antibiotics and vaccines in the late 1940s to 1950s, there were decades when the war against pathogenic microbes was based on avoidance and prevention. This modern era of public hygiene (i.e., municipal sewerage, garbage collection, quarantine, water quality standards, food inspection, and refrigeration), which began in the 1880s, was coupled with a personal hygiene movement. For example, early in the development of germ theory, observations of microscopic germs in house dust led to the notion that house dust, not people, was the main fomite of infectious disease transmission, especially to young children (1). Thus, the common infectious diseases of childhood were

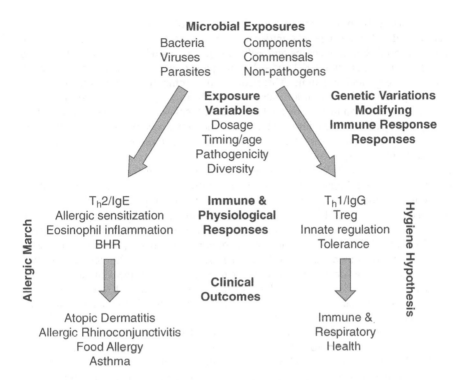

Figure 1 Schema depicting the hygiene hypothesis: how microbial exposures, given the right circumstances, steer immune development away from the allergic march of childhood and toward healthful immune and respiratory outcomes. Key determinants of healthful microbial exposures include (*i*) moderate, nontoxic dosage, (*ii*) early persistent timing, prior to disease development, (*iii*) minimal to no pathogenicity, (*iv*) a diverse microbial burden of exposure, and (*v*) favorable host genetics.

considered to be "house" diseases, and public health campaigns around the turn of the century included in their doctrine the importance of house dust eradication. Together, improved public and personal hygiene greatly reduced microbial burden and improved health.

Through the turn of the 19th to 20th century, the most common causes of death in the United States were infectious diseases (e.g., more than 20% of infants died from infectious diseases) (2). This era of hygiene coincides with the beginning of a dramatic decline in U.S. mortality rates due to infectious diseases. From 1900 to 1980, there was a 95% decline in infectious disease mortality (2). Interestingly, the greatest decline in infectious disease mortality rates came before the widespread implementation of antibiotics and vaccines, and is attributed to improvements in public hygiene. Although the value of hygiene was largely understood by the early 1900s and could be implemented in metropolitan cities by affluent individuals, these measures were unaffordable and not implemented for most of the U.S. population—including the poor, immigrants, and farmers—until the 1930s and 1940s, and after World War II in other countries.

B. Global Rise in Asthma and Allergy Prevalence

Numerous studies from different countries around the world have reported an increase in the prevalence of allergic diseases and asthma (3). These studies are generally limited because they (*i*) began after 1960 and (*ii*) were questionnaire based, without objective measures of allergy and/or asthma. Three studies overcome these limitations. First, one asthma study was performed on a database of all 18- to 19-year-old Finnish men, who undergo a medical examination to establish their fitness for military service (4). This database, going back to 1926, provided not only the prevalence of men with asthma on the basis of physical examination but also the prevalence of those who were exempted or discharged from military service because of the severity of their asthma. A 22-fold rise in asthma prevalence (1961: 0.08% to 1989: 1.79%) began in the 1960s. Prior to that time, asthma in young Finnish men was a rare occurrence. Second, a prospective study of two communities in Australia used objective measures of atopy [i.e., prick skin testing (PST)] and asthma [i.e., bronchial hyperresponsiveness (BHR)] along with questionnaires to determine the prevalence of asthma and allergy in 8- to 10-year-old children in 1982 and 1992 (5). In both locales, asthma and hay fever prevalence increased over the decade. In comparison, prevalence of BHR and inhalant allergen sensitization also increased in both locales, but to a lesser degree. Third, in the United States, the prevalence of allergic sensitization by PST to six common inhalant allergens (alternaria, Bermuda grass, cat, oak, ragweed, and ryegrass) was determined in two nationally representative National Health and Nutrition Examination Surveys (NHANES): NHANES II (1976–1980) and NHANES III (1988–1994) (6). The proportion of the population with sensitization to at least one of the six allergens increased, from 21.8% in NHANES II to 41.9% in NHANES III. These differences were significant for each allergen tested and across all age strata (6–60 years of age). Allergy and asthma prevalence, conservatively estimated from these and other studies, has increased approximately 50% per decade since the 1960s.

C. Population Variance in Allergy and Asthma Prevalence

"Summer catarrh . . . only occurs in the middle or upper classes of society, some indeed of high rank. I have made inquiry at the various dispensaries in London and elsewhere, and I have not heard of a single unequivocal case occurring among the poor" (7).

"It would seem that hay fever has, of late years, been considerably on the increase . . . The persons who are most subjected to the action of the pollen belong to a class which furnishes the fewest cases of the disorder, namely, the farming class" (8).

Population variations in allergy prevalence have a long history. John Bostock, the first to describe a case series of summer catarrh (aka hay fever) sufferers, and Charles Blackley, the first to determine that grass pollens are the inciting agents of hay fever, were intrigued by the paradoxically low occurrence of hay fever in the poor and farmers, those with the greatest exposure to the hay allergen.

Major differences in childhood asthma and allergy prevalence in different locales are apparent today. The International Study of Asthma and Allergies in Childhood (ISAAC), of approximately 500,000 children of 13 to 14 years in 155 centers in 56 different countries, revealed 20- to 60-fold differences in the prevalence of reported asthma, allergic rhinoconjunctivitis, eczema symptoms, and allergic sensitization, among different centers (9,10). Numerous other studies have consistently found that children living in the following two types of locales have a lower prevalence of allergy, asthma, allergic sensitization, and/or BHR than those living in modern metropolitan areas: (*i*) rural areas of developing nations (11–19) and (*ii*) farms (20–26). Possible explanations in the scientific literature include differences in infections and microbial exposures, outdoor and indoor air pollutants (e.g., tobacco smoke), rise in obesity, changes in home environment (more carpeting, "tighter" homes increasing indoor allergens and pollutants), increases in indoor versus outdoor time (less exercise), and dietary changes (i.e., less infant breast-feeding, less vitamin D, more fast food). While the validity of the nonmicrobial factors is beyond the scope of this chapter, it is likely that a combination of factors underlies the observed allergy/asthma prevalence increase over time and differences by locale.

III. Microbes and Less Allergy/Asthma

Serious systemic [e.g., neonatal sepsis (27)] or respiratory tract infections [e.g., tuberculosis (28), measles (29,30)] have been inconsistently associated with less allergic disease and asthma. In a nationwide study in Finland, measles was associated with a slightly increased risk of eczema, allergic rhinitis, and asthma (31). In modernized countries where public hygiene improvements, vaccinations, and antimicrobial therapies are in full force, a lower risk of asthma, BHR, and allergic sensitization with more "viral infections" (e.g., runny nose colds or herpes type infections) in early childhood was observed (32). The longitudinal prospective study design, inclusion of objective disease biomarkers, and greater effect with more viral infections strengthened these findings (e.g., with ≥ 8 viral infections by age three years, odds ratios (OR) of MD-diagnosed asthma and BHR were 0.16 and 0.24, respectively). Neither other types of infections [bacterial, fungal, gastrointestinal (GI)] nor antibiotic courses in the first three years of life altered the risk of asthma or allergic sensitization at age seven years. A large German cohort study linked high exposure to acute respiratory infections in the first nine months of life with reduced odds of subsequent asthma, eczema, hay fever, allergic sensitization, and total IgE when 5 to 14 years old (33).

The above observation about viral infections is consistent with numerous reports over the past decade associating family size (i.e., greater number of older siblings) (34–38) and early day care (39,40) with less allergy and asthma. Indeed, David Strachan's observation of less hay fever and eczema in children with more older siblings is often credited with initiating the current, sustained interest in the hygiene hypothesis (34). Larger families and early day care in early childhood are associated with more respiratory tract illnesses in the first two to three years of life (41–44). They are also associated with higher levels of noninfectious microbial exposures such as endotoxin (45,46), discussed later in this chapter. The idea that these ubiquitous microbial exposures in early childhood may shape immune development and provide respiratory health dividends in later years is also supported by evidence that early day care is associated with a subsequent decreased risk of respiratory illnesses (42), extending through the elementary school years (41).

A variety of GI microbes have been associated with less allergy and asthma. In a study of 1659 male Italian air force cadets, antibody evidence of previous GI tract infections (i.e., hepatitis A, *Toxoplasma gondii, Helicobacter pylori*) was associated with less allergy, asthma, and allergen sensitization (47). Individuals with evidence of two or three of these GI tract infections had a significantly lower likelihood of allergic disease (OR 0.37). Presumably, many of these infections were mild or asymptomatic. In the same study, individual or cumulative antibody evidence of previous measles, mumps, rubella, chicken pox, cytomegalovirus, or herpes simplex virus infection(s) was not associated with less atopy. In a U.S.-wide representative study (NHANES), *H. pylori* seropositivity was inversely related to asthma and allergic rhinitis, especially in child-hood (48). In rural Africa, parasitic infestations with schistosomes (49), ascaris/hookworm (50,51), and *Trichuris trichiura* (52) were associated with less allergen sensitization and asthma. A systematic review and meta-analysis of the epidemiologic studies of parasite infections and the risk of asthma revealed that hookworm infection, which had the strongest protective effect, reduced the odds of asthma significantly (OR 0.50, 9 studies), especially when infection intensity was greater (OR 0.34) (53).

Some investigators identified differences in bacterial microbiota in stool samples from newborns and infants who ultimately go on to develop allergic disease, but there are some inconsistencies in these findings. The GI microbiota of infants who develop allergy had more Clostridia and *Staphylococcus aureus*, while nonallergic infants had more *Enterococci*, *Bifidobacteria*, *Lactobacilli*, and *Bacteroides* (54–57). However, in another study, *Bacteroides* colonization in infants' stools was associated with a higher prevalence of early-onset asthma (58). Using the molecular diversity of 16S rRNA fragments in stool as an indicator of fecal microbiota diversity, the stool of one-week-old infants who subsequently developed atopic eczema was significantly less diverse than that of their noneczema counterparts (59). This is a developing area of investigation with the advent of new molecular techniques to fully speciate microbiota, without the selection biases and limitations of culture-based methods.

Significant differences in microbial exposure have also been associated with fertile soil, rich in nonpathogenic microbes, mostly saprophytic gram-positive bacteria. The microbial ecology of fertile soil is retained in farming and less modernized locales where atopy prevalence is low, but reduced in modern metropolitan settings where atopy prevalence is high (60). In Karelia, Russia, where the prevalence of allergy is low, bacterial genera in house dust were highly diverse, mostly gram-positive bacilli, with more bacterial species associated with animals (61).

To summarize, current evidence suggests that serious, single-event infections do not have a significant protective effect on atopy or asthma development. Instead, fre-quent or persistent, and diverse microbial exposures beginning in early life, typically clinically mild, subclinical, commensal, and/or nonpathogenic, may influence allergic outcomes considerably. While some consistency and replication of observations about microbes, allergy, and asthma exists, they alone cannot establish causation; rather, they have generated a compelling hypothesis (62).

IV. Immunobiology Substantiating the Hygiene Hypothesis
A. The T_h1/T_h2 Paradigm

Immunologically, the hygiene hypothesis is substantiated by a well-known and sim-plistic paradigm that allergic diseases and asthma are the products of T lymphocytes that produce "T_h2" cytokines (i.e., IL-4, IL-5, IL-9, IL-13), which are counterregulated by "T_h1" cytokines (i.e., IFN-γ, IL-12). It appears that the naïve immune system of the newborn is skewed to produce T_h2 cytokines to common environmental allergens (63), presumably because T_h1 cytokine production is inhibited in utero for maintenance of maternal-fetal tolerance (64,65). Longitudinal studies of in vitro T_h1-type cytokine production, in response to nonspecific (66) or allergen-specific (i.e., dust mite allergen) (67) stimuli, have found that children who develop allergic disease produced less in vitro IFN-γ in infancy. Theoretically, microbial exposures in early life may drive early T_h1-type immune development, with a reciprocal inhibition of T_h2-type immune development and ultimately allergies and asthma. In rodent models of atopic asthma, many different types of microbial exposures [e.g., bacterial lipopolysaccharide (LPS) (68,69), Bacille Calmette-Guerin (BCG) (70,71), heat-killed *Lactobacillus* (72), heat-killed *Listeria* (73), *Mycoplasma* (74), bacterial DNA (75–78), and even direct T_h1 cytokine administration (e.g., IFN-γ, IL-12) (79–85)], mitigate the development of the atopic asthma phenotype through T_h1 mechanisms. Importantly, the efficacy of T_h1-type induction (i.e., IL-12, LPS) in mitigating atopy is generally strongest when administered prior to atopy onset (69,86).

B. T_h1-Influenced Repair of Airways Injury

The potential of T_h1-type immune responses to prevent asthma development extends beyond downregulating T_h2-mediated IgE production and preventing allergic sensitization and atopic inflammation in the airways. IFN-γ mitigates the development of other hallmark pathologic features of asthma (87). In in vitro and animal model studies, IFN-γ and IFN-γ-producing T lymphocytes (*i*) decrease mucous gland hypertrophy and hyperplasia (88), (*ii*) inhibit fibroblast proliferation, production of collagen, and differentiation into myofibroblasts (89–92), (*iii*) inhibit mast cell proliferation (93,94), (*iv*) inhibit airway smooth muscle proliferation (95), (*v*) induce epithelial antiviral mechanisms (85) and epithelial/macrophage production of defensins (human β-defensin 2) and collectin (surfactant protein A) production (96–98), and (6) prevent long-term sequelae from respiratory viral infections (99). In humans inoculated with rhinovirus, decreased virus shedding from the airways was associated with increased in vitro IFN-γ production before infection (100). In a human study of infant bronchiolitis and subsequent persistent wheezing (i.e., 5 months later), the peripheral blood of persistent wheezers produced significantly less IFN-γ (101), demonstrating that poor IFN-γ immune responses may underlie persistent wheezing problems, even without concurrent atopy. Therefore, T_h1-type immune responses to injury may be able to prevent most of the pathologic processes observed in asthma.

C. Regulatory T Lymphocytes

Microbial stimulation also induces IL-10 production, which has important immune regulatory and anti-inflammatory actions. The paradox of less atopy in parasite-infested children has excited interest in the potential disease-mitigating role of IL-10-producing cells and parasite-induced immunoregulation (102,103). As discussed earlier, parasitic infestation, a potent T_h2-inducing stimulus, is nevertheless associated with less allergy and asthma. Not only does parasitic infestation induce IgE production and eosinophilia, but it also leads to increased allergen-specific serum IgE levels. In metropolitan locales, these biomarkers are typically associated with allergen sensitization (i.e., skin test sensitivity), allergy, and asthma. However, in locales where parasite infestation is common, there is a disconnection between these classic biomarkers of atopy and allergen sensitization, allergic disease, and asthma. For example, in a study of Gabonese schoolchildren, in whom schistosome infestation was common, 32% had significantly increased serum house-dust mite (HDM) IgE levels (>1 IU/mL), but only 11% had a positive HDM PST (49). In addition, peripheral blood cells from nonallergic patients demonstrated greater in vitro IL-10 production with schistosome antigen-induced stimulation. Mechanistically, IL-10 can differentially regulate IL-4-stimulated B cells to produce IgG_4 instead of IgE (104), block mast cell degranulation, and release of histamine, IL-8, and TNF-a (105), and downregulate IL-4 and IL-5 production from T_h2 clones (106). "Regulatory," IL-10-producing, $CD4^+$ $CD25^+$ T lymphocytes, capable of abrogating autoimmunity and transplant rejection in some model systems, may have a central role in alleviating and preventing atopic inflammatory diseases (107). Clinical observations supporting these mechanisms include the following: allergic asthmatics produce less IL-10 (108), dust mite PST-positive children produce less IL-10 to mite allergen stimulation in vitro, and PST wheal size in mite-sensitized children is negatively correlated with IL-10 (109). Considering these links between IL-10-mediated immune regulation and allergy/asthma development, IL-10, IFN-γ, and IL-12-inducing immune stimuli, such as those provided by microbes, may be a particularly effective combination.

V. Endotoxin: Sterile Microbial Prototype Reveals Key Determinants for the Hygiene Hypothesis

Bacterial endotoxin has been an informative microbial component [i.e., pathogen-associated molecular pattern (PAMP)] and prototypical toll-like receptor (TLR) ligand for study in laboratory and clinical settings. Via endotoxin, we can explore the contribution of sterile (i.e., noninfectious) microbial exposures to allergy/asthma risk reduction in childhood and further understand the mechanisms and key determinants to these beneficial effects.

A. Endotoxin Immunobiology

Endotoxin, a bacterial LPS, comprises most of the outer layer of the outer cell membrane of all gram-negative bacteria. Its potent immune-stimulatory capacity is largely attributed to the lipid A moiety, which is highly conserved across different bacterial species (110). Very small amounts of endotoxin (i.e., picogram amounts of LPS or approximately 10 LPS molecules per cell) are immune stimulatory (111). Endotoxin is also remarkably resilient. For example, rendering glassware "endotoxin-free" requires prolonged baking at high temperatures (e.g., 160°C for 4 hours). Such potency and durability explain endotoxin's persistence as an immune stimulant in our living environment.

The immediate responders of the innate immune system (e.g., monocytes, macrophages, dendritic cells, epithelial cells, neutrophils), as well as many other cell types, recognize endotoxin through TLR4 (112). Cellular sensitivity to endotoxin is, in part, influenced by the TLR4-related enhancer and coreceptor proteins, LPS-binding protein (LBP), CD14, and MD-2. LBP, a soluble protein produced by the liver, shuttles endotoxin to TLR4 (113). CD14, a soluble and cell surface receptor, binds LPS and improves TLR4 sensitivity and detection of endotoxin (114). MD-2, extracellular adapter protein, binds both the hydrophobic portion of LPS and the extracellular domain of TLR4 (115). MD-2 is constitutively associated with TLR4 and is required for TLR4 recognition of and cell activation by endotoxin. Thus, some of the variability of TLR4 sensitivity to endotoxin is attributable to MD-2, LPS BP, and CD14 levels. Other factors that heighten immune cellular sensitivity to endotoxin include priming by innate immune cytokines (e.g., IFNs), low-level endotoxin exposure, or other PAMP exposures (116–118). Conversely, high endotoxin exposure suppresses TLR4-mediated activation (111,118).

B. Key Determinants for Healthful Outcomes

In laboratory models of allergic sensitization and asthma, the *timing, dosage,* and *diversity* of endotoxin and related microbial component exposures affect health/disease outcomes.

Timing

In rodent models, endotoxin exposure prior to or within the first few days of allergen exposure induced a nonpathogenic IgG-specific response. Endotoxin exposure in the later stages of the response amplified pathogenic allergic immune response and BHR upon reexposure to allergen (69). Thus, early timing of endotoxin exposure, prior to development of allergic pathogenic immune responses, was essential for protective benefit. This paradigm of timing was similarly demonstrated for *Mycoplasma pneumoniae* in mouse models of allergic asthma by Chu and Martin (74).

Dosage

In mouse models of asthma, ovalbumin stripped of endotoxin did not induce a persistent immune response; however, ovalbumin with low-level endotoxin induced IgE-mediated allergic sensitization and a T_h2-type allergic inflammatory response (68). Similarly, in vitro TLR4 stimulation of dendritic cells was necessary for pathogenic T_h2 inflammatory responses in the airways (119,120). In contrast, higher levels of endotoxin with ovalbumin led to nonpathogenic IgG and T_h1-type immune responses specific to the allergen (68). Endotoxin in higher concentrations also induced innate antigen-presenting cells, especially dendritic cells, to produce IL-12 and to costimulate T cells to become effector T cells that primarily secrete IFN-γ (121–123). In a murine model, daily intranasal endotoxin or house dust extract blocked T_h2, without blocking ovalbumin-specific IL10 or increasing T_h1, perhaps by inducing IL-10-producing T regulatory lymphocytes (124).

In a final twist of the dose-response relationship of endotoxin with respiratory disease, chronic high-level endotoxin exposure can generate airways fibrosis and progressive airways obstruction. Mice that were chronically exposed to grain dust, which naturally contained endotoxin (4 hr/day, 5 day/wk for 2 months), developed airways inflammation and subepithelial fibrosis around the airways (125).

These studies demonstrate that the dose-response relationship of noninfectious microbial exposures to allergy/asthma is not simply pathogenic or healthful. Instead, moderate doses seem protective, while low and high doses can be pathogenic, although via different mechanisms (low levels are proallergic; chronic high levels are endotoxic). These studies also highlight the essential role of the innate immune system in mediating these allergic or healthful immune responses to microbial exposures like endotoxin.

Diversity

PAMPs, other than endotoxin, have also been tested in murine models of allergic asthma. Unmethylated CpG DNA motifs, unique to microbial DNA, are PAMPs recognized by TLR9 (126). CpG DNA, which activates dendritic cells to induce T-cell proliferation and T_h1 development (127,128), prevented the development of atopic immune responses and allergic asthma or allergic rhinitis in mouse models (129).

In contrast, the bacterial TLR2 ligand peptidoglycan (129) and LPS from *Porphyromonas gingivalis* (130) promoted T_h2 immune responses and allergic inflammation. *P. gingivalis* LPS appears to mediate T_h2 immune responses in dendritic cells via a MyD88-independent, extracellular signaling pathway (131,132). Lipoteichoic acid from *S. aureus* induced an eczematoid inflammatory reaction on murine skin (133). Another *S. aureus* product, Staphylococcal enterotoxin B, conditioned human monocyte–derived dendritic cells to induce T_h2 development in a TLR2-dependent manner, because of induction of IL-2 secretion without IL-12 p70 production (134). Yet, lipotechoic acid and the synthetic TLR2 agonist Pam3CSK4 inhibited dust mite–specific IL-5 and IL-13 responses in peripheral blood mononuclear cells (PBMC) from mite-allergic persons without inducing a strong T_h1 response (135).

To assess the effect of PAMP exposures in a way that better represents what occurs naturally, sterile but unpurified house dust extract was given daily and at low doses to mice. This treatment was potently effective in preventing allergic asthma development, like treating with endotoxin alone (124,136). It also worked in TLR4-deficient mice unable to respond to endotoxin (136).

These rodent model experiments demonstrate the various effects of TLR stimulation of the innate immune system on allergic outcomes. It can cause a pathogenic allergic immune response when exposure is low or when given after the allergic immune response is established. Yet, moderate TLR stimulation, especially from multiple PAMP types, might strongly promote a nonpathogenic immune response.

C. Endotoxin Exposure in Human Health and Allergic/Asthmatic Disease

Timing and Dosage

In humans, endotoxin exposure in early life appears to modify immune development and allergic disease inception. In infants and young children, higher house dust endotoxin levels were associated with less atopic dermatitis (137–139), inhalant allergen sensitization (140–142), allergic rhinitis, and asthma (143–145) in childhood. The strength of this evidence is apparent in multiple longitudinal birth cohort studies (137–139,141,146), as well as in a large European rural farm/nonfarm study where a dose-response relationship between endotoxin exposure and less atopy was shown (144). However, the findings of different studies are not uniformly consistent; for example, some studies found house dust endotoxin to be positively associated with asthma (141,147).

Human studies of immune responses to endotoxin exposure in early life have revealed little IFN-γ from mitogen-stimulated cord blood obtained at birth; however, by three months of age, higher peripheral blood IFN-γ levels were associated with higher home endotoxin levels, as well as living on a farm, and cats and dogs in the home (148). Greater household endotoxin exposure in infancy was also associated with increased proportions of T_h1-type cells (i.e., IFN-γ^+/CD4$^+$ and IFN-γ^+/CD8$^+$ cells) in peripheral blood samples at one to two years of age (140) and increased phytohemagglutinin (PHA)-induced IFN-γ production by PBMC at three years of age (149). However, in the latter study, greater endotoxin exposure was also associated with increased PHA-induced IL-13 levels. In a longitudinal birth cohort study of infants at high risk for asthma and allergy, increased house dust endotoxin levels in the first two to three months of life were associated with decreased IL-13 levels at two to three years of age, in response to whole blood stimulation with cockroach, dust mite, and cat allergens, but not PHA (150). Endotoxin levels were not correlated with allergen- or mitogen-induced IFN-γ, TNF-α, or IL-10. Increased endotoxin levels were associated with decreased cockroach allergen-induced lymphocyte proliferation, suggesting a downregulatory effect of endotoxin exposure in early life. In a large, rural European study inclusive of animal-farming households, where house dust endotoxin levels had a much higher range than what is typically observed in metropolitan homes, endotoxin levels were inversely related to cytokine production by LPS-stimulated whole blood (i.e., TNF-α, IFN-γ, IL-10, IL-12) in a dose-dependent manner (144).

Consistent with microbial induction of regulatory T lymphocyte responses in mouse models, human endotoxin-matured dendritic cells induce $CD4^+$ T lymphocytes to produce not only IFN-γ but also IL-10 and TGF-b, and to express FoxP3 (151). Similarly, human colonic monocytes, when stimulated with endotoxin, induced CD25, IL-10, and FoxP3 expression in lymphocytes (152). In nasal mucosal explanted tissue from toddler-age children, endotoxin induced brisk proliferation of $CD3^+/CD4^+/CD25^+/IL-10^+/TLR4^+$ cells that dominated allergen-induced T_h2 responses in vitro (153). Endotoxin induces the molecular signatures of regulatory T lymphocytes in humans through dendritic cells and monocytes and possibly directly through TLR4-expressing regulatory T lymphocytes that are resident in mucosal tissues.

In contrast to these atopy-protective influences, endotoxin can cause airways disease in endotoxin-hypersensitive individuals, especially when exposure levels are high. In infants and children, higher endotoxin levels were associated with more wheezing, often in the same studies where a protective effect on atopy in early life was concurrently observed (137,139,141,144,154,155). Dose-response endotoxin inhalation studies revealed healthy persons who are hypersensitive to respirable endotoxin at low levels of exposure (156–158). In rural European schoolchildren, very high levels of bed dust endotoxin were associated with an increased prevalence of nonatopic wheeze, while low prevalence of atopy and allergy-associated wheeze were retained (144). In humans, airways hypersensitivity to endotoxin appears to occur in early life and in some individuals. Additionally, chronic high-level exposure in some workplace settings and farm locales can cause nonatopic asthma in susceptible people.

Similar to mouse models showing endotoxin's proinflammatory effects when allergic inflammatory pathways have been established, low-level endotoxin exposure in humans significantly augmented BHR to histamine and increased the airways inflammatory response to allergen exposure in sensitized people with asthma (157–161) or allergic rhinitis (162). When mite-sensitized subjects with allergic rhinitis were challenged with subthreshold doses of mite allergen (100 allergen units of *Dermatophagoides farinae*), simultaneous low-level LPS exposure (1 μg) augmented eosinophilic inflammation in the nasal lavage (162). Endotoxin also augmented the skin test wheal-and-flare responses to allergen (163). Higher dust endotoxin levels in homes (147,163–165) and occupational settings (166,167) have been associated with increased asthma prevalence, severity, and lung dysfunction.

Thus, the dosage and timing relationships between endotoxin and immune development, allergic sensitization, and disease, revealed in rodent models, are recapitulated in human health/disease. However, there are important distinctions; in infancy, the endotoxin exposure levels associated with less atopy also make infant wheezing more likely. Additionally, some adults and children appear susceptible to endotoxin-mediated asthma. These inconsistencies between rodent and human suggest additional key determinants in the real-life circumstances leading to healthful or harmful outcomes from endotoxin exposure.

Microbial Component Diversity

In humans, other PAMP exposures may also protect against the development of allergy and/or asthma. β-1,3-Glucan, a fungal PAMP, was associated with less aeroallergen sensitization in toddler-age children (146). Higher levels of fungal polysaccharides from *Penicillium* and *Aspergillus* in house dust, in addition to endotoxin, were associated with less doctor-diagnosed asthma in young children (145). *N*-acetylmuramic acid, a component of bacterial peptidoglycan and a TLR2 PAMP found in higher levels in farm homes, was associated with less wheezing, but not less allergic sensitization, in school-age children (168). DNA from dust samples from farm homes, farm barns, and rural homes in India had higher proportions of microbial DNA that was presumably rich in TLR9 PAMPs (169). When combined with a small amount of endotoxin, farm barn DNA augmented IL-10 and IL-12 production by PBMC in vitro.

Gene-Environment Interactions with Endotoxin

Polymorphisms in genes encoding proteins that mediate endotoxin recognition can modify endotoxin responsiveness. Heterozygous individuals for either one of two different substitution mutations in TLR4 (+896 A/G; +1196 G/T) demonstrated airways and immune hyporesponsiveness to endotoxin (170,171). Accordingly, healthy adults with TLR4 hyporesponsiveness mutations experienced less lung function decline than nonmutant controls with swine confinement facility exposure, high in respirable endotoxin [change in spirometric forced expiratory volume in the first second (FEV1) -8.5% vs. -11.5%; $p = 0.001$] (172). However, these TLR4 polymorphisms do not exert a consistent effect on asthma prevalence. In an investigation of two North American cohorts, these polymorphisms in the TLR4 gene were not associated with asthma (173). In a small cohort of Swedish children, one of the TLR4 polymorphisms associated with endotoxin hyporesponsiveness (Asp299Gly) was associated with a fourfold higher prevalence of asthma and reduced LPS-induced IL-12p70 and IL-10 release from PBMC (174). In a large population study in Europe, both TLR4 hyporesponsiveness polymorphisms were associated with less BHR and wheeze, but only at moderate levels of endotoxin exposure (175). Taken together, TLR4 polymorphisms do not seem to have a simple effect on allergy or asthma risk. Instead, their effects seem dependent on endotoxin exposure levels.

A common polymorphism in the promoter region (-260C-to-T) of the CD14 gene has been one of the most studied polymorphisms with regard to asthma and allergies. Functionally, the -260CT CD14 promoter polymorphism alters the transcriptional regulation of CD14; the T allele increases CD14 transcription by reducing the binding of proteins that inhibit gene transcription (176). Some studies have found that the C allele of the -260 CD14 promoter polymorphism increases the risk for allergic sensitization (177,178), while others have not (179,180). Furthermore, some studies show this allele to have either protective or risk effects depending on the type of environment in which the individuals live. These discrepancies are likely due to different levels of endotoxin. In infants and young children, only the low responder, "CC" homozygous group demonstrated strong dose-response relationships between higher house dust endotoxin levels and less subsequent allergic sensitization to inhalant allergens, less atopic dermatitis, and more nonatopic wheeze (181). In the study by Eder et al. (182), the C allele was found to be protective in children living in the subset of homes where measured endotoxin levels were high. Conversely, in a study of adult farmers, with presumably greater exposure to endotoxin, the high responder, "TT" homozygous group had significantly lower lung function and a higher prevalence of wheezing (183). Similarly, in an asthma genetics study in Barbados, the TT genotype was an asthma risk factor for individuals with high house dust endotoxin levels (OR, 11.66; 95% CI, 1.03–131.7) while seeming to protect against asthma for individuals with low endotoxin levels (OR, 0.09; 95% CI, 0.03–0.24) (184). These endotoxin receptor complex findings exemplify functional genetic polymorphisms interacting with endotoxin exposure to alter asthma and allergy outcomes and further strengthen the causal inferences of endotoxin in observational studies.

VI. Hygiene Hypothesis Corollaries
A. Protective Microbial Exposures from Animals
Numerous investigations have reported a protective effect of early-life animal exposures—especially to dogs, cows, and pigs—with less atopic dermatitis, allergic sensitization, and/or asthma. Some of these studies are of a longitudinal, prospective study design that is stronger for inferences of causation (185–188). These animals were associated with higher levels of endotoxin in house dust and ambient air samples (189–192). The protective farming lifestyle in European children was also associated with higher peripheral blood expression levels of relevant microbial sensors, CD14 and TLR1, TLR2, TLR4, TLR7, and TLR8 (193,194). Of particular interest, in a large study of farm community children, maternal exposure during pregnancy to increasing numbers of farm animal species was associated with increased PBMC expression of TLR2, TLR4, and CD14 receptors, and less atopic sensitization in their children (195). In rural homes in Kenya, Guinea-Bissau, India, Nepal, and Mongolia, less allergic sensitization and/or less exercise-induced bronchospasm was associated with proximal living with domestic animals (14,19,29,196,197). An attractive hypothesis for the protective effect of proximal living with animals is that greater microbial exposures in early life heighten the expression of relevant microbial sensors, which ready the innate and adaptive immune systems to respond to their environment in a healthful manner.

B. Gut Microbiota and Food Allergy
Murine models of food allergy suggest that endotoxin-mediated TLR stimulation may modify allergic responses to foods. The natural source of TLR ligands in this circumstance is the gut microbiota. In murine studies, IgE-mediated peanut anaphylaxis could be induced in TLR4-deficient mice, or in TLR4-sufficient mice by administering antibiotics in early life to eliminate gut flora (198). TLR4-deficient mice could be protected from the development of peanut allergy by administration of CpG DNA, a TLR9 ligand. The immunologic hallmark of the TLR4-sufficient mice and the TLR9-stimulated mice was a peanut-specific IFN-γ (i.e., T_h1), but not a T_h2 cytokine response, in vitro. In this model of peanut allergy, the findings are similar to the rodent models of allergic asthma: TLR stimulation by gut flora or CpG DNA in early life promoted a nonpathogenic T_h1 immune response to peanut, without peanut allergy.

Interestingly, a mouse model of gut injury revealed a series of important TLR-mediated mechanisms of protection from mucosal injury—the maintenance of intestinal epithelial homeostasis and integrity (199). When given an intestinal epithelial toxicant (dextran sulfate), MyD88-deficient mice (i.e., deficient in signaling via all TLRs) experienced morbidity and mortality, while wild-type control mice did not. Wild-type mice could be rendered vulnerable by pretreatment with antibiotics to eliminate commensal bacteria. However, the antibiotic-treated mice could be rescued by oral administration of endotoxin or lipotechoic acid. TLR4- and TLR2-deficient mice demonstrated an intermediate degree of morbidity but a low degree of mortality. If pretreated with antibiotics, TLR2-deficient, but not TLR4-deficient, mice could be rescued with LPS-treated water, further demonstrating the TLR-dependence of protection from gut injury.

The poor outcomes of the MyD88-deficient mice were not obviously due to differences in immune responses, as no differences in leukocyte infiltration of colonic tissues between deficient and wild-type mice were observed. Instead, intestinal epithelial cells of deficient mice were susceptible to apoptosis, had reduced levels of cytoprotective cytokines (IL-6, TNF, KC-1) and heat shock proteins (HSP25, HSP72), and could not upregulate them in response to injury. In normal conditions, constitutive production of cytoprotective cytokines by gut epithelium appears dependent on TLR signaling via gut flora, because antibiotic treatment eliminated the production of these cytokines in the colon. These recent mouse model studies suggest that compromised TLR-mediated signaling may predispose to peanut and other food allergies by rendering the intestinal epithelium more susceptible to injury and altering the nature of the effector immune response to food allergens from T_h1 to T_h2.

VII. Hygiene Hypothesis: Clinical Implications Today
A. Immunizations, Antibiotic Use, and Allergy/Asthma
The hygiene hypothesis has aroused suspicions that childhood vaccinations and antibiotic usage promote allergies and asthma by reducing early childhood infections.

Immunizations
There is no consistent evidence that the common childhood immunizations, which prevent serious infections, are associated with an increased likelihood of allergy and asthma (200). The ISAAC study group investigated this possibility in their global, comprehensive database and did not find an association between national or local immunization rates (for tuberculosis, diphtheria, tetanus, pertussis, or measles) and prevalence of atopic disease symptoms in children (201). For measles, pertussis, and BCG (for tuberculosis) vaccinations, different research groups have not found an association with an increased likelihood of allergic disease or asthma. On the contrary, in Finland, a slightly increased risk of atopic disease in subjects who had measles was observed (31). Furthermore, some BCG immunization studies have found atopic diseases to be less common in BCG-immunized children (202,203). A large meta-analysis of observational studies found no significant associations for either whole-cell pertussis (seven studies, $n = 186,663$) or BCG (5 studies, $n = 41,479$) vaccinations and incident rates of asthma in children and adolescence (204). It is also important to factor in the risk from immunization exemption in today's world (205). Immunization avoidance still

poses a considerable threat of severe disease; therefore, the balance of evidence strongly favors vaccinating children.

Antibiotic Usage

The common practice of antibiotic administration for common childhood illnesses has also come under suspicion as an antimicrobial practice linked to greater allergy and asthma. A large retrospective study ($n \sim 29,000$) found a significant dose-response relationship between the number of antibiotic courses in the first year of life and diagnosed asthma, eczema, and hay fever (206). However, a large prospective birth cohort study did not find a significant association between antibiotic use and allergic disease or asthma (32). This difference between retrospective and prospective studies continued to be evident in a systematic review and meta-analysis of four retrospective and four prospective studies (207), and a large ($n = 251,817$ live births) prospective study extensively adjusted for potential confounders (208). The retrospective studies continued to demonstrate that antibiotic exposure in the first year of life was associated with subsequently diagnosed asthma in childhood, and this risk increases with the number or courses of antibiotics prescribed. The prospective studies generally did not demonstrate any significant risk, although the largest longitudinal prospective study showed a small but significant risk (hazard ratio 1.12, 95% CI, 1.08–1.16). These studies could not determine if the antibiotic usage could be reducing protective microbial exposures or serving as a proxy for children with susceptibility to respiratory tract infections leading to childhood asthma. Taking into consideration that antibiotic therapy can be essential treatment for bacterial pathogens but overprescribing of antibiotics is associated with increased colonization by antibiotic-resistant bacterial pathogens, judicious use of antibiotics for the treatment of infections is prudent. However, avoiding antibiotics when warranted is an unnecessary risk.

B. Potential for Therapy and Prevention

Already, translational research, supported by public and private sector funding, seeks to bring microbe-derived immune modulators from hypothetical interventions to patient care. These immune modulators are being developed not only for their therapeutic and preventative potential in the allergic diseases and asthma but also as therapeutic agents for intractable infections (i.e., tuberculosis, leprosy) and autoimmune conditions (i.e., inflammatory bowel disease, juvenile type 1 diabetes), and as vaccine adjuvants for infectious diseases and cancer. The development of these products for numerous clinical applications bolsters the likelihood that a clearer picture of the pharmacotherapeutic potential of these products will soon emerge.

One microbe-derived product, BCG, derived from *Mycobacterium bovis*, has been used for many years as a childhood vaccination for tuberculosis and is standard therapy for certain stages of bladder cancer. A study of Japanese schoolchildren (who all received up to 3 BCG immunizations in childhood) revealed that those who had a positive tuberculin response were less likely to develop atopy, allergic disease, or asthma (209). BCG "responders" had more IFN-γ and less T_h2-type cytokines in their serum. There is debate over the meaning of this provocative finding. Is the lower prevalence of atopy and asthma in BCG responders due to (*i*) tuberculosis, leading to a larger tuberculin response and the association with less atopy and asthma or (*ii*) the BCG vaccine itself; (*iii*) or is the tuberculin skin test response serving to identify children with robust IFN-γ responsiveness who are less likely to develop allergy and asthma? While some studies have not confirmed this original compelling observation (210), others have (202). BCG vaccination induces memory T_h1-type immune response in newborns (211) and also improves antibody and cellular responses to other early childhood immunizations (i.e., hepatitis B, oral polio vaccine) (212). In a randomized controlled trial (RCT) of BCG readministration to asthmatic adults, BCG treatment was followed by a reduction in asthma medication use and significant lung function improvement (213).

M. vaccae has been developed as an immune modulator similar to BCG but without antigenic cross-reactivity to *M. tuberculosis*. In a RCT, one intradermal injection of killed *M. vaccae* improved atopic dermatitis in children for three months (214). In contrast, a *M. vaccae* RCT for mite-sensitive asthma did not demonstrate clinical benefit (215). Interestingly, *M. vaccae* clinical trials for psoriasis have also demonstrated sustained improvement, similar to that seen for atopic dermatitis (216,217). Since psoriasis is considered to be a T_h1-mediated disease, this suggests that *M. vaccae* primarily works through neither T_h1 nor T_h2 immune mechanisms but perhaps through regulatory T cells. Preliminary clinical studies with *M. vaccae* have also been published for cancer therapy (i.e., inoperable lung cancer, mesothelioma) (218), multiple sclerosis therapy (219), and pulmonary tuberculosis in several clinical settings: new-onset cases (220,221), multidrug-resistant cases (222), and prevention of HIV-associated tuberculosis (223).

Probiotics

Probiotics, such as *Lactobacillus*, are common bacterial colonizers of the GI tract and induce fermentation in common foods (i.e., yogurt, fermented vegetables). Oral *Lactobacillus* supplementation is currently FDA approved for the prevention of antibiotic-associated diarrhea in children and adults (224,225). Oral *Lactobacillus* RCTs have also demonstrated preventive efficacy for necrotizing enterocolitis in neonatal intensive care unit patients (226), nosocomial diarrhea in hospitalized young children (227) and antibiotic-associated GI side effects of *H. pylori* treatment (228); and therapeutic efficacy for irritable bowel syndrome (229) and acute infectious diarrhea in infants and children (230,231). Other clinical trials with *Lactobacillus* or combined pro/prebiotics demonstrated reduced respiratory infection illnesses in young children (232–234).

Probiotics may also act as an immune modulator to prevent the development of atopy. An initial compelling RCT of oral *Lactobacillus* (beginning with prenatal administration to mothers and continuing in infants or nursing mothers from birth to 6 months postpartum) reduced the relative risk of atopic dermatitis at 2, 4, and 7 years of age (235–237). This same research group found that, in breast-feeding mothers who received *Lactobacillus* supplementation, breast milk had higher concentrations of the anti-inflammatory cytokine TGF-b, and their infants had a reduced relative risk of atopic dermatitis of 0.32 (238). *Lactobacillus* ingestion has also been associated with increased peripheral blood IL-10 production and serum IL-10 levels (239). However, an oral *Lactobacillus* RCT did not demonstrate therapeutic benefits for older patients with birch pollen allergy (240). A meta-analysis of clinical trials for the prevention and treatment of atopic dermatitis in children reported no therapeutic benefit (4 studies) but possibly prevention, with a summary effect size of 0.69 (0.57, 0.83) from six studies (241). A large RCT ($n = 1018$) of pre/probiotic supplementation to prevent allergies found no significant differences in allergic sensitization, eczema, allergic rhinitis, or asthma at five years of age; however, it significantly reduced the OR (0.47) of IgE-associated allergic disease in caesarian-delivered children (242).

Microbe-Enhanced Allergen Immunotherapy
The premise of using microbe-derived immune modulators to enhance the efficacy of allergen-specific immunotherapy (AIT) is also finding its way to clinical investigations. Using a modified "monophosphoryl" version of the immune-stimulatory lipid A component of endotoxin (MPL), an RCT to treat grass pollen rhinoconjunctivitis with grass pollen extract containing MPL (total of 4 preseasonal injections) demonstrated both clinical and immunologic efficacy (243). MPL has also been tested as a vaccine adjuvant for hepatitis B (244) and melanoma (245). Immune-stimulatory DNA (conceptually derived from unmethylated CpG-containing motifs common to microbial DNA) conjugated to the immunodominant ragweed allergen, Amb a1, modified the allergen-induced cytokine response of peripheral blood T cells of allergic subjects from T_h2 to T_h1 (i.e., IFN-γ) (246). This allergen-DNA conjugate was also 30-fold less potent than allergen alone in inducing histamine release from human basophils (247) and much less potent in producing immediate skin test responses (248). A pivotal RCT of CpG-modified Amb a1 AIT in ragweed-allergic subjects revealed long-term (two-year) clinical efficacy, reduction in seasonal Amb a1–specific IgE increases, and less IL-4-positive basophils, with only a six-week regimen (249).

VIII. Concluding Remarks: Back to the Future
Epidemiologic, immunologic, and gene-environment studies by many investigators over the past 20 years provide strong evidence for the hygiene hypothesis. Many of the evidence requirements for causal inference have been investigated and met, including biologic plausibility, longitudinal prospective studies, dose-response relationships, candidate gene-environment interactions, and replication of key observations. The elucidation of the relationships between microbes and allergy/asthma has so far revealed that

- protective microbial exposures can be sterile (e.g., endotoxin);
- while being helpful, microbial exposures can also be harmful;
- key determinants of whether the outcomes of microbial exposures are healthful or harmful include microbial exposure dosage, timing, pathogenicity, diversity, and favorable genetics;
- microbial exposures can induce a spectrum of allergy/asthma-protective mechanisms: innate, T_h1/IFN-γ, Treg/IL-10, antifibrotic; and
- different derivatives of microbes for allergy/asthma therapy and prevention have been tested and shown to have good safety and variable efficacy in humans; these approaches have not yet received commercial attention for complete product development.

A unifying theory proposes that natural variances in microbial exposures and ecology have contributed to the global rise of allergic diseases and asthma, the lower prevalence in farming and rural locales, and the protective effect of living with dogs and domestic animals. Humility comes with the realization that this knowledge has not yet significantly improved human health.

Acknowledgments

The author gratefully acknowledges Ms. Allison Schiltz for her critical review and Ms. Nancy Hafer and Ms. Gabrielle Cheatham for their assistance with the preparation of this manuscript.

References

1. Tomes N. The Gospel of Germs: Men, Women, and the Microbe in American Life. Cambridge, Massachusetts: Harvard University Press, 1999.
2. Armstrong GL, Conn LA, Pinner RW. Trends in infectious disease mortality in the United States during the 20th century. JAMA 1999; 281:61–66.
3. Beasley R, Crane J, Lai CK, et al. Prevalence and etiology of asthma. J Allergy Clin Immunol 2000; 105:466–472.
4. Haahtela T, Lindholm H, Bjorksten F, et al. Prevalence of asthma in Finnish young men. BMJ 1990; 301:266–268.
5. Peat JK, van den Berg RH, Green WF, et al. Changing prevalence of asthma in Australian children. BMJ 1994; 308:1591–1596.
6. Arbes SJ Jr., Sever M, Vaughn B, et al. Feasibility of using subject-collected dust samples in epidemiologic and clinical studies of indoor allergens. Environ Health Perspect 2005; 113:665–669.
7. Bostock J. On the Catarrhus Aestivus or Summer Catarrh. Medico-Chirurgical Transact (London) 1828; xiv:437–446. [From Emanuel MB Clin Allergy 1988.]
8. Blackley C. Experimental Researches on the Causes and Nature of Catarrhus Aestivus (Hay-fever or Hay-asthma). London: Balliere, Tindall & Cox, 1873.
9. Committee IS. Worldwide variation in prevalence of symptoms of asthma, allergic rhino-conjunctivitis, and atopic eczema: ISAAC. Lancet 1998; 351:1225–1232.
10. Weinmayr G, Weiland SK, Bjorksten B, et al. Atopic sensitization and the international variation of asthma symptom prevalence in children. Am J Respir Crit Care Med 2007; 176(6):565–574.
11. Van Niekerk CH, Weinberg EG, Shore SC, et al. Prevalence of asthma: a comparative study of urban and rural Xhosa children. Clin Allergy 1979; 9:319–314.
12. Keeley D, Neill P. Asthma paradox. Lancet 1991; 337(8749):1099.
13. Addo Yobo EO, Custovic A, Taggart SC, et al. Exercise induced bronchospasm in Ghana: differences in prevalence between urban and rural schoolchildren. Thorax 1997; 52(2):161–165.
14. Ng'ang'a LW, Odhiambo JA, Mungai MW, et al. Prevalence of exercise induced bronchospasm in Kenyan school children: an urban-rural comparison. Thorax 1998; 53(11):919–926.
15. Yemaneberhan H, Bekele Z, Venn A, et al. Prevalence of wheeze and asthma and relation to atopy in urban and rural Ethiopia. Lancet 1997; 350(9071):85–90.
16. Waite CA, Eyles EF, Tonkin SL, et al. Asthma prevalence in Tokelauan children in two environments. Clin Allergy 1980; 10:71–75.
17. Lynch NR, Medouze L, Di Prisco-Fuenmayor MC, et al. Incidence of atopic disease in a tropical environment: partial independence from intestinal helminthiasis. J Allergy Clin Immunol 1984; 73(2):229–233.
18. Barnes M, Cullinan P, Athanasaki P, et al. Crete: does farming explain urban and rural differences in atopy? Clin Exp Allergy 2001; 31(12):1822–1828.
19. Vedanthan PK, Mahesh PA, Vedanthan R, et al. Effect of animal contact and microbial exposures on the prevalence of atopy and asthma in urban vs rural children in India. Ann Allergy Asthma Immunol 2006; 96(4):571–578.
20. Braun-Fahrlander C, Gassner M, Grize L, et al. Prevalence of hay fever and allergic sensitization in farmer's children and their peers living in the same rural community. Clin Exp Allergy 1999; 29(1):28–34.

21. Riedler J, Eder W, Oberfeld G, et al. Austrian children living on a farm have less hay fever, asthma and allergic sensitization. Clin Exp Allergy 2000; 30:194–200.

22. von Ehrenstein OS, von Mutius E, Illi S, et al. Reduced risk of hay fever and asthma among children of farmers. Clin Exp Allergy 2000; 30:187–193.

23. Kilpelainen M, Terho EO, Helenius H, et al. Farm environment in childhood prevents the development of allergies. Clin Exp Allergy 2000; 30:201–208.

24. Ernst P, Cormier Y. Relative scarcity of asthma and atopy among rural adolescents raised on a farm. Am J Respir Crit Care Med 2000; 161:1563–1566.

25. Riedler J, Braun-Fahrlander C, Eder W, et al. Exposure to farming in early life and development of asthma and allergy: a cross-sectional survey. Lancet 2001; 358(9288): 1129–1133.

26. Adler A, Tager I, Quintero DR. Decreased prevalence of asthma among farm-reared children compared with those who are rural but not farm-reared. J Allergy Clin Immunol 2005; 115(1):67–73.

27. Cetinkaya F, Uslu HS, Nuhoglu A. Effect of neonatal sepsis on the development of allergies and asthma in later childhood. Int Arch Allergy Immunol 2007; 142(2):145–150.

28. Mungan D, Sin BA, Celik G, et al. Atopic status of an adult population with active and inactive tuberculosis. Allergy Asthma Proc 2001; 22(2):87–91.

29. Shaheen SO, Aaby P, Hall AJ, et al. Measles and atopy in Guinea-Bissau. Lancet 1996; 347:1792–1796.

30. Rosenlund H, Bergstrom A, Alm JS, et al. Allergic disease and atopic sensitization in children in relation to measles vaccination and measles infection. Pediatrics 2009; 123(3): 771–778.

31. Paunio M, Heinonen O, Virtanen M, et al. Measles history and atopic diseases. JAMA 2000; 283:343–346.

32. Illi S, von Mutius E, Lau S, et al. Early childhood infectious diseases and the development of asthma up to school age: a birth cohort study. BMJ 2001; 322(7283):390–395.

33. Zutavern A, von Klot S, Gehring U, et al. Pre-natal and post-natal exposure to respiratory infection and atopic diseases development: a historical cohort study. Respir Res 2006; 7:81.

34. Strachan DP. Hay fever, hygiene, and household size. BMJ 1989; 299(6710):1259–1260.

35. Matricardi PM, Franzinelli F, Franco A, et al. Sibship size, birth order, and atopy in 11,371 Italian young men. J Allergy Clin Immunol 1998; 101:439–444.

36. Rona RJ, Duran-Tauleria E, Chinn S. Family size, atopic disorders in parents, asthma in children, and ethnicity. J Allergy Clin Immunol 1997; 99:454–460.

37. Svanes C, Jarvis D, Chinn S, et al. Childhood environment and adult atopy: results from the European Community Respiratory Health Survey. J Allergy Clin Immunol 1999; 103:415–420.

38. Wickens K, Pearce N, Crane J, et al. Antibiotic use in early childhood and the development of asthma. Clin Exp Allergy 1999; 29:766–771.

39. Ball TM, Castro-Rodriguez JA, Griffith KA, et al. Siblings, day-care attendance, and the risk of asthma and wheezing during childhood. N Engl J Med 2000; 343(8):538–543.

40. Kramer U, Heinrich J, Wjst M, et al. Age of entry to day nursery and allergy in later childhood. Lancet 1999; 353:450–454.

41. Ball TM, Holberg CJ, Aldous MB, et al. Influence of attendance at day care on the common cold from birth through 13 years of age. Arch Pediatr Adolesc Med 2002; 156:121–126.

42. Hurwitz ES, Gunn WJ, Pinsky PF, et al. Risk of respiratory illness associated with day-care attendance: a nationwide study. Pediatrics 1991; 87(1):62–69.

43. Louhiala PJ, Jaakkola N, Ruotsalainen R, et al. Form of day care and respiratory infections among Finnish children. Am J Public Health 1995; 85:1109–1112.

44. Wald ER, Guerra N, Byers C. Frequency and severity of infections in day care: three-year follow-up. J Pediatr 1991; 118:509–514.

45. Rullo VE, Rizzo MC, Arruda LK, et al. Daycare centers and schools as sources of exposure to mites, cockroach, and endotoxin in the city of Sao Paulo, Brazil. J Allergy Clin Immunol 2002; 110(4):582–588.

46. Thorne PS, Cohn RD, Mav D, et al. Predictors of endotoxin levels in U.S. housing. Environ Health Perspect 2009; 117(5):763–771.

47. Matricardi PM, Rosmini F, Riondino S, et al. Exposure to foodborne and orofecal microbes versus airborne viruses in relation to atopy and allergic asthma: epidemiological study. BMJ 2000; 320(7232):412–417.

48. Chen Y, Blaser MJ. Inverse associations of Helicobacter pylori with asthma and allergy. Arch Intern Med 2007; 167(8):821–827.

49. van den Biggelaar AH, van Ree R, Rodrigues LC, et al. Decreased atopy in children infected with Schistosoma haematobium: a role for parasite-induced interleukin-10. Lancet 2000; 356(9243):1723–1727.

50. Scrivener S, Yemaneberhan H, Zebenigus M, et al. Independent effects of intestinal parasite infection and domestic allergen exposure on risk of wheeze in Ethiopia: a nested case-control study. Lancet 2001; 358(9292):1493–1499.

51. Nyan OA, Walraven GE, Banya WA, et al. Atopy, intestinal helminth infection and total serum IgE in rural and urban adult Gambian communities. Clin Exp Allergy 2001; 31(11): 1672–1678.

52. Rodrigues LC, Newcombe PJ, Cunha SS, et al. Early infection with Trichuris trichiura and allergen skin test reactivity in later childhood. Clin Exp Allergy 2008; 38(11):1769–1777.

53. Leonardi-Bee J, Pritchard D, Britton J. Asthma and current intestinal parasite infection: systematic review and meta-analysis. Am J Respir Crit Care Med 2006; 174(5):514–523.

54. Bjorksten B, Naaber P, Sepp E, et al. The intestinal microflora in allergic Estonian and Swedish 2-year old children. Clin Exp Allergy 1999; 29:342–346.

55. Bjorksten B, Sepp E, Julge K, et al. Allergy development and the intestinal microflora during the first year of life. J Allergy Clin Immunol 2001; 108(4):516–520.

56. Kalliomaki M, Kirjavainen P, Eerola E, et al. Distinct patterns of neonatal gut microflora in infants in whom atopy was and was not developing. J Allergy Clin Immunol 2001; 107:129–134.

57. Sjogren YM, Jenmalm MC, Bottcher MF, et al. Altered early infant gut microbiota in children developing allergy up to 5 years of age. Clin Exp Allergy 2009; 39(4):518–526.

58. Vael C, Nelen V, Verhulst SL, et al. Early intestinal Bacteroides fragilis colonisation and development of asthma. BMC Pulm Med 2008; 8:19.

59. Wang M, Karlsson C, Olsson C, et al. Reduced diversity in the early fecal microbiota of infants with atopic eczema. J Allergy Clin Immunol 2008; 121(1):129–134.

60. von Hertzen L, Haahtela T. Disconnection of man and the soil: reason for the asthma and atopy epidemic? J Allergy Clin Immunol 2006; 117:334–344.

61. Pakarinen J, Hyvarinen A, Salkinoja-Salonen M, et al. Predominance of Gram-positive bacteria in house dust in the low-allergy risk Russian Karelia. Environ Microbiol 2008; 10(12):3317–3325.

62. Liu AH, Murphy JR. Hygiene hypothesis: fact or fiction? J Allergy Clin Immunol 2003; 111(3):471–478.

63. Prescott SL, Macaubas C, Holt BJ, et al. Transplacental priming of the human immune system to environmental allergens: universal skewing of initial T cell responses toward the Th2 cytokine profile. J Immunol 1998; 160:4730–4737.

64. Lin H, Mosmann TR, Guilbert L, et al. Synthesis of T Helper 2-type cytokines at the maternal-fetal interface. J Immunol 1993; 151(9):4562–4573.

65. Roth I, Corry DB, Locksley RM, et al. Human placental cytotrophoblasts produce the immunosuppressive cytokine interleukin 10. J Exp Med 1996; 184(2):539–548.

66. Martinez FD, Wright AL, Taussig LM, et al. Asthma and wheezing in the first six years of life. The Group Health Medical Associates. N Engl J Med 1995; 332(3):133–138.
67. Prescott SL, Macaubas C, Smallacombe TB, et al. Development of allergen-specific T-cell memory in atopic and normal children. Lancet 1999; 353:196–200.
68. Eisenbarth SC, Piggott DA, Huleatt JW, et al. Lipopolysaccharide-enhanced, toll-like receptor 4-dependent T helper cell type 2 responses to inhaled antigen. J Exp Med 2002; 196(12):1645–1651.
69. Tulic MK, Wale JL, Holt PG, et al. Modification of the inflammatory response to allergen challenge after exposure to bacterial lipopolysaccharide. Am J Respir Cell Mol Biol 2000; 22:604–612.
70. Erb KJ, Holloway JW, Sobeck A, et al. Infection of mice with Mycobacterium bovis-Bacillus Calmette-Guerin (BCG) suppresses allergen-induced airway eosinophilia. J Exp Med 1998; 187(4):561–569.
71. Herz U, Gerhold K, Gruber C, et al. BCG infection suppresses allergic sensitization and development of increased airway reactivity in an animal model. J Allergy Clin Immunol 1998; 102(5):867–874.
72. Murosaki S, Yamamoto Y, Ito K, et al. Heat-killed Lactobacillus plantarum L-137 suppresses naturally fed antigen-specific IgE production by stimulation of IL-12 production in mice. J Allergy Clin Immunol 1998; 102(1):57–64.
73. Hansen G, Yeung VP, Berry G, et al. Vaccination with heat-killed *Listeria* as adjuvant reverses established allergen-induced airway hyperreactivity and inflammation: role of CD8+ T Cells and IL-18[1]. J Immunol 2000; 164:223–230.
74. Chu HW, Honour JM, Rawlinson CA, et al. Hygiene hypothesis of asthma: a murine asthma model with Mycoplasma pneumoniae infection. Chest 2003; 123(3 suppl):390S.
75. Raz E, Tighe H, Sato Y, et al. Preferential induction of a TH1 immune response and inhibition of specific IgE antibody formation by plasmid DNA immunization. Proc Natl Acad Sci U S A 1996; 93(10):5141–5145.
76. Klinman DM, Yi AK, Beaucage SL, et al. CpG motifs present in bacteria DNA rapidly induce lymphocytes to secrete interleukin 6, interleukin 12, and interferon gamma. Proc Natl Acad Sci U S A 1996; 93(7):2879–2883.
77. Broide D, Schwarze J, Tighe H, et al. Immunostimulatory DNA sequences inhibit IL-5, eosinophilic inflammation, and airway hyperresponsiveness in mice. J Immunol 1998; 161:7054–7062.
78. Kline JN, Waldschmidt TJ, Businga TR, et al. Modulation of airway inflammation by CpG oligodeoxynucleotides in a murine model of asthma. J Immunol 1998; 160:2555–2559.
79. Iwamoto I, Nakajima H, Endo H, et al. Interferon gamma regulates antigen-induced eosinophil recruitment into the mouse airways by inhibiting the infiltration of CD4+ T cells. J Exp Med 1993; 177:573–576.
80. Sur S, Lam J, Bouchard P, et al. Immunomodulatory effects of IL-12 on allergic lung inflammation depend on timing of doses. J Immunol 1996; 157:4173–4180.
81. Schwarze J, Hamelmann E, Cieslewicz G, et al. Local treatment with IL-12 is an effective inhibitor of airway hyperresponsiveness and lung eosinophilia after airway challenge in sensitized mice. J Allergy Clin Immunol 1998; 102:86–93.
82. Kips JC, Brusselle GJ, Joos GF, et al. Interleukin-12 inhibits antigen-induced airway hyperresponsiveness in mice. Am J Respir Crit Care Med 1996; 153:535–539.
83. Gavett SH, O'Hearn DJ, Li X, et al. Interleukin 12 inhibits antigen-induced airway hyperresponsiveness, inflammation, and Th2 cytokine expression in mice. J Exp Med 1995; 182:1527–1536.
84. Lack G, Renz H, Saloga J, et al. Nebulized but not parenteral IFN-gamma decreases IgE production and normalizes airways function in a murine model of allergen sensitization. J Immunol 1994; 152(5):2546–2554.

85. Hogan SP, Foster PS, Tan X, et al. Mucosal IL-12 gene delivery inhibits allergic airways disease and restores local antiviral immunity. Eur J Immunol 1998; 28(2):413–423.
86. Sur S, Crotty TB, Kephart GM, et al. Sudden-onset fatal asthma. A distinct entity with few eosinophils and relatively more neutrophils in the airway submucosa? Am Rev Respir Dis 1993; 148(3):713–719.
87. Liu AH. Endotoxin exposure in allergy and asthma: reconciling a paradox. J Allergy Clin Immunol 2002; 109(3):379–392.
88. Cohn L, Homer RJ, MacLeod H, et al. Th2-induced airway mucus production is dependent on IL-4Ralpha, but not on eosinophils. J Immunol 1999; 162(10):6178–6183.
89. Jimenez SA, Freundlich B, Rosenbloom J. Selective inhibition of human diploid fibroblast collagen synthesis by interferons. J Clin Invest 1984; 74(3):1112–1116.
90. Duncan MR, Berman B. Gamma interferon is the lymphokine and beta interferon the monokine responsible for inhibition of fibroblast collagen production and late but not early fibroblast proliferation. J Exp Med 1985; 162(2):516–527.
91. Goldring MB, Sandell LJ, Stephenson ML, et al. Immune interferon suppresses levels of procollagen mRNA and type II collagen synthesis in cultured human articular and costal chondrocytes. J Biol Chem 1986; 261(19):9049–9055.
92. Diaz A, Jimenez SA. Interferon-gamma regulates collagen and fibronectin gene expression by transcriptional and post-transcriptional mechanisms. Int J Biochem Cell Biol 1997; 29(1):251–260.
93. Kirshenbaum AS, Worobec AS, Davis TA, et al. Inhibition of human mast cell growth and differentiation by interferon gamma-1b. Exp Hematol 1998; 26(3):245–251.
94. Ochi H, Hirani WM, Yuan Q, et al. T helper cell type 2 cytokine-mediated comitogenic responses and CCR3 expression during differentiation of human mast cells in vitro. J Exp Med 1999; 190(2):267–280.
95. Amrani Y, Tliba O, Choubey D, et al. IFN-gamma inhibits human airway smooth muscle cell proliferation by modulating the E2F-1/Rb pathway. Am J Physiol Lung Cell Mol Physiol 2003; 284(6):L1063–L1071.
96. Cole AM, Ganz T, Liese AM, et al. Cutting edge: IFN-inducible ELR-CXC chemokines display defensin-like antimicrobial activity. J Immunol 2001; 167(2):623–627.
97. Becker MN, Diamond G, Verghese MW, et al. CD14-dependent lipopolysaccharide-induced beta-defensin-2 expression in human tracheobronchial epithelium. J Biol Chem 2000; 275(38):29731–29736.
98. Crouch EC. Collectins and pulmonary host defense. Am J Respir Cell Mol Biol 1998; 19:177–201.
99. Sorkness RL, Castleman WL, Kumar A, et al. Prevention of chronic postbronchiolitis airway sequelae with IFN-g treatment in rats. Am J Respir Crit Care Med 1999; 160:705–710.
100. Parry DE, Busse WW, Sukow KA, et al. Rhinovirus-induced PBMC responses and outcome of experimental infection in allergic subjects. J Allergy Clin Immunol 2000; 105(4):692–698.
101. Renzi PM, Turgeon JP, Marcotte JE, et al. Reduced interferon-g production in infants with bronchiolitis and asthma. Am J Respir Crit Care Med 1999; 159:1417–1422.
102. Yazdanbakhsh M, Kremsner PG, van Ree R. Allergy, parasites, and the hygiene hypothesis. Science 2002; 296:490–494.
103. Turner JD, Jackson JA, Faulkner H, et al. Intensity of intestinal infection with multiple worm species is related to regulatory cytokine output and immune hyporesponsiveness. J Infect Dis 2008; 197(8):1204–1212.
104. Jeanin P, Lecoanet S, Delneste Y, et al. IgE versus IgG4 production can be differentially regulated by IL-10. J Immunol 1998; 160(7):3555–3561.
105. Royer B. Inhibition of IgE-induced activation of human mast cells by IL-10. Clin Exp Allergy 2001; 31:694–704.
106. Borish L. IL-10: evolving concepts. J Allergy Clin Immunol 1998; 101:293–297.

107. Hawrylowicz CM, O'Garra A. Potential role of interleukin-10-secreting regulatory T cells in allergy and asthma. Nat Rev Immunol 2005; 5(4):271–283.
108. Borish L, Aarons A, Rumbyrt J, et al. Interleukin-10 regulation in normal subjects and patients with asthma. J Allergy Clin Immunol 1996; 97(6):1288–1296.
109. Macaubas C. Regulation of T-helper cell responses to inhalant allergen during early childhood. Clin Exp Allergy 1999; 29(9):1223–1231.
110. Brigham KL. Endotoxin and the Lungs. New York: Marcel Dekker, Inc., 1994.
111. Pabst MJ, Hedegaard HB, Johnston RB Jr. Cultured human monocytes require exposure to bacterial products to maintain an optimal oxygen radical response. J Immunol 1982; 128(1):123–128.
112. Medzhitov R, Janeway CJ. Innate immunity. N Engl J Med 2000; 343(5):338–344.
113. Wright SD, Tobias PS, Ulevitch RJ, et al. Lipopolysaccharide (LPS) binding protein opsonizes LPS-bearing particles for recognition by a novel receptor on macrophages. J Exp Med 1989; 170(4):1231–1241.
114. Wright SD, Ramos RA, Tobias PS, et al. CD14, a receptor for complexes of lipopolysaccharide (LPS) and LPS binding protein. Science 1990; 249:1431–1433.
115. Visintin A, Iliev DB, Monks BG, et al. MD-2. Immunobiology 2006; 211(6–8):437–447.
116. Pabst MJ, Johnston RB Jr. Increased production of superoxide anion by macrophages exposed in vitro to muramyl dipeptide or lipopolysaccharide. J Exp Med 1980; 151(1):101–114.
117. Forehand JR, Pabst MJ, Phillips WA, et al. Lipopolysaccharide priming of human neutrophils for an enhanced respiratory burst. Role of intracellular free calcium. J Clin Invest 1989; 83(1):74–83.
118. Shnyra A, Brewington R, Alipio A, et al. Reprogramming of lipopolysaccharide-primed macrophages is controlled by a counterbalanced production of IL-10 and IL-12. J Immunol 1998; 160(8):3729–3736.
119. Dabbagh K, Dahl ME, Stepick-Biek P, et al. Toll-like receptor 4 is required for optimal development of Th2 immune responses: role of dendritic cells. J Immunol 2002; 168(9):4524–4530.
120. Piggott DA, Eisenbarth SC, Xu L, et al. MyD88-dependent induction of allergic Th2 responses to intranasal antigen. J Clin Invest 2005; 115(2):459–467.
121. Reis e Sousa C, Hieny S, Scharton-Kersten T, et al. In vivo microbial stimulation induces rapid CD40 ligand-independent production of interleukin 12 by dendritic cells and their redistribution to T cell areas. J Exp Med 1997; 186(11):1819–1829.
122. Macatonia SE, Hosken NA, Litton M, et al. Dendritic cells produce IL-12 and direct the development of Th1 cells from naive CD4+ T cells. J Immunol 1995; 154(10):5071–5079.
123. Hilkens CM, Kalinski P, de Boer M, et al. Human dendritic cells require exogenous interleukin-12-inducing factors to direct the development of naive T-helper cells toward the Th1 phenotype. Blood 1997; 90(5):1920–1926.
124. Ng N, Lam D, Paulus P, et al. House dust extracts have both TH2 adjuvant and tolerogenic activities. J Allergy Clin Immunol 2006; 117(5):1074–1081.
125. George CL, Jin H, Wohlford-Lenane CL, et al. Endotoxin responsiveness and subchronic grain dust-induced airway disease. Am J Physiol Lung Cell Mol Physiol 2001; 280(2):L203–L213.
126. Krieg AM. CpG motifs in bacterial DNA and their immune effects. Annu Rev Immunol 2002; 20:709–760.
127. Boonstra A, Asselin-Paturel C, Gilliet M, et al. Flexibility of mouse classical and plasmacytoid-derived dendritic cells in directing T helper type 1 and 2 cell development: dependency on antigen dose and differential toll-like receptor ligation. J Exp Med 2003; 197(1):101–109.
128. Krug A, Towarowski A, Britsch S, et al. Toll-like receptor expression reveals CpG DNA as a unique microbial stimulus for plasmacytoid dendritic cells which synergizes with CD40 ligand to induce high amounts of IL-12. Eur J Immunol 2001; 31(10):3026–3037.

129. Chisholm D, Libet L, Hayashi T, et al. Airway peptidoglycan and immunostimulatory DNA exposures have divergent effects on the development of airway allergen hypersensitivities. J Allergy Clin Immunol 2004; 113(3):448–454.

130. Pulendran B, Kumar P, Cutler CW, et al. Lipopolysaccharides from distinct pathogens induce different classes of immune responses in vivo. J Immunol 2001; 167(9):5067–5076.

131. Agrawal S, Agrawal A, Doughty B, et al. Cutting edge: different Toll-like receptor agonists instruct dendritic cells to induce distinct Th responses via differential modulation of extracellular signal-regulated kinase-mitogen-activated protein kinase and c-Fos. J Immunol 2003; 171(10):4984–4989.

132. Dillon S, Agrawal A, Van Dyke T, et al. A Toll-like receptor 2 ligand stimulates Th2 responses in vivo, via induction of extracellular signal-regulated kinase mitogen-activated protein kinase and c-Fos in dendritic cells. J Immunol 2004; 172(8):4733–4743.

133. Matsui K, Nishikawa A. Lipoteichoic acid from Staphylococcus aureus induces Th2-prone dermatitis in mice sensitized percutaneously with an allergen. Clin Exp Allergy 2002; 32(5):783–788.

134. Mandron M, Aries M-F, Brehm RD, et al. Human dendritic cells conditioned with Staphylococcus aureus enterotoxin B promote TH2 cell polarization. J Allergy Clin Immunol 2006; 117(5):1141–1147.

135. Taylor RC, Richmond P, Upham JW. Toll-like receptor 2 ligands inhibit TH2 responses to mite allergen. J Allergy Clin Immunol 2006; 117(5):1148–1154.

136. Lam D, Ng N, Lee S, et al. Airway house dust extract exposures modify allergen-induced airway hypersensitivity responses by TLR4-dependent and independent pathways. J Immunol 2008; 181(4):2925–2932.

137. Gehring U, Bolte G, Borte M, et al. Exposure to endotoxin decreases the risk of atopic eczema in infancy: a cohort study. J Allergy Clin Immunol 2001; 108:847–854.

138. Phipatanakul W, Celedon JC, Raby BA, et al. Endotoxin exposure and eczema in the first year of life. Pediatrics 2004; 114(1):13–18.

139. Perzanowski MS, Miller RL, Thorne PS, et al. Endotoxin in inner-city homes: associations with wheeze and eczema in early childhood. J Allergy Clin Immunol 2006; 117(5):1082–1089.

140. Gereda JE, Leung DY, Thatayatikom A, et al. Relation between house-dust endotoxin exposure, type 1 T-cell development, and allergen sensitisation in infants at high risk of asthma. Lancet 2000; 355(9216):1680–1683.

141. Celedon JC, Milton DK, Ramsey CD, et al. Exposure to dust mite allergen and endotoxin in early life and asthma and atopy in childhood. J Allergy Clin Immunol 2007; 120(1):144–149.

142. Gehring U, Spithoven J, Schmid S, et al. Endotoxin levels in cow's milk samples from farming and non-farming families—the PASTURE study. Environ Int 2008; 34(8):1132–1136.

143. Gehring U, Bischof W, Fahlbusch B, et al. House dust endotoxin and allergic sensitization in children. Am J Respir Crit Care Med 2002; 166(7):939–944.

144. Braun-Fahrlander C, Riedler J, Herz U, et al. Environmental exposure to endotoxin and its relation to asthma in school-age children. N Engl J Med 2002; 347(12):869–877.

145. Douwes J, Siebers R, Wouters I, et al. Endotoxin, (1−>3)-beta-D-glucans and fungal extracellular polysaccharides in New Zealand homes: a pilot study. Ann Agric Environ Med 2006; 13(2):361–365.

146. Gehring U, Heinrich J, Hoek G, et al. Bacteria and mould components in house dust and children's allergic sensitisation. Eur Respir J 2007; 29(6):1144–1153.

147. Thorne PS, Kulhankova K, Yin M, et al. Endotoxin exposure is a risk factor for asthma: the national survey of endotoxin in United States housing. Am J Respir Crit Care Med 2005; 172(11):1371–1377.

148. Roponen M, Hyvarinen A, Hirvonen M-R, et al. Change in IFN-g-producing capacity in early life and exposure of environmental microbes. J Allergy Clin Immunol 2005; 116: 1048–1052.

149. Bufford JD, Reardon CL, Li Z, et al. Effects of dog ownership in early childhood on immune development and atopic diseases. Clin Exp Allergy 2008; 38(10):1635–1643.

150. Abraham JH, Finn PW, Milton DK, et al. Infant home endotoxin is associated with reduced allergen-stimulated lymphocyte proliferation and IL-13 production in childhood. J Allergy Clin Immunol 2005; 116(2):431–437.

151. Verhasselt V, Vosters O, Beuneu C, et al. Induction of FOXP3-expressing regulatory CD4pos T cells by human mature autologous dendritic cells. Eur J Immunol 2004; 34(3): 762–772.

152. Shirai Y, Hashimoto M, Kato R, et al. Lipopolysaccharide induces CD25-positive, IL-10-producing lymphocytes without secretion of proinflammatory cytokines in the human colon: low MD-2 mRNA expression in colonic macrophages. J Clin Immunol 2004; 24(1):42–52.

153. Tulic MK, Fiset PO, Manoukian JJ, et al. Role of toll-like receptor 4 in protection by bacterial lipopolysaccharide in the nasal mucosa of atopic children but not adults. Lancet 2004; 363(9422):1689–1697.

154. Park JH, Gold DR, Spiegelman DL, et al. House dust endotoxin and wheeze in the first year of life. Am J Respir Crit Care Med 2001; 163(2):322–328.

155. Gillespie J, Wickens K, Siebers R, et al. Endotoxin exposure, wheezing, and rash in infancy in a New Zealand birth cohort. J Allergy Clin Immunol 2006; 118(6):1265–1270.

156. Kline JN, Cowden JD, Hunninghake GW, et al. Variable airway responsiveness to inhaled lipopolysaccharide. Am J Respir Crit Care Med 1999; 160(1):297–303.

157. Michel O, Ginanni R, Le Bon B, et al. Inflammatory response to acute inhalation of endotoxin in asthmatic patients. Am Rev Respir Dis 1992; 146:352–357.

158. Michel O, Duchateau J, Sergysels R. Effect of inhaled endotoxin on bronchial reactivity in asthmatic and normal subjects. J Appl Physiol 1989; 66:1059–1064.

159. Michel O. Systemic and local airways inflammatory response to endotoxin. Toxicology 2000; 152:25–30.

160. Hunt LW, Gleich GJ, Ohnishi T, et al. Endotoxin contamination causes neutrophilia following pulmonary allergen challenge. Am J Respir Crit Care Med 1994; 149:1471–1475.

161. Boehlecke B, Hazucha M, Alexis NE, et al. Low-dose airborne endotoxin exposure enhances bronchial responsiveness to inhaled allergen in atopic asthmatics. J Allergy Clin Immunol 2003; 112(6):1241–1243.

162. Eldridge MW, Peden DB. Allergen provocation augments endotoxin-induced nasal inflammation in subjects with atopic asthma. J Allergy Clin Immunol 2000; 105:475–481.

163. Michel O, Ginanni R, Le Bon B, et al. Effect of endotoxin contamination on the antigenic skin test response. Ann Allergy 1991; 66:39–42.

164. Rabinovitch N, Liu AH, Zhang L, et al. Importance of the personal endotoxin cloud in school-age children with asthma. J Allergy Clin Immunol 2005; 116:1053–1057.

165. Michel O, Kips J, Duchateau J, et al. Severity of asthma is related to endotoxin in house dust. Am J Respir Crit Care Med 1996; 154(6 pt 1):1641–1646.

166. Christiani DC, Ye TT, Zhang S, et al. Cotton dust and endotoxin exposure and long-term decline in lung function: results of a longitudinal study. Am J Ind Med 1999; 35(4):321–331.

167. Rylander R. Endotoxin and occupational airway disease. Curr Opin Allergy Clin Immunol 2006; 6(1):62–66.

168. van Strien RT, Engel R, Holst O, et al. Microbial exposure of rural school children, as assessed by levels of N-acetyl-muramic acid in mattress dust, and its association with respiratory health. J Allergy Clin Immunol 2004; 113(5):860–867.

169. Roy SR, Schiltz AM, Marotta A, et al. Bacterial DNA in house and farm barn dust. J Allergy Clin Immunol 2003; 112(3):571–578.

170. Arbour NC, Lorenz E, Schutte BC, et al. TLR4 mutations are associated with endotoxin hyperresponsiveness in humans. Nat Genet 2000; 25(2):187–191.

171. Michel O, LeVan TD, Stern D, et al. Systemic responsiveness to lipopolysaccharide and polymorphisms in the toll-like receptor 4 gene in human beings. J Allergy Clin Immunol 2003; 112(5):923–929.
172. Senthilselvan A, Dosman JA, Chenard L, et al. Toll-like receptor 4 variants reduce airway response in human subjects at high endotoxin levels in a swine facility. J Allergy Clin Immunol 2009; 123(5):1034–1040, 1040.e1–e2.
173. Raby BA, Klimecki WT, Laprise C, et al. Polymorphisms in toll-like receptor 4 are not associated with asthma or atopy-related phenotypes. Am J Respir Cell Mol Biol 2002; 166(11):1449–1456.
174. Fageras Bottcher M, Hmani-Aifa M, Lindstrom A, et al. A TLR4 polymorphism is associated with asthma and reduced lipopolysaccharide-induced interleukin-12(p70) responses in Swedish children. J Allergy Clin Immunol 2004; 114(3):561–567.
175. Werner M, Topp R, Wimmer K, et al. TLR4 gene variants modify endotoxin effects on asthma. J Allergy Clin Immunol 2003; 112:323–330.
176. LeVan TD, Bloom JW, Bailey TJ, et al. A common single nucleotide polymorphism in the CD14 promoter decreases the affinity of Sp protein binding and enhances transcriptional activity. J Immunol 2001; 167(10):5838–5844.
177. Baldini M, Lohman IC, Halonen M, et al. A Polymorphism* in the 5' flanking region of the CD14 gene is associated with circulating soluble CD14 levels and with total serum immunoglobulin E. Am J Respir Cell Mol Biol 1999; 20(5):976–983.
178. Koppelman GH, Reijmerink NE, Colin Stine O, et al. Association of a promoter polymorphism of the CD14 gene and atopy. Am J Respir Crit Care Med 2001; 163(4):965–969.
179. Litonjua AA, Belanger K, Celedon JC, et al. Polymorphisms in the 5' region of the CD14 gene are associated with eczema in young children. J Allergy Clin Immunol 2005; 115(5):1056–1062.
180. Ober C, Tsalenko A, Parry R, et al. A second-generation genomewide screen for asthma-susceptibility alleles in a founder population. Am J Hum Genet 2000; 67(5):1154–1162.
181. Simpson A, John SL, Jury F, et al. Endotoxin exposure, CD14, and allergic disease: an interaction between genes and the environment. Am J Respir Crit Care Med 2006; 174(4):386–392.
182. Eder W, Klimecki W, Yu L, et al. Opposite effects of CD 14/-260 on serum IgE levels in children raised in different environments. J Allergy Clin Immunol 2005; 116(3):601–607.
183. LeVan TD, Von Essen S, Romberger DJ, et al. Polymorphisms in the CD14 gene associated with pulmonary function in farmers. Am J Respir Crit Care Med 2005; 171(7):773–779.
184. Zambelli-Weiner A, Ehrlich E, Stockton ML, et al. Evaluation of the CD14/-260 polymorphism and house dust endotoxin exposure in the Barbados Asthma Genetics Study. J Allergy Clin Immunol 2005; 115(6):1203–1209.
185. Ownby DR, Johnson CC, Peterson EL. Exposure to dogs and cats in the first year of life and risk of allergic sensitization at 6 to 7 years of age. JAMA 2002; 288(8):963–972.
186. Remes ST, Castro-Rodriguez JA, Holberg CJ, et al. Dog exposure in infancy decreases the subsequent risk of frequent wheeze but not of atopy. J Allergy Clin Immunol 2001; 108:509–515.
187. Gern JE, Reardon CL, Hoffjan S, et al. Effects of dog ownership and genotype on immune development and atopy in infancy. J Allergy Clin Immunol 2004; 113:307–314.
188. Leynaert B, Guilloud-Bataille M, Soussan D, et al. Association between farm exposure and atopy, according to the CD14 C-159T polymorphism. J Allergy Clin Immunol 2006; 118(3): 658–665.
189. Gereda JE, Klinnert MD, Price MR, et al. Metropolitan home living conditions associated with indoor endotoxin levels. J Allergy Clin Immunol 2001; 107:790–796.
190. Gereda JE, Leung DYM, Liu AH. House-dust endotoxin is higher in rural homes in developing countries and farm homes, where asthma is less prevalent. JAMA 2000; 284(13):1652–1653.
191. Rabinovitch N, Liu AH, Zhang L, et al. Increased personal respirable endotoxin exposure with furry pets. Allergy 2006; 61(5):650–651.

192. Waser M, Schierl R, von Mutius E, et al. Determinants of endotoxin levels in living environments of farmers' children and their peers from rural areas. Clin Exp Allergy 2004; 34(3):389–397.
193. Lauener RP, Birchler T, Adamski J, et al. Expression of CD14 and Toll-like receptor 2 in farmers' and non-farmers' children. Lancet 2002; 360(9331):465–466.
194. Ege MJ, Frei R, Bieli C, et al. Not all farming environments protect against the development of asthma and wheeze in children. J Allergy Clin Immunol 2007; 119(5):1140–1147.
195. Ege M, Bieli C, Frei R, et al. Prenatal farm exposure is related to the expression of receptors of the innate immunity and to atopic sensitization in school-age children. J Allergy Clin Immunol 2006; 117(4):817–823.
196. Viinanen A, Munhbayarlah S, Zevgee T, et al. The protective effect of rural living against atopy in Mongolia. Allergy 2007; 62(3):272–280.
197. Melsom T, Brinch L, Hessen JO, et al. Asthma and indoor environment in Nepal. Thorax 2001; 56(6):477–481.
198. Bashir ME, Louie S, Shi HN, et al. Toll-like receptor 4 signaling by intestinal microbes influences susceptibility to food allergy. J Immunol 2004; 172(11):6978–6987.
199. Rakoff-Nahoum S, Paglino J, Esilami-Varzaneh F, et al. Recognition of commensal microflora by toll-like receptors is required for intestinal homeostasis. Cell 2004; 118:229–241.
200. Gruber C, Nilsson L, Bjorksten B. Do early childhood immunizations influence the development of atopy and do they cause allergic reactions? Pediatr Allergy Immunol 2001; 12:296–311.
201. Anderson HR, Poloniecki JD, Strachan DP, et al. Immunization and symptoms of atopic disease in children: results from the international study of asthma and allergies in childhood. Am J Public Health 2001; 91:1126–1129.
202. Aaby P, Shaheen SO, Heyes CB, et al. Early BCG vaccination and reduction in atopy in Guinea-Bissau. Clin Exp Allergy 2000; 30:644–650.
203. Gruber C, Kulig M, Bergmann R, et al. Delayed hypersensitivity to tuberculin, total immunoglobulin E, specific sensitization, and atopic manifestation in longitudinally followed early Bacille Calmette-Guerin-vaccinated and nonvaccinated children. Pediatrics 2001; 107(3):E36.
204. Balicer RD, Grotto I, Mimouni M, et al. Is childhood vaccination associated with asthma? A meta-analysis of observational studies. Pediatrics 2007; 120(5):e1269–c1277.
205. Feikin DR, Lezotte DC, Hamman RF, et al. Individual and community risks of measles and pertussis associated with personal exemptions to immunization. JAMA 2000; 284:3145–3150.
206. McKeever TM, Lewis SA, Smith C, et al. Early exposure to infections and antibiotics and the incidence of allergic disease: a birth cohort study with the West Midlands General Practice Research Database. J Allergy Clin Immunol 2002; 109(1):43–50.
207. Marra F, Lynd L, Coombes M, et al. Does antibiotic exposure during infancy lead to development of asthma? A systematic review and metaanalysis. Chest 2006; 129(3):610–618.
208. Marra F, Marra CA, Richardson K, et al. Antibiotic use in children is associated with increased risk of asthma. Pediatrics 2009; 123(3):1003–1010.
209. Shirakawa T, Enomoto T, Shimazu S, et al. The inverse association between tuberculin responses and atopic disorder. Science 1997; 275:77–79.
210. Alm JS, Lilja G, Pershagen G, et al. Early BCG vaccination and development of atopy. Lancet 1997; 350:400–403.
211. Marchant A, Goetghebuer T, Ota MO, et al. Newborns develop a Th1-type immune response to Mycobacterium bovis bacillus Calmette-Guerin vaccination. J Immunol 1999; 163(4):2249–2255.
212. Ota MO, Vekemans J, Schlegel-Haueter SE, et al. Influence of Mycobacterium bovis bacillus Calmette-Guerin on antibody and cytokine responses to human neonatal vaccination. J Immunol 2002; 168(2):919–925.

213. Choi IS, Koh YI. Therapeutic effects of BCG vaccination in adult asthmatic patients: a randomized, controlled trial. Ann Allergy 2002; 88(6):584–591.
214. Arkwright PD, David TJ. Intradermal administration of a killed mycobacterium vaccae suspension (SRL 172) is associated with improvement in atopic dermatitis in children with moderate-to-severe disease. J Allergy Clin Immunol 2001; 107(3):531–534.
215. Shirtcliffe PM, Easthope SE, Cheng S, et al. The effect of delipidated deglycolipidated (DDMV) and heat-killed Mycobacterium vaccae in asthma. Am J Respir Crit Care Med 2001; 163:1410–1414.
216. Balagon MV, Tan PL, Prestidge R, et al. Improvement in psoriasis after intradermal administration of delipidated, deglycolipidated mycobacterium vaccae (PVAC): results of an open-label trial. Clin Exp Dermatol 2001; 26(3):233–241.
217. Lehrer A, Bressanelli A, Wachsmann V, et al. Immunotherapy with Mycobacterium vaccae in the treatment of psoriasis. FEMS Immunol Med Microbiol 1998; 21(1):71–77.
218. O'Brien ME, Saini A, Smith IE, et al. A randomized phase II study of SRL172 (Mycobacterium vaccae) combined with chemotherapy in patients with advanced inoperable non-small-cell lung cancer and mesothelioma. Br J Cancer 2000; 83(7):853–857.
219. Ristori G, Buzzi MG, Sabatini U, et al. Use of Bacille Calmette-Guerin (BCG) in multiple sclerosis. Neurology 1999; 53:1588–1589.
220. Group DIT. Immunotherapy with Mycobacterium vaccae in patients with newly diagnosed pulmonary tuberculosis: a randomized controlled trial. Lancet 1999; 354(9173):116–119.
221. Johnson JL, Kamya RM, Okwera A, et al. Randomized controlled trial of Mycobacterium vaccae immunotherapy in non-human immunodeficiency virus-infected Ugandan adults with newly diagnosed pulmonary tuberculosis. The Uganda-Case Western Reserve University Research Collaboration. J Infect Dis 2000; 181(4):1304–1312.
222. Stanford JL, Stanford CA, Grange JM, et al. Does immunotherapy with heat-killed mycobacterium vaccae offer hope for the treatment of multi-drug-resistant pulmonary tuberculosis? Respir Med 2001; 95(6):444–447.
223. Waddell RD, Chintu C, Lein AD, et al. Safety and immunogenicity of a five-dose series of inactivated Mycobacterium vaccae vaccination for the prevention of HIV-associated tuberculosis. Clin Infect Dis 2000; 30(suppl 3):S309–S315.
224. Arvola T, Laiho K, Torkkeli S, et al. Prophylactic Lactobacillus GG reduces antibiotic-associated diarrhea in children with respiratory infections: a randomized study. Pediatrics 1999; 104(5):e64.
225. Vanderhoof JA, Whitney DB, Antonson DL, et al. Lactobacillus GG in the prevention of antibiotic-associated diarrhea in children. J Pediatr 1999; 135(5):564–568.
226. Hoyos AB. Reduced incidence of necrotizing enterocolitis associated with enteral administration of lactobacillus acidophilus and Bifidobacterium infantis to neonates in an intensive care unit. Int J Infect Dis 1999; 3(4):197–202.
227. Szajewska H, Kotowska M, Mrukowicz JZ, et al. Efficacy of Lactobacillus GG in prevention of nosocomial diarrhea in infants. J Pediatr 2001; 138(3):361–365.
228. Armuzzi A, Cremonini F, Ojetti V, et al. Effect of Lactobacillus GG supplementation on antibiotic-associated gastrointestinal side effects during Helicobacter pylori eradication therapy: a pilot study. Digestion 2001; 63(1):1–7.
229. Niedzielin K, Kordecki H, Birkenfeld B. A controlled, double-blind, randomized study on the efficacy of Lactobacillus plantarum 299V in patients with irritable bowel syndrome. Eur J Gastroenterol Hepatol 2001; 13(10):1135–1136.
230. Szajewska H, Mrukowicz JZ. Probiotics in the treatment and prevention of acute infectious diarrhea in infants and children: a systematic review of published randomized, double-blind, placebo-controlled trials. J Pediatr Gastroenterol Nutr 2001; 33(suppl 2):S17–S25.
231. Van Niel CW, Feudtner C, Garrison MM, et al. Lactobacillus therapy for acute infectious diarrhea in children: a meta-analysis. Pediatrics 2002; 109(4):678–684.

232. Hatakka K, Savilahti E, Ponka A, et al. Effect of long term consumption of probiotic milk on infections in children attending day care centers: double blind, randomized trial. BMJ 2001; 322:1–5.

233. Kukkonen K, Savilahti E, Haahtela T, et al. Long-term safety and impact on infection rates of postnatal probiotic and prebiotic (synbiotic) treatment: randomized, double-blind, placebo-controlled trial. Pediatrics 2008; 122(1):8–12.

234. Rautava S, Salminen S, Isolauri E. Specific probiotics in reducing the risk of acute infections in infancy—a randomised, double-blind, placebo-controlled study. Br J Nutr 2009; 101(11):1722–1726.

235. Kalliomaki M, Salminen S, Arvilommi H, et al. Probiotics in primary prevention of atopic disease: a randomized placebo-controlled trial. Lancet 2001; 357(9262):1076–1079.

236. Kalliomaki M, Salminen S, Poussa T, et al. Probiotics and prevention of atopic disease: 4-year follow-up of a randomised placebo-controlled trial. Lancet 2003; 361(9372):1869–1871.

237. Kalliomaki M, Salminen S, Poussa T, et al. Probiotics during the first 7 years of life: a cumulative risk reduction of eczema in a randomized, placebo-controlled trial. J Allergy Clin Immunol 2007; 119(4):1019–1021.

238. Rautava S, Kalliomaki M, Isolauri E. Probiotics during pregnancy and breast-feeding might confer immunomodulatory protection against atopic disease in the infant. J Allergy Clin Immunol 2002; 109(1):119–121.

239. Pessi T, Sutas Y, Hurme M, et al. Interleukin-10 generation in atopic children following oral Lactobacillus rhamnosus GG. Clin Exp Allergy 2000; 30(12):1804–1808.

240. Helin T, Haahtela S, Haahtela T. No effect of oral treatment with an intestinal bacterial strain, Lactobacillus rhamnosus (ATCC 53103), on birch-pollen allergy: a placebo-controlled double-blind study. Allergy 2002; 57(3):243–246.

241. Lee J, Seto D, Bielory L. Meta-analysis of clinical trials of probiotics for prevention and treatment of pediatric atopic dermatitis. J Allergy Clin Immunol 2008; 121(1):116–121 e11.

242. Kuitunen M, Kukkonen K, Juntunen-Backman K, et al. Probiotics prevent IgE-associated allergy until age 5 years in cesarean-delivered children but not in the total cohort. J Allergy Clin Immunol 2009; 123(2):335–341.

243. Drachenberg KJ, Wheeler AW, Stuebner P, et al. A well-tolerated grass pollen-specific allergy vaccine containing a novel adjuvant, monophosphoryl lipid A, reduces allergic symptoms after only four preseasonal injections. Allergy 2001; 56:498–505.

244. Ambrosch F, Wiedermann G, Kundi M, et al. A hepatitis B vaccine formulated with a novel adjuvant system. Vaccine 2000; 18:2095–2101.

245. Schultz N, Oratz R, Chen D, et al. Effect of DETOX as an adjuvant for melanoma vaccine. Vaccine 1995; 13:503–508.

246. Marshall JD, Abtahi S, Elden JJ, et al. Immunostimulatory sequence DNA linked to the Amb a 1 allergen promotes T_H1 cytokine expression while downregulating T_H2 cytokine expression in PBMCs from human patients with ragweed allergy. J Allergy Clin Immunol 2001; 108:191–197.

247. Tighe H, Takabayashi K, Schwartz D, et al. Conjugation of immunostimulatory DNA to the short ragweed allergen amb a 1 enhances its immunogenicity and reduces its allergenicity. J Allergy Clin Immunol 2000; 106:124–134.

248. Creticos PS, Eiden JJ, Balcer SL, et al. Immunostimulatory oligodeoxynucleotides conjugated to Amb a 1: safety, skin test reactivity, and basophil histamine release. J Allergy Clin Immunol 2000; 105:S70 (abstr).

249. Creticos PS, Schroeder JT, Hamilton RG, et al. Immunotherapy with a ragweed-toll-like receptor 9 agonist vaccine for allergic rhinitis. N Engl J Med 2006; 355(14):1445–1455.

4

Asthma Exacerbation Induced by Virus and Bacteria

KAHARU SUMINO and MICHAEL J. WALTER
Washington University School of Medicine, St. Louis, Missouri, U.S.A.

I. Introduction

Asthma is a chronic inflammatory disorder of the airways that is characterized by variable and recurring symptoms (wheezing, shortness of breath, and chest tightness), airflow obstruction, and bronchial hyperresponsiveness. An asthma exacerbation is defined as an episode of progressively worsening symptoms that is associated with a decrease in expiratory airflow (1,2). In the United States, asthma exacerbations occur frequently, with 56% of asthmatics reporting that they had one or more asthma exacerbation in the preceding 12 months (3). These exacerbations range in severity from mild to life threatening, and contribute greatly to the morbidity, mortality, and total cost of the disease (4,5). An asthma exacerbation can be triggered by exposure to a variety of insults including respiratory tract infections, allergens, chemicals, ozone, pollutants, tobacco smoke, and cold air. Collectively, respiratory infections have been identified as the most common precipitant of asthma exacerbation in both children and adults (6). In this chapter, we will review the role of viral and bacterial infections in the precipitation of an asthma exacerbation. First, since infections are the most common etiology of asthma exacerbations, we will review the data examining the susceptibility of asthmatics to becoming infected with a virus or bacteria. Second, we will discuss the data identifying respiratory viral infection as the most prevalent cause for an asthma exacerbation. Third, we will highlight the data identifying bacterial infections as a trigger for an asthma exacerbation. Fourth, we will describe pathophysiologic alterations in animal models and humans that occur in an infection-induced asthma exacerbation. Fifth, specific treatment options for a respiratory infection during an asthma exacerbation will be reviewed. We will conclude with a brief summary and future research directions that will be required for the development of individualized treatment strategies to prevent or treat infection-induced asthma exacerbations.

II. Susceptibility to Respiratory Infection in Patients with Asthma

Given that the airways of asthmatic patients are chronically inflamed and that many asthmatics are treated with local or systemic glucocorticoids, it is possible that asthmatic patients may be more susceptible to respiratory infections. To address this issue, prospective longitudinal studies comparing infection rates between asthmatic children and their nonasthmatic siblings (7) or between asthmatic adults and their nonasthmatic partners have been performed (8,9). This cohabiting cohort study design attempts to ensure that similar pathogen exposures, identical illness screening protocols, and the same pathogen detection methods are used on both asthmatics and nonasthmatics and thus allows for valid comparisons of incidence rates between the cohorts.

In the childhood study, 16 asthmatics and 15 nonasthmatic siblings were prospectively tested for bacterial and viral infection during a seven-month follow-up period that began in the end of October (7). Although there was no difference in the incidence of total detectable respiratory infections (viral, bacterial, and unknown etiology) between the asthmatics and nonasthmatic siblings (5.6 vs. 4.9 per 7 months, respectively), the asthmatics demonstrated a higher incidence of confirmed viral infections (3.4 vs. 2.3 per 7 months, $p < 0.01$). This higher incidence of viral infection in asthmatics was driven largely by an increased detection rate of rhinovirus. It is noteworthy that the incidence of total detectable respiratory infections per year of follow-up was very high in this asthmatic cohort (approximating 10 viral illnesses per year) and that the asthmatic cohort also had a somewhat lower incidence of bacterial infections.

While this report suggests that asthmatic children may be more susceptible to viral infection, data from two adult studies suggested asthmatics were not more susceptible to respiratory viral infections. In the first study, 20 married couples with one asthmatic and one nonasthmatic partner were prospectively followed for 12 months (9). The asthmatics had a nonsignificant increase in the incidence of total cold episodes; however, they actually had a statistically significant lower incidence of confirmed viral infections. There were no differences in cold frequencies between asthmatics taking and not taking glucocorticoids and no differences in bacterial infection rates. In a more recent three-month longitudinal cohort study, the frequency, severity, and duration of rhinovirus infection were assessed in 76 cohabiting couples consisting of one atopic asthmatic and one nonasthmatic partner (8). This study used a more sensitive reverse transcription polymerase chain reaction (RT-PCR) assay to identify rhinovirus, and asthmatics were not more susceptible to rhinovirus infection compared with nonasthmatics [for asthmatics odds ratio (OR) = 1.15; 95% confidence interval (CI), 0.71–1.87]. Although there was no increased susceptibility to acquisition of the rhinoviral infection, the asthmatic patients developed more severe and longer-lasting lower respiratory tract symptoms as well as a greater fall in their peak expiratory flow (PEF) rates compared with the nonasthmatics. These increased lower tract symptoms may reflect increased viral replication or an inability to prevent viral spread from the upper airways to the lower airways.

In regard to susceptibility for bacterial infection, asthma was identified as an independent risk factor for the development of invasive pneumococcal disease. This nested case-control study of patients enrolled in Tennessee's Medicaid program utilized multivariable models to demonstrate that asthma was an independent risk factor for invasive pneumococcal disease (adjusted OR 2.4; 95% CI, 1.9–3.1) (10). Using a similar approach, asthma was also identified as a risk factor for serious pneumococcal disease (invasive pneumococcal disease plus pneumococcal pneumonia) in patients living in Minnesota and for invasive pneumococcal disease in patients living in Puerto Rico (11,12). These studies suggest that asthmatics are more susceptible to invasive pneumococcal disease, and one possible explanation is that asthmatic patients may have a decreased capacity in preventing hematogenous spread following an initial infection of their respiratory tract.

Collectively, these findings suggest that asthmatics may be more susceptible to certain respiratory infections. This may be due to the underlying chronic airway inflammation or an inappropriate immune response to the infection. For example, an inadequate immune response in asthmatics may allow for an otherwise subclinical pneumococcal infection to become invasive or for increased rhinoviral replication to result in a more widespread infection that involves the lower airways. In the case of rhinoviral infection, mechanisms supporting this possibility have been identified. Compared with primary bronchial epithelial cells from normal controls, rhinoviral infection of cells from asthmatic patients resulted in enhanced viral replication and secretion of approximately sevenfold more progeny virus. In asthmatic cells, this enhanced viral replication was associated with impaired induction of the antiviral proteins interferon (IFN)-β, IFN-$\lambda 1$, and IFN-$\lambda 2/3$. Interestingly, impaired induction of IFN-λ was also observed in bronchoalveolar lavage cells infected with rhinovirus or stimulated with LPS, suggesting the possibility of a more global defect in the innate immune response in asthmatics (13,14).

III. Prevalence of Viral Infection and Individual Viruses in Asthma Exacerbations

The clinical association between respiratory infection and worsening of asthma symptoms has been observed for many years, and recently, the use of more sensitive diagnostic techniques has identified respiratory viral infections as the most common etiology of an asthma exacerbation. The first descriptions of asthma in the English language noted that infections were one of many conditions that were associated with worsening asthma symptoms (15). Studies from the early 1920s classified the etiology of asthma according to clinical characteristics and noted that in a subset of patients, their asthma was related to infections, a group they referred to as having bacterial asthma (16,17). Shortly thereafter, active infections were also identified at the time of autopsy in some asthmatics with a fatal asthma exacerbation (18). To better establish a relationship between infections and asthma exacerbations, cross-sectional prevalence studies and prospective cohort studies that employed viral surveillance in children and adults were performed. In these earlier studies, viral infections were identified using nonmolecular diagnostic strategies such as cell culture, immunofluorescent labeling of viral proteins on respiratory cells, and measurement of viral specific acute and convalescent antibodies in the serum (19). These studies demonstrated that approximately 30% of childhood and 15% of adult asthma exacerbations were associated with viral infection. Similar studies have been repeated more recently using RT-PCR assays to identify viral nucleotides in biologic specimens. Using this more sensitive diagnostic approach for viral detection, these reports have demonstrated that respiratory viral infections are the most common etiology of asthma exacerbations.

Multiple reports have examined the association between respiratory viruses (identified by RT-PCR) and asthma exacerbations. It is somewhat challenging to make direct comparisons between these studies because of differences in study design, study populations, geographic location, season of follow-up, inclusion criteria, clinical setting, severity of asthma exacerbation, source of respiratory specimens, viral detection assays, and definitions of an asthma exacerbation. Over the last 15 years, multiple prospective longitudinal cohort studies, cross-sectional prevalence studies, and case-control cohort studies have been performed in both children and adults with asthma. These studies have been performed in many countries around the world, span follow-up throughout all seasons of the year, include exacerbations of all severities (mild to life threatening), and have tested a variety of biologic samples (nasal swab, throat swab, nasal wash, bronchoalveolar lavage). For this current section on viral-induced asthma exacerbations, we have limited our discussion to reports that included patients with a known diagnosis of asthma, RT-PCR detection of respiratory viruses (with or without concurrent non-molecular testing), and defined an asthma exacerbation (Table 1). Collectively, in these 9 studies with 11 distinct asthmatic populations, there were 798 asthma exacerbations tested for virus and 447 (56%) were associated with the detection of one or more viruses. In general, the prevalence was slightly higher in children compared with that in adults. Despite the many differences between these studies, the results were relatively consistent, with a range of 26% to 80% of all asthma exacerbations associated with a virus.

To examine the prevalence of individual viruses detected during a viral-induced exacerbation, we limited the studies to those that gave a distinct breakdown of the viral detection rates for the exacerbations and also tested for picornaviruses (Table 2). When a virus was identified during an exacerbation, the picornaviruses were the most prevalent. Approximately two-thirds of viral-induced exacerbations were associated with picornaviruses, and when both human rhinovirus and enterovirus were individually detected, rhinovirus accounted for approximately 93% to 100% of these picornaviral infections (26,28). Given that about half of all exacerbations are associated with virus infection and approximately 60% of these are caused by rhinovirus, it is estimated that rhinovirus causes approximately 30% of all asthma exacerbations. This estimate has been confirmed in three adult cohort studies that restricted the RT-PCR viral detection to rhinovirus and found evidence of rhinovirus in 21% and 35% of all exacerbations (29–31). However, this estimate may be conservative for children as studies that employed selective testing for rhinovirus in childhood asthma exacerbations found that 82% and 79% of all exacerbations were associated with rhinovirus (32,33). Coronavirus was the second most prevalent virus identified (18%), followed by influenza, which accounted for approximately 11% of all viral-induced exacerbations. The estimate of 7% of viral-induced asthma exacerbations being associated with metapneumovirus (MPV) is similar to the prevalence rates reported in three other studies that utilized a more restricted viral detection protocol in either asthmatic children (2–6%) or adults (7%) (27,30,32). We note that another report detected a much higher rate of MPV-induced asthma exacerbation in children (13% of all exacerbations); however, this higher rate may be due to the inclusion of known asthmatics as well as wheezing infants and children (34). Bocavirus was not identified in a childhood case cohort study that tested samples for multiple respiratory viruses but was identified in a childhood cross-sectional study of inpatient hospitalization for an asthma exacerbation (14% of total exacerbations) and acute expiratory wheezing (39% of total), so additional studies will be required to better define the true prevalence of this virus in asthma exacerbations (26,27,35).

In addition to identifying respiratory viral infections as the most common etiology of an asthma exacerbation, the longitudinal cohort studies have compared baseline characteristics and the severity of the asthma exacerbation between viral- and nonviral-induced exacerbations. In a childhood case-control cohort study by Khetsuriani et al., there were 41 viral-induced exacerbations and 24 nonviral-induced exacerbations. Comparison of baseline demographic and clinical characteristics between these cohorts did not identify any features that were more frequent in the exacerbation cohort with a

Table 1 Prevalence of Viral-Induced Asthma Exacerbations

Author (reference number)	Year	Study design	Age range	Source of cases	Conv	RT-PCR detection	Exacerbation criteria	Exacerbations tested for virus	Any virus detected during exacerbation[a]
Nicholson (20)	1993	Longitudinal cohort	19–46	Outpatient	Yes	Picornavirus (HRV)	Fall in PEF	61	26 (43)
Johnston (21)	1995	Longitudinal cohort	9–11	Outpatient	Yes	Picornavirus (HRV and EV), HCV (OC43 and 229)	Fall in PEF	157	126 (80)
Atmar (22)	1998	Longitudinal cohort	19–50	Outpatient	Yes	Picornavirus (HRV and EV), HCV (OC43), IFV A	Wheezing and/or dyspnea	137	60 (44)
Atmar (22)	1998	Cross-sectional	17–77	Emergency department	Yes	Picornavirus (HRV and EV), HCV (OC43), IFV A	Wheezing and/or dyspnea	148	82 (55)
Green (23)	2002	Case-control cohort	17–50	Inpatient	No	Picornavirus (HRV and EV), HCV (OC43 and 229), RSV-A and RSV-B, PIV 1-3, IFV A and B, AD	Clinical	61	16 (26)
Tan (24)	2003	Cross-sectional	42 ± 15[b]	Inpatient	No	Picornavirus, RSV, PIV, IFV A and B, AD	Clinical	17	10 (59)
Tan (24)	2003	Cross-sectional	42 ± 15[b]	Intensive care unit	No	Picornavirus, RSV, PIV, IFV A and B, AD	Clinical	29	12 (41)

Johnston (25)	2005	Case-control cohort	5–15	Emergency department	No	Picornavirus (HRV and EV), HCV (OC43 and 229), RSV-A and RSV-B, PIV 1–3, IFV A and B, AD	Clinical	52	32 (62)
Khetsuriani (26)	2007	Case-control cohort	2–17	Inpatient and outpatient	No	Picornavirus (HRV and EV), HCV (OC43 and 229), RSV, PIV 1–3, IFV A and B, AD, MPV, bocavirus	Sx, meds, and unscheduled visit	65	41 (63)
Gendrel (27)	2007	Cross-sectional	2–15	Inpatient	No	RSV, PIV, IFV A and B, AD, MPV, bocavirus	Clinical	50	26 (52)
Kistler (28)	2008	Longitudinal cohort	>18	Outpatient	Yes	Pan-viral microarray assay with confirmatory RT-PCR	Sx, meds, and fall in PEF or FEV$_1$	21	16 (76)
Total								798	447 (56)

[a]Data presented as *n* (%). Percent calculated as the number of viral-induced exacerbations divided by the number of exacerbations tested multiplied by 100.
[b]Data presented as mean ± SD.
Abbreviations: Conv, detection of virus using nonmolecular techniques such as cell culture, immunofluorescent labeling, and/or serologic assays; RT-PCR, reverse transcription polymerase chain reaction; HRV, human rhinovirus; HCV, human coronavirus; IFV, influenza virus; EV, enterovirus; RSV, respiratory syncytial virus; PIV, parainfluenza virus; AD, adenovirus; MPV, metapneumovirus; Sx, asthma symptoms (cough, wheeze, shortness of breath, or chest tightness); meds, increased use of short-acting β-agonists and increased use of controller medication; FEV$_1$, forced expiratory volume in one second.

Table 2 Prevalence of Individual Viruses Detected During a Viral-Induced Asthma Exacerbation

Author (reference)	Total viruses identified	Picornavirus	Coronavirus	IFV	PIV	RSV	AD	MPV	Boca	Other	2 Viruses detected	3 Viruses detected
Nicholson (20)	27	17 (63)	5 (19)	1 (4)	3 (11)	1 (4)	0	ND	ND	0	1	0
Atmar (22)	63	24 (38)	10 (16)	11 (17)	16 (25)	0 (0)	1 (2)	ND	ND	0	3	0
Atmar (22)	94	53 (56)	21 (22)	12 (13)	0	4 (4)	1 (1)	ND	ND	3 (4)[a]	10	1
Green (23)	16	6 (38)	10 (63)	0	0	0	0	ND	ND	ND	0	0
Tan (24)	13	8 (62)	ND	1 (8)	0	0	4 (31)	ND	ND	ND	3	0
Tan (24)	15	8 (53)	ND	6 (40)	0	0	1 (7)	ND	ND	ND	3	0
Johnston (25)	32	27 (84)	0	0	1 (3)	4 (13)	0	ND	ND	ND	3	0
Khetsuriani (26)	43	39 (91)	0	0	0	1 (2)	0	3 (7)	0	ND	4	0
Kistler (28)	18	10 (56)	4 (22)	1 (6)	0	3 (17)	0	0	0	0	2	0
Total	321	192 (60)	50 (17)[b]	32 (10)	20 (6)	18 (6)	7 (2)	3 (5)[b]	0	3 (1)[b]	26 (4)[c]	1 (0.2)[c]

Data presented as *n* (%). Percent values calculated as the times an individual virus was detected divided by the total number of viruses identified multiplied by 100.

[a]Cytomegalovirus.

[b]Total number of viruses identified adjusted downward as some studies did not test for all viruses. Coronavirus, 293; MPV, 61; other, 202.

[c]Percent values calculated as the times two or three viruses were detected divided by the total number of exacerbations tested multiplied by 100. Total exacerbations tested = 591.

Abbreviations: IFV, influenza virus; RSV, respiratory syncytial virus; PIV, parainfluenza virus; AD, adenovirus; MPV, metapneumovirus; Boca, bocavirus; ND, detection assay for individual virus not done.

viral pathogen detected. Variables tested include demographic and socioeconomic features (age, race, parental educational level, and family income), atopy, history of allergen exposure, asthma severity estimates (prior health care visits, hospitalizations, and ICU admissions in last 12 months), and medications (inhaled corticosteroids or montelukast) (26). Two reports have identified that lower lung function at baseline was associated with a viral-induced exacerbation, and one demonstrated that patients with a viral-induced asthma exacerbation were less bronchodilator responsive than those without an identified viral pathogen (36,37). However, three different reports did not demonstrate that a viral-induced exacerbation was more severe than a nonviral-induced exacerbation. Severity of an exacerbation was assessed by fall in PEF (approximately 100 L/min decrease on day 2 to 3), the subsequent use of oral corticosteroids (38%), the subsequent use of antibiotics (33%), exacerbation duration, chance of being admitted to the hospital, and the duration of hospitalization (4.9 ± 2.7 days with virus vs. 4.0 ± 2.0 without virus, $p = 0.23$) (20–22). Interestingly, infection with coronavirus was associated with a less severe exacerbation, as evidenced by a smaller decrease in PEF and fewer lower respiratory tract symptoms when compared with all other viruses (21). Collectively, this data suggests that asthma patients with low function may be more likely to have a virus identified during an exacerbation but that identification of a respiratory virus during an exacerbation does not necessarily indicate a more severe subsequent exacerbation.

Two studies have analyzed respiratory viral infection as a specific risk factor for an asthma exacerbation that results in hospitalization (23,26). Khetsuriani and colleagues noted that in a multivariable logistic regression model, the detection of a respiratory virus was a significant risk factor for an asthma exacerbation (OR = 5.5; 95% CI, 2.5–12.3). Green et al. identified 61 adult cases of asthma exacerbations admitted to the hospital. At the time of admission, nasal washings were collected for viral detection and skin prick testing for nine aeroallergens was performed to determine allergen sensitization. To estimate level of antigen exposure at the time of the exacerbation, dust samples were collected from the participant's house and allergen concentrations were quantified. For all the exacerbations, the authors noted a relatively low prevalence of viral-induced asthma exacerbation (26%), and a disproportionately high proportion of these viral-induced exacerbations were associated with coronavirus (62.5% coronavirus and 37.5% picornavirus). Sensitization and exposure to high concentrations of allergen were identified in 40% of exacerbations. Univariate logistic regression models for the asthma exacerbation end point determined that being both sensitized and exposed to high level of allergen was an independent risk factor for hospitalized asthma exacerbation (OR = 3.22; 95% CI, 1.47–705), whereas the presence of viral infection was not (OR =1.67; 95% CI, 0.69–4.07). It is possible that the low viral prevalence in this study and the high frequency of coronavirus diminished the risk attributable to respiratory virus. In a multivariable logistic regression model, the presence of a viral infection and being both sensitized and exposed to high level of allergen increased the risk of hospitalization from an asthma exacerbation (OR=8.4; 95% CI, 2.1–32.8). Likewise, Murray and coworkers used multivariable logistic regression models and reported that viral infection and being both sensitized and exposed to allergen were significant risk factors for a subsequent asthma exacerbation (38). Taken together, these three studies support a role for viral infection as a risk factor for subsequent asthma exacerbations.

The use of RT-PCR assays to detect viral nucleotides in respiratory specimens indicates that over half of all exacerbations are associated with the presence of virus. Since most of these asthma exacerbations were associated with upper and lower respiratory tract infectious symptoms, a cause-and-effect relationship has been assumed to exist. However, detecting viral nucleotides by RT-PCR in respiratory samples from asymptomatic asthmatics and normal control subjects as well as from asthmatics long after their infectious symptoms have resolved has raised some concern that RT-PCR may overestimate the true prevalence of viral-induced asthma exacerbations.

To determine the overall prevalence of viral detection in asymptomatic asthmatics and healthy normal controls using RT-PCR, a number of study populations have been examined (Table 3). The overall estimate from these studies indicated that respiratory viral nucleotides are detected in approximately 25% of all asymptomatic asthmatics, with a range from 12% to 41%. We note that the highest prevalence of 41% was observed in a study that collected biologic specimens from children during September, a month that was chosen because it was historically associated with very high viral detection rates. As with viral-induced asthma exacerbations, the prevalence in asymptomatic asthmatics is generally higher in children than that in adults. The prevalence of the individual viruses parallels that seen in viral-induced asthma exacerbations, with picornavirus accounting for 78% of all viruses, coronavirus accounting for approximately 10%, and fewer cases of respiratory syncytial virus (RSV) and MPV. In these studies of asymptomatic asthmatics, influenza, parainfluenza, adenovirus, and bocavirus were not detected. The detection of respiratory viral nucleotides is approximately two to three times lower in asymptomatic normal subjects than that in asymptomatic asthmatics, with an overall prevalence of about 10% in asymptomatic normals. In normals, picornaviruses was again the most prevalent virus, accounting for approximately 80% of all detected viruses, with coronavirus detected in about 20% of the cases, and minimal detection of the other respiratory viruses. The very low frequencies of RSV, MPV, and bocavirus in normals have been confirmed in additional studies that employed a more restricted viral detection protocol for these viruses (43,44). Collectively, these studies indicate that viral nucleotides can be detected in biologic samples from approximately one-fourth of asymptomatic asthmatics and one-tenth of asymptomatic normals.

Possible explanation for the detection of viral nucleotides in asymptomatic asthmatics and normals includes misclassification of symptomatic subjects as asymptomatic, false-positive results due to RT-PCR contamination, the detection of virus prior to the development of infectious symptoms, persistence of viral nucleotides from a previous infection after resolution of symptoms, and the presence of a low-level subclinical infection. Reporting of respiratory symptoms is subjective and can be difficult to ascertain especially in young children, so it is possible that some truly symptomatic subjects may have been misclassified as asymptomatic. Although false-positive RT-PCR results can arise from a variety of reasons, most reports included negative controls to minimize this possibility. In longitudinal studies with serial surveillance protocols, it has been demonstrated that viral nucleotides are detected during an asymptomatic period that may last for days to a week prior to the development of the clinical symptoms of the cold. Two studies have demonstrated that 14% to 38% of asymptomatic subjects with detectable rhinoviral nucleotides developed a respiratory illness in the following one to two weeks (45,46). In some individuals with asthma, continued surveillance for rhinovirus following an initial infection revealed virus could be identified five weeks later in

Table 3 Prevalence of Viral Detection in Asymptomatic Asthmatics and Normal Subjects

Author (reference)	Year	Age range	Asymptomatic subjects	Conv	RT-PCR	Samples tested for virus	Detection of any virus[a]	Picornavirus[b]	Coronavirus[b]	IFV[b]	PIV[b]	RSV[b]	AD[b]	MPV[b]	Boca[b]
Johnston (21)	1995	9–11	Asthma	No	Picornavirus (HRV and EV)	65	8 (12)	8 (100)	ND	ND	ND	ND	ND	ND	ND
Green (23)	2002	17–50	Asthma	No	Picornavirus (HRV and EV), HCV (OC43 and 229), RSV-A and RSV-B, PIV 1–3, IFV A and B, AD	57	10 (18)	2 (20)	8 (80)	0	0	0	0	ND	ND
Rawlinson (32)	2004	2–17	Asthma	No	Picornavirus (HRV and EV), MPV	29	6 (21)	6 (100)	ND	ND	ND	ND	ND	0	ND
Kling (33)	2005	4–12	Asthma	No	Picornavirus (HRV), RSV	9	2 (22)	2 (100)	ND	ND	ND	0	ND	ND	ND
Johnston (25)	2005	5–15	Asthma	No	Picornavirus (HRV and EV), HCV (OC43 and 229), RSV-A and RSV-B, PIV 1–3, IFV A and B, AD	150	62 (41)	43 (69)	0	2 (3)	0	16 (26)	0	ND	ND
Khetsuriani (26)	2007	2–17	Asthma	No	Picornavirus (HRV and EV), HCV (OC43 and 229), RSV, PIV 1–3, IFV A and B, AD, MPV, bocavirus	77	18 (23)	15 (83)	1 (6)	0	0	1 (6)	0	2 (11)	0
Harju (36)	2008	43 ± 13	Asthma	No	Picornavirus (HRV and EV), RSV, AD	103	14 (14)	14 (100)	ND	ND	ND	0	0	ND	ND
Total						490	120 (24)	93 (78)	9 (10)[c]	2 (2)[c]	0	17 (9)[c]	0	2 (8)[c]	0

(*Continued*)

Table 3 Prevalence of Viral Detection in Asymptomatic Asthmatics and Normal Subjects (*Continued*)

Author (reference)	Year	Age range	Asymptomatic subjects	Conv	RT-PCR	Samples tested for virus	Detection of any virus[a]	Picornavirus[b]	Coronavirus[b]	IFV[b]	PIV[b]	RSV[b]	AD[b]	MPV[b]	Boca[b]
Johnston (39)	1993	<65	No asthma	Yes	Picornavirus (HRV and EV)	53	2 (4)	2 (100)	0	0	0	0	0	ND	ND
Green (23)	2002	17–50	No asthma	No	Picornavirus (HRV and EV), HCV (OC43 and 229), RSV-A and RSV-B, PIV 1–3, IFV A and B, AD	59	5 (9)	2 (40)	3 (60)	0	0	0	0	ND	ND
Nokso-Koivisto (40)	2002	0.1–16	No asthma	No	Picornavirus (HRV and EV), HCV (OC43 and 229)	30	5 (17)	5 (100)	0	ND	ND	ND	ND	ND	ND
van Gageldonk-Lafeber (41)	2005	0–87	No asthma	No	Picornavirus (HRV and EV), HCV, RSV, PIV 1–3, IFV A and B, AD, MPV	541	94 (17)	67 (71)	21 (22)	3 (3)	0	3 (3)	0	0	ND
Winther (42)	2006	1–9	No asthma	No	Picornavirus (HRV and EV)	740	37 (5)	37 (100)	ND	ND	ND	ND	ND	ND	ND
Harju (36)	2008	39 ± 14	No asthma	No	Picornavirus (HRV and EV), RSV, AD	30	4 (13)	4 (100)	ND	ND	ND	0	0	ND	ND
Total						1453	147 (10)	117 (80)	24 (23)[d]	3 (3)[d]	0	3 (2)[d]	0	0	0

[a]Data presented as *n* (%). Percent calculated as number of times any virus detected divided by number of samples tested for virus multiplied by 100.
[b]Data presented as *n* (%). Percent calculated as number of times an individual virus was detected divided by the total number of viruses detected multiplied by 100.
[c]For some viruses, the total number of viruses identified adjusted downward as some studies did not test for all viruses. Coronavirus, 90; IFV, 90; RSV, 195; MPV, 24.
[d]For some viruses, the total number of viruses identified adjusted downward as some studies did not test for all viruses. Coronavirus, 106; IFV, 101; RSV, 131.
Abbreviations: Conv, detection of virus using nonmolecular techniques such as cell culture, immunofluorescent labeling, and/or serologic assays; RT-PCR, reverse transcription polymerase chain reaction; HRV, human rhinovirus; HCV, human coronavirus; IFV, influenza virus; EV, enterovirus; RSV, respiratory syncytial virus; PIV, parainfluenza virus; AD, adenovirus; MPV, metapneumovirus; Boca, bocavirus; ND, detection assay for individual virus not done.

one study and for six months in another study (33,46). Although these studies did not perform strain identification to exclude reinfection, in immunocompromised lung transplant recipients, persistent rhinoviral infection has been confirmed by genetic sequencing of sequential isolates grown from airway specimens (47).

Since viral nucleotides are present in asymptomatic asthmatics, it is important to directly compare the viral detection rates in asthma exacerbations and asymptomatic asthmatics to confirm an association between respiratory viral infections and exacerbations. Ideally, this comparison is done using a case-control cohort study design so as to ensure identical viral detection techniques between the cohorts. We identified five reports that compared viral nucleotide detection during an exacerbation with asymptomatic asthmatics, and in all five, there was a statistically significant higher proportion of viral detection rates during an exacerbation (22,23,25,26,32). Accordingly, this data supports a definite association between respiratory viral infection and asthma exacerbations. However, it remains unclear how the prevalence of virus in asymptomatic asthmatics affects the reported estimate that over half of all exacerbations are due to respiratory viral infections.

IV. Prevalence of Bacterial Infection in Asthma Exacerbations

Over the years, bacterial infections have also been associated with asthma exacerbations. While early reports noted that bacterial infections were associated with asthma in a subset of patients and that bacterial infections were present in the airways of patients at autopsy for asthma exacerbations (16,17), a stronger association between bacterial sinusitis and exacerbations was later described (48). Initially, bacteria that commonly caused sinusitis were explored as triggers for asthma exacerbations, but as culture techniques and alternative diagnostic tests for atypical bacteria were developed, it became apparent that *Mycoplasma pneumoniae* and *Chlamydophila pneumoniae* (formerly *Chlamydia pneumoniae*) were the most common bacterial precipitants of an exacerbation (49). The true prevalence of bacterial-induced asthma exacerbations is challenging to calculate because of difficulties in culturing certain bacteria, practical limitations of obtaining lower respiratory tract specimens during an exacerbation, inability to discriminate bacterial colonization from true infection, high seroreactivity due to prior infections, differences in laboratory-specific diagnostic techniques, and the poor concordance between different diagnostic tests. To help minimize these limitations in estimating a prevalence of *C. pneumoniae*– and *M. pneumoniae*–induced asthma exacerbations, we have restricted the discussion to case cohort studies that included patients with a diagnosis of asthma as well as an asymptomatic control cohort. This allows for more robust comparisons of samples obtained during asthmatic exacerbations with those from asymptomatic asthmatics or asymptomatic subjects without asthma.

We identified 11 case-control cohort studies in children and adults that examined the prevalence of *C. pneumoniae*–induced asthma exacerbations (Table 4). Overall, the estimated prevalence of a *C. pneumoniae*–induced asthma exacerbation was approximately 10% of all asthma exacerbations. These studies showed variable results, with the prevalence ranging from 0% to 36%. This variability may reflect differences in patient populations or alternative diagnostic tests used to identify an acute infection [culture, serologic, or polymerase chain reaction (PCR) based]. In studies that performed multiple

Table 4 Prevalence of *Chlamydophila pneumoniae* Detection in Case-Control Studies of Asthma Exacerbations

Author (reference)	Year	Age range	Source of cases	Asymptomatic controls	CP detection method	Exacerbation criteria	Exacerbations tested for CP	CP detected during exacerbation[a]	Asymptomatic controls tested for CP	CP detected in asymptomatic controls[a]
Emre (50)	1994	5–18	Emergency department	No asthma	Culture	Wheezing	138	13 (11)	41	2 (5)
Teichtahl (51)	1997	17–69	Emergency department	Asthma	Culture, serology	Clinical	79	0	54	0
Cunningham (52)	1998	9–11	Outpatient	Asthma	Nasal aspirate IgA, PCR	Symptoms and or fall in PEF	292	68 (23)	65	18 (28)
Miyashita (53)	1998	16–80	Inpatient	No asthma	Culture, serology, PCR	Wheezing	168	15 (9)	108	3 (3)
Cook (54)	1998	15–88	Emergency department	Asthma / No asthma	Serology	Wheezing	123	7 (6)	46 asthma / 1518 no asthma	2 (4) asthma / 87 (6) no asthma
Green (23)	2002	17–50	Inpatient	Asthma / No asthma	PCR	Clinical	61	0	58 asthma / 59 no asthma	0 / 0
Lieberman (55)	2003	18–78	Inpatient	No asthma	Serology	Dyspnea	100	8 (8)	100	6 (6)
Betsou (56)	2003	17–68	Not described	No asthma	Serology	Clinical	160	11 (7)	88	13 (15)
Biscardi (57)	2004	2–15	Inpatient	Asthma and or rhinitis	Serology	Clinical	119	4 (3)	120	3 (3)
Johnston (25)	2005	5–15	Emergency department	Asthma	PCR	Clinical	52	2 (4)	150	6 (4)
Kocabas (58)	2008	33.2 ± 9.1[b]	Not described	Asthma / No asthma	Serology, PCR	Clinical	22	8 (36)	84 asthma / 34 no asthma	30 (36) asthma / 9 (26) no asthma
Total							1314	134 (10)	2525	179 (7)

[a]Data presented as *n* (%). Percent calculated as number of times CP detected divided by number of samples tested for CP multiplied by 100.
[b]Data presented as mean ± SD.
Abbreviations: CP, *Chlamydophila pneumoniae*; IgA, immunoglobulin A; PCR, polymerase chain reaction; PEF, peak expiratory flow rate.

diagnostic tests on the same subject, PCR detection is generally more sensitive than culture and appears to correlate with chronic infection (58). In a large study in children, *C. pneumoniae* detection by PCR was similar between 292 samples taken during an exacerbation compared with 65 samples from an asymptomatic period (23% vs. 28%), but *C. pneumoniae*–specific secretory immunoglobulin A antibodies in the serum were more than seven times greater in subjects who reported four or more exacerbations compared with those with just one exacerbation ($p = 0.02$) (52). In these same studies, the overall prevalence of *C. pneumoniae* in the control subjects is estimated at about 7%. In most, but not all of these studies, there was an increased prevalence of *C. pneumoniae* in the subjects with an exacerbation compared with the control cohort; however, this difference was statistically significant in only one study (53).

M. pneumoniae has also been associated with asthma exacerbations, although the overall prevalence appears to be lower than that in *C. pneumoniae*. In six case-control cohort studies, acute *M. pneumoniae* infection was identified in approximately 7% of all exacerbations (Table 5). When compared with controls, two of these six studies found a statistically increased rate of acute *M. pneumoniae* infection in asthma exacerbations compared with controls. In one study of hospitalized adults, *M. pneumoniae* infection was found in 18% of asthma exacerbations compared with only 3% in a hospitalized control cohort ($p = 0.0006$). There were no differences in the frequency of *Streptococcus pneumoniae*, *Legionella*, *Coxiella burnetii*, or *C. pneumoniae* infection between these cohorts (55). A second study of 119 hospitalized preschool and school-age asthma children found a significantly higher frequency of acute *M. pneumoniae* infection asthma exacerbations compared with a cohort of outpatient controls with stable asthma or rhinitis (20% compared with 5%, $p < 0.005$). There were no differences in the frequency of *Bordetella pertussis* or *C. pneumoniae* infection between these cohorts (57). Three studies did not find any statistical differences between acute *M. pneumoniae* infection during an exacerbation compared with control cohorts (23,49,51), and one study observed a nonsignificant higher rate of infection in the control cohort compared with those with an asthma exacerbation (52). Collectively, in these studies, the overall prevalence of *M. pneumoniae* infection in asymptomatic control subjects is estimated at about 2%.

Taken together, it appears that infections with *C. pneumoniae* and *M. pneumoniae* do induce asthma exacerbations but that their prevalence is substantially lower than viral-induced exacerbations. Additional studies will need to be performed to identify demographic features, clinical characteristics, and biologic markers that help predict an exacerbation caused by these atypical bacterial infections and to determine if the clinical course is more or less severe in an exacerbation because of infection with these organisms.

V. Inflammatory Cells and Mediators of an Infection-Induced Asthma Exacerbation

Both in vitro and in vivo experiments have provided insight into the biochemical pathways and inflammatory proteins that mediate a postinfectious asthma exacerbation. The in vitro responses of epithelial cells to infectious microbes and the in vivo host defense responses will be addressed in subsequent chapters of this book. To fully understand the pathophysiologic mechanisms and inflammatory mediators that underlie

Table 5 Prevalence of *Mycoplasma pneumoniae* Detection in Case-Control Studies of Asthma Exacerbations

Author (reference)	Year	Age range	Source of cases	Asymptomatic controls	MP detection method	Exacerbation criteria	Exacerbations tested for MP	MP detected during exacerbation[a]	Asymptomatic controls tested for MP	MP detected in asymptomatic controls[a]
Teichtahl (51)	1997	17–69	Emergency department	No asthma	Culture, serology	Clinical	79	1 (1)	54	0
Cunningham (52)	1998	9–11	Outpatient	Asthma	PCR	Symptoms and or fall in PEF	292	2 (0.7)	65	2 (3%)
Green (23)	2002	17–50	Inpatient	Asthma No asthma	PCR	Clinical	61	0	58 asthma 59 no asthma	0 0
Lieberman (55)	2003	18–78	Inpatient	No asthma	Serology	Dyspnea	100	18 (18)	100	3 (3)
Biscardi (57)	2004	2–15	Inpatient	Asthma and or rhinitis	Serology	Clinical	119	24 (20)	152	8 (5)
Johnston (25)	2005	5–15	Emergency department	Asthma	PCR	Clinical	52	0	150	0
Total							673	45 (7)	638	13 (2)

[a]Data presented as *n* (%). Percent calculated as number of times MP detected divided by number of samples tested for MP multiplied by 100.
Abbreviations: **MP**, *Mycoplasma pneumoniae*; **PCR**, polymerase chain reaction; **PEF**, peak expiratory flow rate.

a viral- or bacterial-induced asthma exacerbation, comparisons will need to be made between allergic inflammatory models with and without a superimposed infection. It is likely that the inflammatory response to an infection is different in the setting of chronic asthmatic inflammation. Accordingly, in this section, we will focus on animal studies that have investigated viral and bacterial infections in the setting of an established allergic inflammatory response and human studies that have investigated inflammatory mechanisms in asthmatics during a naturally occurring infection.

To recreate an infectious asthma exacerbation model in animals, researchers have superimposed an airway infection (both viral and bacterial) on an underlying allergic inflammatory response. Three groups have examined the effects of a respiratory viral infection during or immediately after the development of an allergic airway inflammation response (induced by prior allergen sensitization and challenge) (59–62). All of these studies have been performed in female BALB/c mice; however, the specific allergen sensitization and challenge protocol, as well as the viral infection protocol, differed among the studies. The first study compared mice that were only infected with RSV-A with those that were only ovalbumin sensitized and challenged to those that were infected with RSV-A during the ovalbumin challenge (59). Viral infection occurring during the ovalbumin challenge resulted in an exaggerated inflammatory response manifested as a prolonged phase of airway hyperreactivity to methacholine, increased peribronchiolar lymphocyte accumulation, and increased mucous production (i.e., PAS-positive airway epithelial cells); however, no differences in eosinophil accumulation were observed 15 days following viral infection. In a subsequent study, using the same protocol, this group demonstrated that RSV-A infection given during the ovalbumin challenge also resulted in the prolonged expression of the proteins Muc5ac (a specific mucin gene), gob-5 (a calcium-dependent chloride channel that is expressed in airway goblet cells), and IL-17 (an inducer of Muc5ac expression) (61). These exaggerated responses seen when combining allergic inflammation and RSV-A infection were only observed for the first two weeks after infection, suggesting that the exaggerated inflammatory response prolonged these asthma phenotypes but did not necessarily result in a long-lasting exaggerated response.

Similar results have been described in a second report that used RSV-A to infect *Dermatophagoides farinae*–sensitized mice one day after they had been challenged with this allergen (60). Compared with RSV-A-infected or *D. farinae*–sensitized and *D. farinae*–challenged mice, combining RSV-A infection after the challenge resulted in exaggerated airway hyperreactivity to methacholine, increased IFN-γ production, and a trend toward increased production of IL-4 and IL-5 from *D. farinae*–stimulated thoracic lymph node mononuclear cells. In the allergen-challenged and infected mice, airway eosinophils (measured on an hematoxylin and eosin-stained lung section) were increased at day 4 following the viral infection. Another study in ovalbumin-sensitized mice tested the effects of rhinovirus-1B infection given immediately after the last ovalbumin challenge (62). Compared with rhinoviral-1B infection alone and ovalbumin sensitization and challenge alone, the combination resulted in an increased accumulation of neutrophils in the BAL, airway hyperreactivity to methacholine, the production of IL-4, IL-13, and IFN-γ at day 1 after infection, increased eosinophils and Muc5ac in the BAL at day 7, and increased lymphocyte accumulation in the BAL at days 3 through 14. Collectively, these animal studies indicate that respiratory viral infection superimposed on an allergic inflammatory response results in an exaggerated neutrophilic, lymphocytic, and eosinophilic immune response that is associated with enhanced cytokine production (IL-4, IL-13, and IFN-γ), augmented mucous gene induction and goblet cell metaplasia, and increased airway hyperreactivity. These phenotypes resemble the response that is observed in an asthma exacerbation, and additional studies will be required to identify the specific inflammatory cells and mediators responsible for the exaggerated immune response seen when combining a respiratory viral infection and allergic airway inflammation.

One animal study has evaluated the role of a bacterial infection with *M. pneumoniae* in the setting of allergic airway inflammation in mice (63). In this study, ovalbumin-sensitized BALB/c mice were infected with *M. pneumoniae* two days following the last ovalbumin challenge. Compared with ovalbumin-sensitized and ovalbumin-challenged mice that were inoculated with saline, the ovalbumin-sensitized and ovalbumin-challenged mice inoculated with *M. pneumoniae* demonstrated an early decrease in airway hyperresponsiveness to methacholine at day 3, which was followed by a later increase at days 7 and 14. These changes in airway hyperresponsiveness were associated with a parallel early decrease and later increase in BAL concentrations of IL-4. As opposed to IL-4, the opposite trend was observed for BAL concentrations of IFN-γ, higher levels at day 3 and lower levels at day 7. Examination of the inflammatory cells that accumulated in the BAL demonstrated a trend toward more neutrophils at day 3 and more total cells seven days following the infection. This study suggests that bacterial infection in the setting of allergic airway inflammation can also exaggerate airway inflammation and airway hyperresponsiveness, and additional studies will be required to further understand the pathophysiologic changes seen with other pathogens, such as *C. pneumoniae*, in the setting of allergic airway inflammation.

In humans, it is challenging to study the pathophysiology and biologic mediators of an infection-induced asthma exacerbation because these exacerbations are sporadic, safety concerns limit the availability of biologic specimens to the upper airway and peripheral blood, and the variability in the host response to the viral infection. Nevertheless, studies have compared inflammatory characteristics in serum, induced sputum, and nasal washes in patients with a viral-induced exacerbation with those with a nonviral-induced exacerbation.

To characterize the airway inflammation during a viral-induced asthma exacerbation, the cellular constituents and concentrations of inflammatory mediators in induced sputum have been examined by one group in two studies (64,65). In the first study, 49 adult patients who presented to the emergency department with an acute asthma exacerbation were tested for 10 common respiratory viruses by RT-PCR. Compared with sputum from patients with a nonviral-induced asthma exacerbation, the viral-induced asthma exacerbations had higher total cell counts, neutrophil counts, neutrophil elastase levels, and lactate dehydrogenase concentrations and a lower percentage of eosinophils and IL-5-positive cells. There were no differences in total eosinophil count, concentrations of IL-8, or levels of eosinophil cationic protein (65). In the second study, induced sputum was examined from five cohorts: inpatient viral-induced asthma exacerbations ($n = 46$), inpatients with a nonviral-induced asthma exacerbation ($n = 13$), outpatients with stable asthma without a respiratory viral infection ($n = 14$), outpatient healthy controls without a respiratory viral infection (16), and outpatient healthy control with a respiratory viral infection ($n = 15$) (64). Respiratory viral infection was diagnosed using RT-PCR detection of six common respiratory viruses. Comparing inpatients with and without a viral-induced asthma exacerbation, the virus-positive group had a trend toward a lower forced expiratory volume in one second (FEV_1) at the time of exacerbation, a 4-fold increase in total neutrophils, and a 10-fold increase in total lymphocytes. In the viral-induced asthma exacerbation, there was a predominant accumulation of neutrophils (54% of the total cells), whereas in the remaining four cohorts (including the nonviral-induced exacerbation), the predominant cell was the macrophage. Cytokine expression in the induced sputum was measured with quantitative RT-PCR and demonstrated a significant increase in CCL5 (RANTES) and a trend toward significance in IL-10 in the inpatients with a viral-induced asthma exacerbation compared with the inpatients with a nonviral-induced asthma exacerbation. No significant differences between these groups were detected for IL-8 and MIP-1α, whereas IL-5 and eotaxin-1 mRNA levels were not consistently detected in the induced sputum.

Another study has measured serum cytokine concentrations from a group of 26 adult asthmatics with a viral-induced asthma exacerbation and a group of 10 adult patients with a nonviral-induced exacerbation (65). All these patients presented to the emergency department for an asthma exacerbation and provided post-bronchodilator spirometry to assess airflow obstruction, serum for cytokine measurements, and throat swab for RT-PCR detection of eight common respiratory viruses. The patients with viral-induced exacerbations were less responsive to bronchodilators than those with the nonviral-induced exacerbation. Serum concentrations of the chemokine IFN-γ induced protein 10 (IP-10, CXCL10) were significantly higher in the subjects with viral-induced asthma exacerbation compared with the group with a nonviral-induced exacerbation. This finding suggests that serum IP-10 levels may be useful in distinguishing patients with and without a viral-induced asthma exacerbation, and a concentration above a cut point of 168 pg/mL yielded a sensitivity of 95% and specificity of 70% for the diagnosis of a viral-induced asthma exacerbation. There was a trend toward lower serum concentration of TNF-α in the viral-induced asthma exacerbation cohort ($p = 0.07$), whereas there were no differences between the groups with respect to serum IL-6 or IL-8 concentrations, and CCL5 (RANTES) was below the level of detection for the majority of the specimens. To our knowledge, measurements of inflammatory cells or mediators during a bacterial-induced asthma exacerbation have not been performed.

Collectively, these human studies indicate that a viral-induced asthma exacerbation is characterized by an exaggerated inflammatory response compared with a nonviral-induced asthma exacerbation. Consistent with the inflammatory pattern seen during a viral infection in an allergic animal, asthmatics with a viral-induced exacerbation also demonstrated an exaggerated accumulation of neutrophils and, to a lesser extent, lymphocytes. Additional animal and human translational studies will be required to further identify the critical inflammatory mediators that drive the accumulation of neutrophils, as well as the exaggerated inflammatory response seen in a viral-induced asthma exacerbation.

VI. Specific Treatments for Viral- or Bacterial-Induced Asthma Exacerbation

Specific treatment strategies that have been evaluated for a viral-induced asthma exacerbation include administration of oseltamivir for viral symptoms, an early increase in corticosteroids for viral symptoms, and the use of influenza vaccine to prevent influenza-induced asthma exacerbation. In a placebo-controlled, randomized, double-blind trial in asthmatic children, the administration of oseltamivir (2 mg/kg twice a day for five days) did not shorten the time to freedom from illness (the primary end point); however, treatment did significantly improve symptom scores, FEV_1 at day 6, and the frequency of exacerbations (defined as a >20% decrease in PEF from baseline). Furthermore, these improvements were greater when treatment was started within the first 24 hours of symptoms (66).

Three placebo-controlled studies in asthmatics have examined the ability of inhaled corticosteroids at the initial signs of an upper respiratory tract infection to improve subsequent asthma-related outcomes (67–69). All of these studies have been performed in asthmatic children with a prior history of upper respiratory tract infection–related wheezing episodes; two were randomized, double-blind, placebo-controlled crossover studies (67,68), and one was a randomized, double-blind, placebo-controlled parallel group trial (69). The major limitation for all of these studies is that no microbiologic testing for the presence of virus or bacteria was performed. Accordingly, it is impossible to make specific conclusions regarding early glucocorticoids' use for a viral- or bacterial-induced exacerbation. With this limitation in mind, the early initiation of inhaled corticosteroids was associated with less asthma symptoms in one study (69), less asthma symptoms in a subgroup of patients in the second study (67), and no difference in the third study (68). There were no beneficial effects in the number of exacerbations requiring oral prednisone, emergency department visits, or hospitalizations. One childhood study has demonstrated that initiation of prednisone (1 mg/kg/day) at the onset of symptoms of an upper respiratory tract infection decreased asthma attacks, emergency room visits, and hospitalizations; however, this was an unblinded study with a relatively small sample size ($n = 16$) that did not test for viral infection, so firm conclusions related to the role of early prednisone for a viral-induced asthma exacerbation cannot be made at this time (70).

The ability of influenza vaccine to prevent influenza-induced asthma exacerbations was evaluated in a randomized, double-blind, placebo-controlled trial in children (71). Patients received either placebo or influenza vaccine and were followed prospectively for infectious episodes, asthma exacerbations, and concurrent influenza infection (detected by cell culture, RT-PRC, and serology). Compared with placebo, influenza vaccine did not decrease the number or severity of influenza-induced asthma exacerbations. There was a trend toward a shorter duration of the influenza-induced asthma exacerbations in the vaccinated group, but this did not reach statistical significance ($p = 0.06$). In a follow-up report, the vaccinated group had an improved health-related quality of life score during the influenza-induced asthma exacerbation; however, there were no differences in the upper or lower respiratory tract symptom scores (72).

Although there have been multiple reports on the use of antibiotics during an acute asthma exacerbation, there were only two randomized, double-blind, placebo-controlled studies that met the selection criteria of the most recent Cochrane review of antibiotics use in asthma exacerbation (73). In the first study, amoxicillin or placebo was added to bronchodilators and corticosteroids in 60 adult patients admitted to the hospital with an acute asthma exacerbation. No benefit was seen in lung function or the number of days for participants to achieve 50% improvement with antibiotics (74). In the second study, the efficacy of hetacillin was examined in 37 children aged between 1 and 18 years admitted to the hospital with an acute asthma exacerbation. The addition of antibiotics to standard of care (aminophylline and oral corticosteroids) did not show any benefit in lung function or hospital course (75). Importantly, these studies were conducted several decades ago with a total of 97 patients, and they did not attempt to stratify treatment or results according to the presence of a bacterial infection. Additionally, they used amoxicillin or hetacillin, which have no activity against *C. pneumoniae* and *M. pneumoniae*, the two most common bacterial infections that induce asthma exacerbations. Current guidelines recommend the use of antibiotics during an asthma exacerbation for patients with fever and purulent secretions, pneumonia, and if bacterial sinusitis is strongly suspected (1).

A recent randomized, multicenter, double-blind, placebo-controlled study evaluated the role of telithromycin, a ketolide antibiotic with activity against *C. pneumoniae* and *M. pneumoniae*, in patients with an acute asthma exacerbation (76). The Telithromycin, Chlamydia, and Asthma Trial (TELICAST) evaluated 278 adult asthmatic patients with moderate to severe acute exacerbation that required short-term medical care. Patients received standard treatment for an asthma exacerbation (bronchodilators and corticosteroids) and were randomly assigned to receive telithromycin 800 mg daily or matching placebo for 10 days. There were mixed findings for the two coprimary end points: patients treated with telithromycin had significantly greater improvement in asthma symptoms during the treatment period but did not have an improvement in morning PEF. Telithromycin demonstrated a benefit for a number of secondary outcomes including: change in FEV_1 from baseline to the end of treatment, proportion of symptom-free days during the treatment period, and mean decrease in asthma symptoms scores from baseline to the end of treatment. A total of 61% of patients met at least one criterion for infection with *C. pneumoniae*, *M. pneumoniae*, or both, with most being positive by serology. The improvement of FEV_1 after treatment with telithromycin was only significant in the subgroup of 131 patients who were positive for infection (0.67 L in the treatment group vs. 0.38 L in the placebo group) but not in the 82 patients without infection (0.58 L vs. 0.46 L). The study indicates that telithromycin provides a benefit in symptoms in patients with acute asthma exacerbation and a benefit in FEV_1 improvement in those with *C. pneumoniae* or *M. pneumoniae* infection. It is important to mention that telithromycin was later discovered to be associated with serious liver toxicity, and although it is still approved for the treatment of community-acquired pneumonia of mild to moderate severity, the FDA removed the approval for acute bacterial sinusitis and acute bacterial exacerbations of chronic bronchitis. Taken together, an individualized treatment strategy for a viral- or bacterial-induced asthma exacerbation has not been identified, and in general, treatment of an infection-induced exacerbation should follow the same general principles as treatment for a noninfectious exacerbation (1,2).

VII. Summary and Future Directions

Collectively, respiratory viral and bacterial infections are associated with asthma exacerbations with viral infections causing over half of all exacerbations and the combination of *C. pneumoniae* and *M. pneumoniae* infection causing approximately another one-tenth of all exacerbations. Animal models that combine respiratory infection and allergic airway inflammation and human studies of biologic samples obtained during as asthma exacerbation suggest that infection amplifies the expression of inflammatory mediators resulting in an exaggerated neutrophilic inflammatory response that likely culminates in an exacerbation (i.e., worsening of clinical symptoms and airflow obstruction). Although individualized treatment strategies for infection-induced asthma exacerbation have not been clearly identified, the early use of anti-microbial agents, such as oseltamivir for influenza infection or macrolides for atypical bacteria, may prevent or attenuate a subsequent infection-induced asthma exacerbation.

An ideal individualized treatment strategy for an infection-induced asthma exacerbation will require the rapid diagnosis of a specific acute infection in a patient at risk for a postcold asthma exacerbation followed by specific treatment with an effective anti-microbial. Along these lines, new assays have been developed that can rapidly identify up to 17 community-acquired respiratory viruses from noninvasive respiratory specimens using a multiplexed RT-PCR assay to amplify viral nucleotides followed by a sensitive flow cytometry–based detection assay (77). To identify patients at risk for an infection-induced asthma exacerbation, early predictors of worsening postcold asthma control have been identified. These include quantifying cold severity within the first 48 hours after symptoms with a relatively simple questionnaire (78), and quantification of the chemokine IP-10 in the serum (37). These tools will be useful in designing future randomized, placebo-controlled trials to test the efficacy of current or newly developed antimicrobial agents in preventing or treating specific viral- and bacterial-induced asthma exacerbations.

References
1. National Heart, Lung, and Blood Institute National Asthma Education and Prevention Program, Expert Panel Report 3: Guidelines for the diagnosis and management of asthma, 2007. Available at: http://www.nhlbi.nih.gov/guidelines/asthma.
2. Global strategy for asthma management and prevention, 2006. Available at: http://www.ginasthma.org.
3. Moorman J, Rudd R, Johnson C, et al. National surveillance for asthma-United States, 1980–2004. MMWR Surveill Summ 2007; 56(SS08):1–14, 8–54. Available at: http://www.cdc.gov/mmwr/preview/mmwrhtml/ss5608a1.htm.
4. Awadh Behbehani N, Grunfeld A, FitzGerald JM. Health care costs associated with acute asthma: a prospective economic analysis. Can Respir J 1999; 6(6):521–525.
5. Akinbami L. Asthma prevalence, health care use and mortality: United States, 2003–05. 2006. Available at: http://www.cdc.gov/nchs/products/pubs/pubd/hestats/ashtma03-05/asthma03-05.htm.
6. Sykes A, Johnston SL. Etiology of asthma exacerbations. J Allergy Clin Immunol 2008; 122 (4):685–688.
7. Minor TE, Dick EC, DeMeo AN, et al. Viruses as precipitants of asthmatic attacks in children. JAMA 1974; 227(3):292–298.
8. Corne JM, Marshall C, Smith S, et al. Frequency, severity, and duration of rhinovirus infections in asthmatic and non-asthmatic individuals: a longitudinal cohort study. Lancet 2002; 359(9309):831–834.
9. Tarlo S, Broder I, Spence L. A prospective study of respiratory infection in adult asthmatics and their normal spouses. Clin Allergy 1979; 9(3):293–301.
10. Talbot TR, Hartert TV, Mitchel E, et al. Asthma as a risk factor for invasive pneumococcal disease. N Engl J Med 2005; 352(20):2082–2090.
11. Juhn YJ, Kita H, Yawn BP, et al. Increased risk of serious pneumococcal disease in patients with asthma. J Allergy Clin Immunol 2008; 122(4):719–723.

12. Rivera-Matos IR, Rios-Olivares E. A multicenter hospital surveillance of invasive Strepto-coccus pneumoniae, Puerto Rico, 2001. P R Health Sci J 2005; 24(3):185–189.
13. Contoli M, Message SD, Laza-Stanca V, et al. Role of deficient type III interferon-lambda production in asthma exacerbations. Nat Med 2006; 12(9):1023–1026.
14. Wark PA, Johnston SL, Bucchieri F, et al. Asthmatic bronchial epithelial cells have a deficient innate immune response to infection with rhinovirus. J Exp Med 2005; 201(6):937–947.
15. Sakula A. A history of asthma. The FitzPatrick lecture 1987. J R Coll Physicians Lond 1988; 22(1):36–44.
16. Rackemann FM. A clinical classification of asthma based upon a review of six hundred and forty-eight cases. Am J Med Sci 1921; clxii:802–811.
17. Walker IC. A clinical study of 400 patients with bronchial asthma. Boston Med Surg J 1918; clxxix:288–300.
18. Huber HL, Koessler KK. The pathology of bronchial asthma. Arch Intern Med 1922; 30: 689–760.
19. Pattemore PK, Johnston SL, Bardin PG. Viruses as precipitants of asthma symptoms. I. Epidemiology. Clin Exp Allergy 1992; 22(3):325–336.
20. Nicholson KG, Kent J, Ireland DC. Respiratory viruses and exacerbations of asthma in adults. BMJ 1993; 307(6910):982–986.
21. Johnston SL, Pattemore PK, Sanderson G, et al. Community study of role of viral infections in exacerbations of asthma in 9–11 year old children. BMJ 1995; 310(6989):1225–1229.
22. Atmar RL, Guy E, Guntupalli KK, et al. Respiratory tract viral infections in inner-city asthmatic adults. Arch Intern Med 1998; 158(22):2453–2459.
23. Green RM, Custovic A, Sanderson G, et al. Synergism between allergens and viruses and risk of hospital admission with asthma: case-control study. BMJ 2002; 324(7340):763.
24. Tan WC, Xiang X, Qiu D, et al. Epidemiology of respiratory viruses in patients hospitalized with near-fatal asthma, acute exacerbations of asthma, or chronic obstructive pulmonary disease. Am J Med 2003; 115(4):272–277.
25. Johnston NW, Johnston SL, Duncan JM, et al. The September epidemic of asthma exacer-bations in children: a search for etiology. J Allergy Clin Immunol 2005; 115(1):132–138.
26. Khetsuriani N, Kazerouni NN, Erdman DD, et al. Prevalence of viral respiratory tract infections in children with asthma. J Allergy Clin Immunol 2007; 119(2):314–321.
27. Gendrel D, Guedj R, Pons-Catalano C, et al. Human bocavirus in children with acute asthma. Clin Infect Dis 2007; 45(3):404–405.
28. Kistler A, Avila PC, Rouskin S, et al. Pan-viral screening of respiratory tract infections in adults with and without asthma reveals unexpected human coronavirus and human rhinovirus diversity. J Infect Dis 2007; 196(6):817–825.
29. Ferreira A, Williams Z, Donninger H, et al. Rhinovirus is associated with severe asthma exacerbations and raised nasal interleukin-12. Respiration 2002; 69(2):136–142.
30. Williams JV, Crowe JE Jr., Enriquez R, et al. Human metapneumovirus infection plays an etiologic role in acute asthma exacerbations requiring hospitalization in adults. J Infect Dis 2005; 192(7):1149–1153.
31. Venarske DL, Busse WW, Griffin MR, et al. The relationship of rhinovirus-associated asthma hospitalizations with inhaled corticosteroids and smoking. J Infect Dis 2006; 193(11): 1536–1543.
32. Rawlinson WD, Waliuzzaman Z, Carter IW, et al. Asthma exacerbations in children asso-ciated with rhinovirus but not human metapneumovirus infection. J Infect Dis 2003; 187(8): 1314–1318.
33. Kling S, Donninger H, Williams Z, et al. Persistence of rhinovirus RNA after asthma exacerbation in children. Clin Exp Allergy 2005; 35(5):672–678.
34. Ong BH, Gao Q, Phoon MC, et al. Identification of human metapneumovirus and Chla-mydophila pneumoniae in children with asthma and wheeze in Singapore. Singapore Med J 2007; 48(4):291–293.

35. Allander T, Jartti T, Gupta S, et al. Human bocavirus and acute wheezing in children. Clin Infect Dis 2007; 44(7):904–910.
36. Harju TH, Leinonen M, Nokso-Koivisto J, et al. Pathogenic bacteria and viruses in induced sputum or pharyngeal secretions of adults with stable asthma. Thorax 2006; 61(7):579–584.
37. Wark PA, Bucchieri F, Johnston SL, et al. IFN-gamma-induced protein 10 is a novel bio-marker of rhinovirus-induced asthma exacerbations. J Allergy Clin Immunol 2007; 120(3): 586–593.
38. Murray CS, Poletti G, Kebadze T, et al. Study of modifiable risk factors for asthma exac-erbations: virus infection and allergen exposure increase the risk of asthma hospital admis-sions in children. Thorax 2006; 61(5):376–382.
39. Johnston SL, Sanderson G, Pattemore PK, et al. Use of polymerase chain reaction for diagnosis of picornavirus infection in subjects with and without respiratory symptoms. J Clin Microbiol 1993; 31(1):111–117.
40. Nokso-Koivisto J, Kinnari TJ, Lindahl P, et al. Human picornavirus and coronavirus RNA in nasopharynx of children without concurrent respiratory symptoms. J Med Virol 2002; 66(3): 417–420.
41. van Gageldonk-Lafeber AB, Heijnen ML, Bartelds AI, et al. A case-control study of acute respiratory tract infection in general practice patients in The Netherlands. Clin Infect Dis 2005; 41(4):490–497.
42. Winther B, Hayden FG, Hendley JO. Picornavirus infections in children diagnosed by RT-PCR during longitudinal surveillance with weekly sampling: association with symptomatic illness and effect of season. J Med Virol 2006; 78(5):644–650.
43. Falsey AR, Criddle MC, Walsh EE. Detection of respiratory syncytial virus and human metapneumovirus by reverse transcription polymerase chain reaction in adults with and without respiratory illness. J Clin Virol 2006; 35(1):46–50.
44. Brieu N, Guyon G, Rodiere M, et al. Human bocavirus infection in children with respiratory tract disease. Pediatr Infect Dis J 2008; 27(11):969–973.
45. Jartti T, Lee WM, Pappas T, et al. Serial viral infections in infants with recurrent respiratory illnesses. Eur Respir J 2008; 32(2):314–320.
46. Jartti T, Lehtinen P, Vuorinen T, et al. Persistence of rhinovirus and enterovirus RNA after acute respiratory illness in children. J Med Virol 2004; 72(4):695–699.
47. Kaiser L, Aubert JD, Pache JC, et al. Chronic rhinoviral infection in lung transplant recip-ients. Am J Respir Crit Care Med 2006; 174(12):1392–1399.
48. Friedman R, Ackerman M, Wald E, et al. Asthma and bacterial sinusitis in children. J Allergy Clin Immunol 1984; 74(2):185–189.
49. Johnston SL, Martin RJ. Chlamydophila pneumoniae and Mycoplasma pneumoniae: a role in asthma pathogenesis? Am J Respir Crit Care Med 2005; 172(9):1078–1089.
50. Emre U, Roblin PM, Gelling M, et al. The association of Chlamydia pneumoniae infection and reactive airway disease in children. Arch Pediatr Adolesc Med 1994; 148(7):727–732.
51. Teichtahl H, Buckmaster N, Pertnikovs E. The incidence of respiratory tract infection in adults requiring hospitalization for asthma. Chest 1997; 112(3):591–596.
52. Cunningham AF, Johnston SL, Julious SA, et al. Chronic Chlamydia pneumoniae infection and asthma exacerbations in children. Eur Respir J 1998; 11(2):345–349.
53. Miyashita N, Kubota Y, Nakajima M, et al. Chlamydia pneumoniae and exacerbations of asthma in adults. Ann Allergy Asthma Immunol 1998; 80(5):405–409.
54. Cook PJ, Davies P, Tunnicliffe W, et al. Chlamydia pneumoniae and asthma. Thorax 1998; 53(4):254–259.
55. Lieberman D, Lieberman D, Printz S, et al. Atypical pathogen infection in adults with acute exacerbation of bronchial asthma. Am J Respir Crit Care Med 2003; 167(3):406–410.
56. Betsou F, Sueur JM, Orfila J. Anti-Chlamydia pneumoniae heat shock protein 10 antibodies in asthmatic adults. FEMS Immunol Med Microbiol 2003; 35(2):107–111.

57. Biscardi S, Lorrot M, Marc E, et al. Mycoplasma pneumoniae and asthma in children. Clin Infect Dis 2004; 38(10):1341–1346.
58. Kocabas A, Avsar M, Hanta I, et al. Chlamydophila pneumoniae infection in adult asthmatics patients. J Asthma 2008; 45(1):39–43.
59. Peebles RS Jr., Sheller JR, Johnson JE, et al. Respiratory syncytial virus infection prolongs methacholine-induced airway hyperresponsiveness in ovalbumin-sensitized mice. J Med Virol 1999; 57(2):186–192.
60. Matsuse H, Behera AK, Kumar M, et al. Recurrent respiratory syncytial virus infections in allergen-sensitized mice lead to persistent airway inflammation and hyperresponsiveness. J Immunol 2000; 164(12):6583–6592.
61. Hashimoto K, Graham BS, Ho SB, et al. Respiratory syncytial virus in allergic lung inflammation increases Muc5ac and gob-5. Am J Respir Crit Care Med 2004; 170(3):306–312.
62. Bartlett NW, Walton RP, Edwards MR, et al. Mouse models of rhinovirus-induced disease and exacerbation of allergic airway inflammation. Nat Med 2008; 14(2):199–204.
63. Chu HW, Honour JM, Rawlinson CA, et al. Effects of respiratory Mycoplasma pneumoniae infection on allergen-induced bronchial hyperresponsiveness and lung inflammation in mice. Infect Immun 2003; 71(3):1520–1526.
64. Grissell TV, Powell H, Shafren DR, et al. Interleukin-10 gene expression in acute virus-induced asthma. Am J Respir Crit Care Med 2005; 172(4):433–439.
65. Wark PA, Johnston SL, Moric I, et al. Neutrophil degranulation and cell lysis is associated with clinical severity in virus-induced asthma. Eur Respir J 2002; 19(1):68–75.
66. Johnston SL, Ferrero F, Garcia ML, et al. Oral oseltamivir improves pulmonary function and reduces exacerbation frequency for influenza-infected children with asthma. Pediatr Infect Dis J 2005; 24(3):225–232.
67. Connett G, Lenney W. Prevention of viral induced asthma attacks using inhaled budesonide. Arch Dis Child 1993; 68(1):85–87.
68. Svedmyr J, Nyberg E, Asbrink-Nilsson E, et al. Intermittent treatment with inhaled steroids for deterioration of asthma due to upper respiratory tract infections. Acta Paediatr 1995; 84 (8):884–888.
69. Svedmyr J, Nyberg E, Thunqvist P, et al. Prophylactic intermittent treatment with inhaled corticosteroids of asthma exacerbations due to airway infections in toddlers. Acta Paediatr 1999; 88(1):42–47.
70. Brunette MG, Lands L, Thibodeau LP. Childhood asthma: prevention of attacks with short-term corticosteroid treatment of upper respiratory tract infection. Pediatrics 1988; 81(5):624–629.
71. Bueving HJ, Bernsen RM, de Jongste JC, et al. Influenza vaccination in children with asthma: randomized double-blind placebo-controlled trial. Am J Respir Crit Care Med 2004; 169 (4):488–493.
72. Bueving HJ, van der Wouden JC, Raat H, et al. Influenza vaccination in asthmatic children: effects on quality of life and symptoms. Eur Respir J 2004; 24(6):925–931.
73. Graham V, Lasserson T, Rowe BH. Antibiotics for acute asthma. Cochrane Database Syst Rev 2001; (3):CD002741.
74. Graham VA, Milton AF, Knowles GK, et al. Routine antibiotics in hospital management of acute asthma. Lancet 1982; 1(8269):418–420.
75. Shapiro GG, Eggleston PA, Pierson WE, et al. Double-blind study of the effectiveness of a broad spectrum antibiotic in status asthmaticus. Pediatrics 1974; 53(6):867–872.
76. Johnston SL, Blasi F, Black PN, et al. The effect of telithromycin in acute exacerbations of asthma. N Engl J Med 2006; 354(15):1589–1600.
77. Nolte FS, Marshall DJ, Rasberry C, et al. MultiCode-PLx system for multiplexed detection of seventeen respiratory viruses. J Clin Microbiol 2007; 45(9):2779–2786.
78. Walter MJ, Castro M, Kunselman SJ, et al. Predicting worsening asthma control following the common cold. Eur Respir J 2008; 32(6):1548–1554.

5
Interaction Between Allergen and Bacteria in Chronic Asthma

RICHARD J. MARTIN
National Jewish Health, Denver, Colorado, U.S.A.

I. Introduction

Acute exacerbations of asthma have been linked to viral infections in approximately 50% of asthmatic patients (1). However, pathogens playing a role in the pathobiology of chronic asthma has only recently been scientifically investigated in both human and murine models. Infection of the lower respiratory tract with the atypical bacteria *Mycoplasma pneumoniae* and *Chlamydophila (Chlamydia) pneumoniae* has emerged as a clinical issue of importance in chronic asthmatic patients. A growing body of both clinical and basic science implicates these pathogens as potentially important factors in asthma; however, the exact contribution of atypical bacterial infection to asthma pathobiology and phenotype still remains to be determined.

There are multiple challenges that need to be faced to elucidate the relationship between atypical or other bacterial infections and chronic asthma. Robust animal models of chronic atypical bacterial infections are still being developed. Detection of atypical bacteria in humans is difficult, with many techniques being either insensitive or nonspecific. Reliable detection of lower respiratory tract infection typically requires invasive diagnostic procedures such as bronchoscopy with lavage, brush, and biopsy. Furthermore, since asthma is not a specific disease but rather a syndrome that is influenced by a host of intrinsic and acquired factors, determining the importance of infectious agents relative to other risk factors in the pathogenesis and prognosis of chronic asthma poses a challenge. In fact, infection more than likely interacts with other risk factors, for example, allergens, to have a synergistic effect on asthma pathobiology.

II. Asthma: *Mycoplasma pneumoniae* and *Chlamydophila pneumoniae* Association

M. pneumoniae, which is a common cause of atypical pneumonia and tracheobronchitis (2), attaches to ciliated airway epithelial cells by means of a terminal organelle, infecting the cell and causing epithelial damage and ciliary dysfunction (3). Evidence linking *M. pneumoniae* to new-onset wheezing, exacerbations of persistent asthma, and long-term decrements in lung function suggests that this organism can play an important role in asthma.

Although sporadic case reports (4) have suggested that antecedent *mycoplasma* infection can be associated with the subsequent development of asthma, a stronger and

84

perhaps more clinically relevant association is the importance of *M. pneumoniae* as a precipitant of exacerbations in asthmatic subjects. One example of this is the report by Lieberman and colleagues (5) of a prospective study of atypical bacterial infections in patients hospitalized with acute asthma exacerbation that demonstrated serologic evidence of acute *M. pneumoniae* infection in 18% of patients with an asthma exacerbation, compared with a prevalence of 3% in a matched control group ($p = 0.0006$). In an earlier series (6) of children with preexisting asthma, *M. pneumoniae* infection was similarly seen in 7 of 40 episodes (18%) of acute exacerbation.

In addition to causing a decrement in pulmonary function during acute infection, *M. pneumoniae* might also be associated with the long-term impairment of pulmonary function in both asthmatic subjects and nonasthmatic subjects. In a series of 108 children with lower respiratory tract infection caused by *M. pneumoniae* (detected by increased complement fixation titers), 40% of subjects presented with wheezing as an initial clinical finding. At both three months and three years of age, there were decrements in forced vital capacity (FVC) (93.1% vs. 100.8% of predicted, $p < 0.01$) and forced expiratory volume in one second (FEV_1) (94.5% vs. 100.6% of predicted, $p < 0.02$) in infected nonasthmatic subjects compared with control subjects (7). The reported strength of this association is, however, variable, as a separate series of 50 children evaluated 1.5 to 9.5 years after clinical and radiographic recovery from *M. pneumoniae* pneumonia did not demonstrate persistent reductions in FVC or FEV_1 (8). A report by Kim and colleagues suggested a potential anatomic substrate for impaired lung function after acute *M. pneumoniae* pneumonia, in that high-resolution chest CT scanning performed in 37 children at a mean interval of 1.5 years after the episode of pneumonia demonstrated findings such as bronchial wall thickening, mosaic perfusion, and air trapping, features that were not seen in control population of 17 children with *mycoplasma* upper airway infection (9).

C. pneumoniae, also classified as an "atypical" bacterial pathogen, is a common cause of bronchitis and atypical pneumonia, may result in chronic infection (10), and like *M. pneumoniae*, has been associated with subsequent wheezing illness. *C. pneumoniae* also causes exacerbations of preexisting asthma, as reported in case series such as that of Allegra and colleagues, where in a cohort of seventy adults presenting with asthma exacerbation, 10% were shown by serology to be acutely infected with *C. pneumoniae* (11). In a community-based cohort of 365 patients with lower respiratory tract illness, 47% of patients with acute *C. pneumoniae* infection were found to wheeze during the course of the infection, with statistically significant dose-response relationship between the level of *C. pneumoniae* IgG titer and prevalence of wheezing in the cohort. There was also an association of *C. pneumoniae* antibody titers and subsequent development of "asthmatic bronchitis" after the acute illness, which was seen in 32% of cases (odds ratio = 7.2, 95% CI, 2.2–23.4) (12).

In 2001, Martin and colleagues (13) published the first systemic evaluation of *mycoplasma* and *chlamydophila* infection in the upper and lower airways of adults with chronic, stable asthma. The investigators evaluated 55 stable asthmatic subjects and 11 healthy control subjects for the presence of *M. pneumoniae* and *C. pneumoniae*, performing serology, cultures, and polymerase chain reaction (PCR) for these organisms on specimens obtained from the nasopharynx and oropharynx, bronchoalveolar lavage (BAL), and endobronchial biopsy. *M pneumoniae* or *C. pneumoniae* was detected by PCR in 56% of asthmatic subjects, compared with 9% of control subjects ($p = 0.02$). Culture findings for both organisms were negative in all subjects. A total of 18 asthmatic subjects and 1 healthy control subject had serologic results that were positive for *C. pneumoniae*. Of these 18 asthmatic subjects, 10 had positive results by IgG criteria and 5 had positive results by IgM criteria, with 3 of the subjects demonstrating both positive IgG and positive IgM criteria. However, only seven subjects had PCR results that were positive for *C. pneumoniae*; of these, only three subjects had serologic results that were positive for *C. pneumoniae*. On the basis of these data, the authors concluded that a majority of stable adults with chronic asthma are chronically infected with *M. pneumoniae*, with a significantly greater frequency than that for nonasthmatic subjects, and that serologic evaluation does not reliably indicate lower airway PCR status (13). At this time, more study is needed to evaluate whether *mycoplasma* or *chlamydophila* infection is a pathogenic factor in asthma or merely an epiphenomenon that is somehow related to the enhanced airway inflammation seen in subjects with chronic asthma.

III. Hygiene Hypothesis in Asthma

In the study by Martin and colleagues (13), a characteristic that separated the asthmatic subjects who were positive for *M. pneumoniae* and *C. pneumoniae* from asthmatic subjects who were negative for these bacteria was the mast cell number found on biopsy tissue. Those who were positive had about a fourfold increased tissue mast cell number (Fig. 1). This suggests that either there exists a link between infection and an allergic process and/or the mast cells are also participating in host defense (14,15).

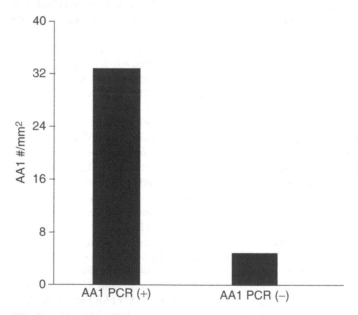

Figure 1 The phenotypic characteristic that appears to separate *mycoplasma-* and *chlamydophila-*positive [PCR (+)] from *mycoplasma-* and *chlamydophila-*negative [PCR (−)] subjects is the number of mast cells (AA1) on endobronchial biopsies. *Abbreviation*: PCR, polymerase chain reaction. *Source*: From Ref. 13.

The hygiene hypothesis of asthma suggests that the immune system in newborn infants is skewed toward T_h2 cells and needs timely and appropriate environmental stimuli (e.g., infection) to create a balanced immune response. Thus, if newborns, or perhaps even prior in utero, are exposed to infection or endotoxins [lipopolysaccharide (LPS)] prior to allergen exposure, the prevalence of allergy and asthma are decreased, whereas if allergen exposure precedes the infection or LPS exposure, then there is profound T_h2 response and increase in allergy and asthma.

The hygiene hypothesis predicts that the "cleaner" the environment, the more allergy and asthma will be seen, and vice versa. Two quotes from well over a century ago emphasize this point (16,17):

Summer catarrh ... only occurs in the middle or upper classes of society, some indeed of high rank. I have made inquiry at the various dispensaries in London and elsewhere, and I have not heard of a single unequivocal case occurring among the poor.

J. Bostuck 1828

It would seem that hay-fever has, of late years, been considerably on the increase ... the persons who are most subjected to the action of the pollen belong to a class which furnishes the fewest cases of the disorder; namely, the farming class.

CH Blackley 1873

In a cross-sectional survey of rural areas of Austria, Germany, and Switzerland, 75% of 3504 parents completed a standardized questionnaire on asthma, hay fever, and atopic eczema (18). All had children 6 to 13 years of age: children from farming families and a random sample of nonfarmers' children had samples obtained for specific serum IgE antibodies to common allergens ($n = 901$). Children who were less than one year of age and at that time exposed to stables and used farm milk in their diet had a lower frequency of asthma: 1% (3/218) versus 11% (115/138) of nonexposure children. Additionally, hay fever and atopic sensitization were also reduced: 3% (7/218) versus 13% (18/138) and 12% (27/218) versus 29% (40/138), respectively. Of interest, the protection against the development of asthma was independent of the effect on atopic sensitization. Furthermore, continued exposure to stables until five years of age was associated with the lowest frequency of asthma (<1%), hay fever (<1%), and atopic sensitization (8%). Thus, long-term early-life exposure to stables (microses, endotoxin) and farm milk induces a strong protective immune response against the induction of asthma and allergic disease.

Multiple other studies investigating the difference between rural and urban living or certain types of early exposures produce similar data as the above described study (19–24).

A similar finding can be associated with sibling rank and day care attendance. The more the number of siblings in the family, the less the occurrence of asthma and atopy in the younger siblings (25). Additionally, children attending day care who are less than one year of age also have decreased prevalence of asthma/allergy (26).

In a BALB/c mouse model of the hygiene hypothesis, Chu and colleagues (27) demonstrated that respiratory infection with *M. pneumoniae* prior to allergen sensitization and challenge produced a suppression of airway hyperresponsiveness to methacholine. This was associated with a shift to a T_h1 (nonallergic) response and away from a T_h2 (allergic) response. Thus, interferon (IFN)-γ in the BAL was increased, while interleukin (IL)-4 was decreased compared with that in a saline control group (Fig. 2A). However, when mice were initially sensitized and challenged to an allergen followed by a *mycoplasma* respiratory infection, in the longer term, the reverse occurred. Acute (day 3 postinfection) suppression of airway hyperresponsiveness occurred with a T_h1 response taking place. However, over time, hyperresponsiveness increased (days 7, 14, and 21 postinfection), while a T_h2 response took over, that is, a shift to T_h2 cytokines (Fig. 2B). Of interest, by day 21, the ratio of T_h1/T_h2 (INF-γ/IL-4) was approximately the same. This suggests that another process, such as airway remodeling, was accounting for the noted increase in hyperresponsiveness in the chronic state (see the following text).

IV. Effect of Bacterial Infection Without Allergen Interaction

It would be very difficult, if not impossible, to answer the question of how a bacterium would affect asthma control and outcomes in humans. We do know that the atypical bacteria cause about 25% of all community-acquired pneumonia (28). Furthermore, in many individuals, these atypical bacteria persist for months following recovery from the pneumonia with lung function being decreased and/or having increased airway hyperresponsiveness (29).

Using murine models, many questions can be directly answered. A mouse model of *mycoplasma* respiratory infection demonstrated that airway hyperresponsiveness was markedly increased at day 3 with a slow return to baseline by day 21 (30). Airway function, measured by lung resistance, was inversely correlated to the T_h1 response ($r = -0.5$, $p = 0.02$). Again, moving away from a T_h1 response worsens lung function. Decrements in airway function, that is, increasing airway resistance, was also positively correlated to the lung tissue inflammation score ($r = 0.79$, $p = <0.0001$).

Thus, in the absence of an allergic background, *mycoplasma* can increase lung reactivity and decrease lung function. However, in the presence of an allergic background, *mycoplasma* (perhaps many other bacteria) further accelerates the T_h2 inflammatory cascade.

Endotoxin, a LPS, comprises most of the outer layer of the outer cell membrane of all gram-negative bacteria. Its potent immune stimulator capacity is largely attributed to the lipid A moiety of endotoxin, which is highly conserved across different bacterial species (31). Endotoxin has also been attributed to the decrease in allergy and asthma in farming children compared with nonfarming households in rural areas of central Europe (32). In this cross-sectional study of 812 children between 6 and 13 years old, endotoxin levels found in mattress dust demonstrated a relationship between higher levels of endotoxin in the dust and a decreased frequency of allergic sensitization, hay fever, and asthma in this group of children.

Endotoxin levels vary widely but are usually the highest in areas where farm animals are located. Figure 3 demonstrates the various levels of endotoxin measured in multiple different locations (33–39). The levels are measured by dosimetry, which takes into account concentration × respiratory ventilation × duration. In its airborne form, endotoxin can be inhaled or swallowed and is a potent immunostimulatory process via the lipid A moiety. Signaling occurs through CD14 and toll-like receptor (TLR)4. Other molecules of the innate immune process, for example, MyD88 and TLR9, are also activated.

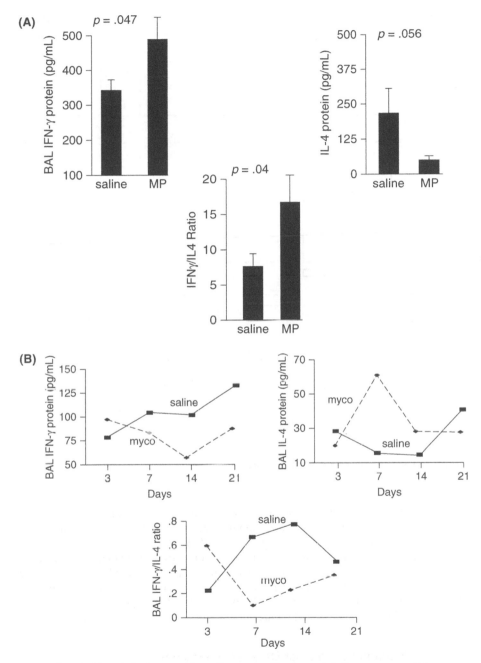

Figure 2 (**A**) Myco infection preceding allergen sensitization and challenge causes a T$_h$1 response with increase in IFN-γ and decrease in IL-4. (**B**) Myco infection following acute allergen sensitization and challenge (day 3 postinfection) produces a T$_h$1 response; however, a more chronic (days 7 and 14) time course produces a switch to a T$_h$2 response. Although by day 21 the response is similar to control, airway hyperreactivity is still elevated. *Abbreviations*: BAL, bronchoalveolar lavage; IFN, interferon; IL, interleukin; MP, *Mycoplasma pneumoniae*; myco, *mycoplasma*. *Source*: From Ref. 27.

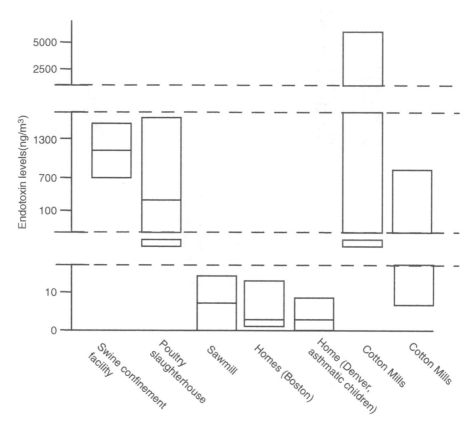

Figure 3 Endotoxin exposures. Mean and range are given (no means for cotton mills). See text for discussion.

Of interest, low levels of endotoxin serve as a potent inducer of IL-12 and IFN-γ. These cytokines stimulate T_h1-mediated immune response while decreasing production of T_h2 (allergic) cytokines, for example, IL-4, IL-5, and IL-13. However, at high doses, endotoxin can yield a hypersensitivity pneumonitis with marked inflammatory response (40). Thus, exposure dose and perhaps duration are important in determining if a shift to a protective T_h1 pattern or an overwhelming inflammatory response will take place. Also, timing in a human life may be important in the response to endotoxin, as demonstrated in children raised in farming homes, particularly in the first year of life (32).

V. Deficiencies in Host Defense That Allow Asthma-Associated Characteristics to Develop and Decreased Bacterial Clearance

Innate immunity against pathogens covers a wide range of responses, which far exceeds this brief description. Since, to the present date, it appears that the atypical bacteria are involved in chronic asthma (12,13), the focus of the innate response deficiencies will be for these bacteria. Again, mouse models of *mycoplasma* infection without and with allergen interactions help to understand potential human deficiencies.

IFN-γ is a key T_h1 cytokine produced by multiple cells [CD4, CD8, $\gamma\delta$-T cells, and natural killer (NK) cells] and is upregulated in response to infections such as the atypical bacteria (41,42). IFN-γ activates alveolar macrophages, which enhances antimicrobial activities through nitric oxide production and oxygen radicals (43). If the allergic T_h2 cytokines are upregulated, these will then produce a downregulation of antimicrobial activities and impair clearance of microbes, which could allow a persistent airway infection to develop.

Bakshi and colleagues used T-bet-deficient (T-bet$^{-/-}$) strain of mice to determine the effect of *mycoplasma* infection in an asthmatic environment (44). T-bet is a member of the T-box family of transcription factors, and mice deficient in T-bet develop an asthma-like phenotype probably secondarily to downregulation of TFN-γ (45,46) and from overproduction of IL-13 by CD4 cells (46). In human asthmatics, T-bet expression is significantly decreased compared with nonasthmatics (45). The T-bet$^{-/-}$ mice had an inability to mount an effective immune response to defend against a *mycoplasma* infection and allowed colonization of microbes to occur. Then, innate immune response was through a decrease in TFN-γ, while T_h2 cytokine production as well as IgE increased (44).

The mast cell appears to be a bidirectional cell with respect to participating in the T_h2 allergic paradigm, which would enhance the asthmatic response (47), and as a host defense cell against bacteria (14,15), which would then dampen the asthmatic response. As stated above, a phenotypic characteristic that separated the asthmatic subjects who were positive and negative for the atypical bacteria was the mast cell. Asthmatics who were positive had about a fourfold increase in the number of tissue mast cells found on a lung biopsy (13). The question here would be if the mast cells were pro-T_h2 inflammation or pro-host defense.

Xu and colleagues in a mouse model demonstrated that mast cells are protective against *mycoplasma* infection (48). Wild-type and mast cell-deficient mice were given a respiratory infection with *Mycoplasma pulmonis*. A sham infection control group was also evaluated. The results demonstrated that the mast cell-deficient group, compared with the other groups, lost more weight and were more likely to die, had a greater lung *Mycoplasma* burden, developed larger bronchial lymph nodes, had a progressive pneumonia and airway occlusion with neutrophil exudates, and developed angiogenesis and lymphangiogenesis. Thus, mast cells appear to be important in innate immunity and recovery from a respiratory *mycoplasma* infection but also have a marked effect on T_h2 inflammation.

A key factor in *mycoplasma* respiratory infections is with regard to TLR2 signaling. In a series of experiments from the Denver group, this signaling mechanism appears to be a critical factor (49–51). Since excessive airway mucin production contributes to airway obstruction in lung diseases such as asthma and chronic obstructive pulmonary disease, Chu and colleagues (49) showed that TLR2 signaling is critical in *M. pneumoniae*-induced airway mucin expression in mice and human lung epithelial cells. In BALB/c mice, *mycoplasma* activated TLR2 signaling and increased airway mucin production. A TLR2-neutralizing antibody significantly reduced mucin expression and was abolished in TLR2 gene-deficient C57BL/6 mice. Furthermore, *mycoplasma* increased human lung A549 epithelial cell mucin expression, which was inhibited by the overexpression of a human TLR2-dominant negative mutant. These results clearly demonstrate that a respiratory *mycoplasma* infection increases airway mucin expression, which is dependent on the activation of TLR2 signaling.

As discussed above with regard to the hygiene hypothesis of asthma, a respiratory infection prior to allergen sensitization causes suppression of the allergic response, while a respiratory infection post allergen sensitization will amplify the allergic response. Wu and colleagues first demonstrated the molecular mechanism involved in an infection-allergen sequence with respect to mucin production (50). Using wild-type and TLR2-deficient mice with *M. pneumoniae* infection preceding allergen challenge again demonstrated the importance of TLR2 signaling pathways in IFN-γ production and mucin control. In wild-type mice, there was a significant reduction in airway mucin associated with an increased IFN-γ level. In contrast, TLR2-deficient mice had an increase in mucin protein without a change in IFN-γ. Additionally, in cultures of mouse primary tracheal epithelial cells, IFN-γ was shown to directly inhibit mucin expression in a dose-dependent manner. Thus, a bacterial infection in asthmatic patients with weakened TLR2-IFN-γ signaling may result in increased airway mucin production, which can be a major complaint in these patients.

In the third experimental study, involving TLR-2 signaling, mice were initially sensitized and challenged to an allergen and then given a *M. pneumoniae* respiratory infection (51). The objective was to test whether the established allergic airway inflammation compromises host innate immunity (TLR2) to hinder the elimination of *M. pneumoniae* from the lungs. With establishment of allergic airway inflammation (T_h2 cytokines IL-4 and IL-13) or inhibition of TLR2 expression, all led to impaired host defense against *mycoplasma* clearance. Additionally, studies in IL-6 knockout mice indicate that IL-6 directly promotes *mycoplasma* clearance from the lungs. IL-4 and IL-13 directly induced suppression of TLR2, which was mediated by inhibiting nuclear factor-κB via signal transducer and activator of transcription 6 (STAT6) signaling pathway. Thus, in an established allergic airway with the T_h2 inflammatory environment impairment of TLR2 expression and host defense, cytokine IL-6 production occurs with resultant decreases in bacterial clearance. For asthma, these findings could lead to future novel therapeutic strategies of increasing TLR2 by TLR2 ligands and/or blocking IL-4 and IL-13 with resultant improved bacterial clearance.

VI. Allergen-Bacteria Interaction: Potential for Airway Remodeling in Chronic Asthma

Airway remodeling in asthma is a concept that helps to explain why all patients cannot achieve normal lung function and airway reactivity. However, there are multiple causes for this remodeling including, but not limited to, collagen deposition, smooth muscle hypertrophy, mucous gland hyperplasia, inflammation, edema, and elastolysis. A prominent feature in asthma can be the collagen deposition, that is, fibrosis, in the subbasement membrane area. In a mouse study of allergic inflammation with a subsequent *M. pneumoniae* infection, a chronic model of airway remodeling via collagen deposition was demonstrated (52). In allergen-naive mice, *mycoplasma* did not alter airway wall collagen. In allergen-challenged mice, the *mycoplasma* infection in the more acute setting (14 days) also showed no change in collagen deposition, but more chronically (42 days postinfection), there was a significant increase in airway collagen deposition. This increase in collagen was accompanied by increased transforming growth factor (TGF)-β1 protein in the airway wall. Again, the important allergen-bacteria interaction is observed, and in this study, it produces a chronic change seen in clinical asthma.

VII. Bacteria-Virus Interaction

Although this chapter has emphasized the allergen-bacteria interaction producing or perpetuating asthma, it appears that another interaction is important. One such inter-action is between *mycoplasma* and virus. Schoeb and Lindsey (53) infected mice with *M. pulmonis* and allowed the mice to recover. They then introduced sialodacryoadenitis virus into this group versus a group without the prior *mycoplasma* infection. The group of mice that had the prior bacterial infection had greater airways inflammation and a protracted course compared with the viral-only infected group. Perhaps in viral-induced acute exacerbations of asthma, this interaction may be involved.

VIII. Bacterial Respiratory Load

In human asthmatics, rarely are the atypical bacteria cultured, rather, PCR genetic testing is needed. There are two potential reasons for this. The organisms are difficult to culture even if high concentrations are present such as with a true pneumonia. Since a true pneumonia is not occurring in these asthmatic patients, the respiratory load is small.

Giving different concentrations of *M. pneumoniae* to mice in an allergic milieu produces different eosinophil and IL-4 (T_h2) cytokine responses (Fig. 4A, B). The lowest load of organisms, 10^3, produces the highest eosinophil and IL-4 response in the BAL fluid. There is a reverse dose response seen as the high respiratory *mycoplasma* load produces the lowest eosinophil counts and lowest levels of IL-4. At 10^9 and 10^8 con-centrations, *mycoplasma* can be cultured, whereas at 10^5 and 10^3, they need to be detected by PCR analysis. This is similar to what may be occurring in human asthma as a low load of organisms in the lung bypass host defense but propagates the T_h2 immune responses.

IX. Treatment

Treatment of atypical bacteria in asthma patients has not been extensively evaluated, particularly decreasing T_h2 cytokines with intervention to determine if this will clear the bacteria from the lungs.

Kraft and colleagues did demonstrate that if patients have proven respiratory positivity to *mycoplasma* or *chlamydophila*, then these individuals do improve lung function on macrolide antimicrobial therapy (54). This study was a double-blind, placebo-controlled trial that randomized asthmatic subjects into PCR-positive and PCR-negative groups. Although macrolides have anti-inflammatory properties unto themselves, if this was the only factor that accounted for improved lung function, then all asthmatics should have improved. Thus, it appears from this study that the presence of the atypical bacteria in the respiratory track is needed for the antimicrobial therapy to be successful. This study was "only" six weeks in duration. On a clinical basis, we have found that six months of therapy is needed to produce close to maximum benefit in most patients.

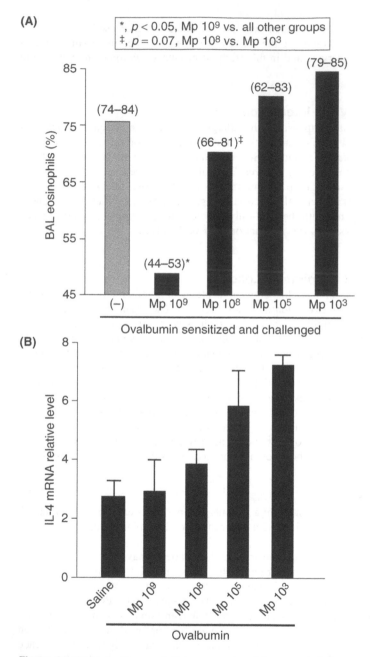

Figure 4 (**A**) In an allergen challenge mouse model, a reverse dose response with respect to the percent of eosinophils in the BAL fluid occurs in response to the load of MP respiratory infection. (**B**) Similar to Figure 4A, a reverse dose response occurs in that a lower load of MP (10^3) produces the highest concentration of IL-4. *Abbreviations*: BAL, bronchoalveolar lavage; MP, *Mycoplasma pneumoniae*; IL, interleukin.

In a large multinational study, Black and colleagues (55) showed minimal improvement with macrolide therapy. A problem with this study could have been that serology was used as a marker of positivity. This can give you false positives or negatives compared with bronchoscopy with lavage, brushing, and biopsy using PCR analysis (13).

Inhaled corticosteroids are the mainstay of asthma treatment to suppress the eosinophilic and T_h2 inflammatory responses. However, these agents also stimulate host defense mechanisms (56–58). Thus, corticosteroids suppress adaptive immunity while simultaneously enhancing innate immunity. The host defense mechanism of nebulized corticosteroids was demonstrated by Chu and colleagues in a mouse model of *M. pneumoniae* respiratory infection without an allergic background (59). These investigators demonstrated that nebulized fluticasone propionate significantly decreases the lung tissue load of *mycoplasma* as well as the related inflammatory response compared with control mice. Thus, in asthmatic patients, inhaled corticosteroids may well play a role in innate immunity.

References

1. Nicholson KG, Kent J, Ireland DC. Respiratory viruses and exacerbations of asthma in adults. BMJ 1993; 307:982–986.
2. Baseman JB, Tully JG. Mycoplasmas: sophisticated, reemerging, and burdened by their notoriety. Emerg Infect Dis 1997; 3:21–32.
3. Andersen P. Pathogenesis of lower respiratory tract infections due to Chlamydia, Mycoplasma, Legionella and viruses. Thorax 1998; 53:302–307.
4. Yano T, Ichikawa Y, Komatu S, et al. Association of Mycoplasma pneumoniae antigen with initial onset of bronchial asthma. Am J Respir Crit Care Med 1994; 149:1348–1353.
5. Lieberman D, Printz S, Ben-Yaakov M, et al. Atypical pathogen infection in adults with acute exacerbation of bronchial asthma. Am J Respir Crit Care Med 2003; 167:406–410.
6. Berkovich S, Millian SJ, Snyder RD. The association of viral and mycoplasma infections with recurrence of wheezing in the asthmatic child. Ann Allergy 1970; 28:43–49.
7. Sabato AR, Martin AJ, Marmion BP, et al. Mycoplasma pneumoniae: acute illness, antibiotics, and subsequent pulmonary function. Arch Dis Child 1984; 59:1034–1037.
8. Mok JY, Waugh PR, Simpson H. Mycoplasma pneuminia infection. A follow-up study of 50 children with respiratory illness. Arch Dis Child 1979; 54:506–511.
9. Kim CK, Chung CY, Kim JS, et al. Late abnormal findings on high-resolution computed tomography after Mycoplasma pneumonia. Pediatrics 2000; 105:372–378.
10. Grayston JT, Kuo CC, Wang SP, et al. A new Chlamydia psittaci strain, TWAR, isolated in acute respiratory tract infections. N Engl J Med 1986; 315:161–168.
11. Allegra L, Blasi F, Centanni S, et al. Acute exacerbations of asthma in adults: role of Chlamydia pneumoniae infection. Eur Respir J 1994; 7:2165–2168.
12. Hahn DL, Dodge RW, Golubjatnikov R. Association of Chlamydia pneumoniae (strain TWAR) infection with wheezing, asthmatic bronchitis, and adult-onset asthma. JAMA 1991; 266:225–230.
13. Martin RJ, Kraft M, Chu HW, et al. A link between chronic asthma and chronic infection. J Allergy Clin Immunol 2001; 107:595–601.
14. Malaviya R, Ikeda T, Ross E, et al. Mast cell modulation of neutrophil influx and bacterial clearance at sites of infection through TNF-alpha. Nature 1996; 381:77–80.
15. Echtenacher B, Mannel DN, Hultner L. Critical protective role of mast cells in a model of acute septic peritonitis. Nature 1996; 381:75–77.

16. Bostock J. On the Catarrhus Aestivus or Summer Catarrh. London: Medico-Chirurgical Transactions, 1828.
17. Blackley C. Experimental Researches on the Causes and Nature of Catarrhus Aestivus (Hay-Fever or Hay-Asthma). London: Balliere, Tindall and Cox, 1873.
18. Riedler J, Braun-Fahrlander C, Eder W, et al. Exposure to farming in early life and development of asthma and allergy: a cross-sectional survey. Lancet 2001; 358:1129–1133.
19. Braun-Fahrlander C, Gassner M, Grize L, et al. Prevalence of hay fever and allergic sensitization in farmer's children and their peers living in the same rural community. SCARPOL team. Swiss Study on Childhood Allergy and Respiratory Symptoms with Respect to Air Pollution. Clin Exp Allergy 1999; 29:28–34.
20. Riedler J, Eder W, Oberfeld G, et al. Austrian children living on a farm have less hay fever, asthma and allergic sensitization. Clin Exp Allergy 2000; 30:194–200.
21. Von Ehrenstein OS, Von Mutius E, Illi S, et al. Reduced risk of hay fever and asthma among children of farmers. Clin Exp Allergy 2000; 30:187–193.
22. Kilpelainen M, Terho EO, Helenius H, et al. Farm environment in childhood prevents the development of allergies. Clin Exp Allergy 2000; 30:201–208.
23. Ernst P, Cormier Y. Relative scarcity of asthma and atopy among rural adolescents raised on a farm. Am J Respir Crit Care Med 2000; 161:1563–1566.
24. von Mutius E, Braun-Fahrlander C, Schierl R, et al. Exposure to endotoxin or other bacterial components might protect against the development of atopy. Clin Exp Allergy 2000; 30: 1230–1234.
25. Strachan DP. Hay fever, hygiene, and household size. BMJ 1989; 299:1259–1260.
26. Celedon JC, Wright RJ, Litonjua AA, et al. Day care attendance in early life, maternal history of asthma, and asthma at the age of 6 years. Am J Respir Crit Care Med 2003; 167:1239–1243.
27. Chu HW, Honour JM, Rawlinson CA, et al. Effects of respiratory Mycoplasma pneumoniae infection on allergen-induced bronchial hyperresponsiveness and lung inflammation in mice. Infect Immun 2003; 71:1520–1526.
28. Cassell GH. Severe Mycoplasma disease—rare or underdiagnosed? West J Med 1995; 162:172–175.
29. Melbye H, Kongerud J, Vorland L. Reversible airflow limitation in adults with respiratory infection. Eur Respir J 1994; 7:1239–1245.
30. Martin RJ, Chu HW, Honour JM, et al. Airway inflammation and bronchial hyperresponsiveness after Mycoplasma pneumoniae infection in a murine model. Am J Respir Cell Mol Biol 2001; 24:577–582.
31. Brigham KL. Endotoxin and the Lungs. New York: Marcel Dekker, Inc., 1994.
32. Braun-Fahrlander C, Riedler J, Herz U, et al. Environmental exposure to endotoxin and its relation to asthma in school-age children. N Engl J Med 2002; 347:869–877.
33. Zhiping W, Malmberg P, Larsson BM, et al. Exposure to bacteria in swine-house dust and acute inflammatory reactions in humans. Am J Respir Crit Care Med 1996; 154:1261–1266.
34. Park JH, Spiegelman DL, Gold DR, et al. Predictors of airborne endotoxin in the home. Environ Health Perspect 2001; 109:859–864.
35. Rabinovitch N, Liu AH, Zhang L, et al. Importance of the personal endotoxin cloud in school-age children with asthma. J Allergy Clin Immunol 2005; 116:1053–1057.
36. Castellan RM, Olenchock SA, Kinsley KB, et al. Inhaled endotoxin and decreased spirometric values. An exposure-response relation for cotton dust. N Engl J Med 1987; 317:605–610.
37. Rylander R, Haglind P, Lundholm M. Endotoxin in cotton dust and respiratory function decrement among cotton workers in an experimental cardroom. Am Rev Respir Dis 1985; 131:209–213.
38. Hagmar L, Schutz A, Hallberg T, et al. Health effects of exposure to endotoxins and organic dust in poultry slaughter-house workers. Int Arch Occup Environ Health 1990; 62:159–164.

39. Douwes J, McLean D, van der Maarl E, et al. Worker exposures to airborne dust, endotoxin and beta(1,3)-glucan in two New Zealand sawmills. Am J Ind Med 2000; 38:426–430.
40. Liu AH. Endotoxin exposure in allergy and asthma: reconciling a paradox. J Allergy Clin Immunol 2002; 109:379–392.
41. Jones HP, Tabor L, Sun X, et al. Depletion of CD8+ T cells exacerbates CD4+ Th cell-associated inflammatory lesions during murine mycoplasma respiratory disease. J Immunol 2002; 168:3493–3501.
42. Dalton DK, Pitts-Meek S, Keshav S, et al. Multiple defects of immune cell function in mice with disrupted interferon-gamma genes. Science 1993; 259:1739–1742.
43. Moncada S, Higgs EA. Endogenous nitric oxide: physiology, pathology and clinical relevance. Eur J Clin Invest 1991; 21:361–374.
44. Bakshi CS, Malik M, Carrico PM, et al. T-bet deficiency facilitates airway colonization by Mycoplasma pulmonis in a murine model of asthma. J Immunol 2006; 177:1786–1795.
45. Finotto S, Neurath MF, Glickman JN, et al. Development of spontaneous airway changes consistent with human asthma in mice lacking T-bet. Science 2002; 295:336–338.
46. Finotto S, Hausding M, Doganci A, et al. Asthmatic changes in mice lacking T-bet are mediated by IL-13. Int Immunol 2005; 17:993–1007.
47. Metcalfe DD, Corta JJ, Burd PR. Mast cells and basophils. In: Gallin JI, Goldstein IM, Synderman R, eds. Inflammation: Basic Principals and Clinical Correlates. 2nd ed. New York: Raven Press, 1992.
48. Xu X, Zhang D, Lyubynska N, et al. Mast cells protect mice from Mycoplasma pneumonia. Am J Respir Crit Care Med 2006; 173:219–225.
49. Chu HW, Jeyaseelan S, Rino JG, et al. TLR2 signaling is critical for Mycoplasma pneumoniae-induced airway mucin expression. J Immunol 2005; 174:5713–5719.
50. Wu Q, Martin RJ, Rino JG, et al. A deficient TLR2 signaling promotes airway mucin production in Mycoplasma pneumoniae-infected allergic mice. Am J Physiol Lung Cell Mol Physiol 2007; 292:L1064–L1072.
51. Wu Q, Martin RJ, Lafasto S, et al. Toll-like receptor 2 down-regulation in established mouse allergic lungs contributes to decreased mycoplasma clearance. Am J Respir Crit Care Med 2008; 177:720–729.
52. Chu HW, Rino JG, Wexler RB, et al. Mycoplasma pneumoniae infection increases airway collagen deposition in a murine model of allergic airway inflammation. Am J Physiol Lung Cell Mol Physiol 2005; 289:L125–L133.
53. Schoeb TR, Lindsey JR. Exacerbation of murine respiratory mycoplasmosis by sialodacryoadenitis virus infection in gnotobiotic F344 rats. Vet Pathol 1987; 24:392–399.
54. Kraft M, Cassell GH, Pak J, et al. Mycoplasma pneumoniae and Chlamydia pneumoniae in asthma: effect of clarithromycin. Chest 2002; 121:1782–1788.
55. Black PN, Blasi F, Jenkins CR, et al. Trial of roxithromycin in subjects with asthma and serological evidence of infection with Chlamydia pneumoniae. Am J Respir Crit Care Med 2001; 164:536–541.
56. Schleimer RP. Glucocorticosteroids. Part A: Mechanisms of Action in Allergic Diseases. St. Louis: Mosby, 2003.
57. Heasman SJ, Giles KM, Ward C, et al. Glucocorticoid-mediated regulation of granulocyte apoptosis and macrophage phagocytosis of apoptotic cells: implications for the resolution of inflammation. J Endocrinol 2003; 178:29–36.
58. Liu Y, Cousin JM, Hughes J, et al. Glucocorticoids promote nonphlogistic phagocytosis of apoptotic leukocytes. J Immunol 1999; 162:3639–3646.
59. Chu HW, Campbell JA, Rino JG, et al. Inhaled fluticasone propionate reduces concentration of Mycoplasma pneumoniae, inflammation, and bronchial hyperresponsiveness in lungs of mice. J Infect Dis 2004; 189:1119–1127.

6
Viral-Allergy Interactions

JONATHAN D. R. MACINTYRE, ANNEMARIE SYKES,
and SEBASTIAN L. JOHNSTON
National Heart and Lung Institute, Imperial College London, London, U.K.

I. Introduction

Respiratory virus infections, in particular rhinoviruses (RV), are the most frequently identified precipitants of asthma exacerbations in all age groups. Approximately 80% of exacerbations are related to respiratory viral infections, with RV being responsible for about two-thirds (1,2). The importance of allergen sensitization in asthma is also well recognized; it is the major risk factor for asthma, and sensitization and exposure to allergens are associated with increased risk of asthma exacerbations. Approximately 50% to 90% of adult asthmatics are atopic (3), and in these patients, it is increasingly recognized that an interaction between virus infection and allergy occurs. An asthmatic with a cold continues to be exposed to airborne allergens, and there is evidence of a synergistic interaction between virus infection and allergen exposure in increasing risk of asthma exacerbations in sensitized individuals.

There is also evidence of a role of allergen exposure and virus infections in influencing the risk of the development of asthma and allergy in childhood. Certain viral infections are associated with increased risk of development of asthma, while a greater overall load of infection appears protective. Similarly, there are studies reporting both increased and decreased risks of asthma in relation to early-life allergen exposure. The mechanisms of these interactions are not well understood, and a greater understanding of these viral-allergy interactions may identify areas for novel therapeutic targets.

II. Evidence of Viral-Allergen Interaction in Early Life
A. The Importance of Allergens in the Development of Asthma and Allergy

Many studies have addressed the importance of allergen exposure in the first two years of life and the development of asthma. A prospective study of British children with a family history of allergy investigated the relationship between exposure and sensitization to house-dust mite (HDM) allergen and the development of asthma (4). All but one of the asthmatic children studied at the age of 11 had been exposed to greater than 10 μg of Der p I per gram of dust. The age of first onset of wheeze was inversely correlated to the level of Der p I exposure at one year of age, particularly in atopic children. The authors concluded that early exposure to HDM allergens is a significant factor in sensitization and the development of asthma, but it remains difficult to define the age at which immunopathological responses occur. Similarly, Peat et al. examined the relationship of atopy with airway hyperresponsiveness (AHR) and respiratory symptoms in a population of schoolchildren (5). They found that early-onset atopy was an important risk factor for the development of asthma, continuing into later childhood years.

HDM have been considered as one of the most important indoor allergens associated with asthma. More than 50% of children and adolescents with asthma are sensitized to HDM (6), and studies have demonstrated a linear dose-response relationship between the dose of exposure and allergic symptoms (7). However, recent work by Tovey et al. showed a nonlinear relationship between HDM concentration at home and the development of asthma at five years of age in a high-risk cohort of children (8). This study showed trends of increased prevalence of sensitization and asthma correlating with HDM exposure up to a critical point, then sharply dropping at the highest level of exposure. In contrast to studies showing an association with HDM and subsequent development of asthma and allergy, Torrent et al. performed a prospective multicenter trial of a general population cohort and found no relationship between house HDM levels and allergic sensitization or asthma (9). Subgroup analysis of high-risk infants was also unremarkable. A recent Cochrane meta-analysis of reducing HDM in homes of asthmatics concluded that no clinical benefits were achieved irrespective of reduction in HDM concentration through chemical and/or physical methods (10). In cross-sectional studies of farming communities, where exposure to HDM are considerably higher than nonfarming dwellings, HDM sensitization rates were similar or higher among farmers' children compared with other children, but the occurrence of atopic diseases was lower in children living on farms compared with children not living on farms (11).

Other allergens are also of importance, particularly pet allergens, and there is evidence to suggest both a causative and a protective effect in the development of asthma and allergy. Data from the Asthma Multicentre Infant Cohort Study suggests a nonlinear relationship between cat allergen exposure and the development of asthma and sensitization (9). Counter to this, some studies have shown that exposure to cats exerts a slight protective effect on asthma (12). Similarly, Perzanowski et al. showed that living with a cat was inversely related to having a positive skin prick test to cat and incidence of physician-diagnosed asthma (13). Custovic et al. showed that the prevalence of sensitization to cat is decreased in groups with a high cat allergen exposure (14). More recently, a longitudinal study of cat allergen exposure and asthma development suggested that cat allergen exposure in infancy increases the risk of sensitization in early childhood but not in school-age children (15). Clearly, the question of whether cat allergens have a causative or protective effect on asthma development is still to be fully answered.

High exposure to aeroallergens is also associated with increased pediatric asthma-related hospitalizations. A relationship has been demonstrated between acute asthma admissions and daily airborne concentrations of pollen, fungal spores, air pollutants, and weather factors in Mexico City (16). Aeroallergens were more strongly associated with asthma admissions than pollutants. Asthma-related hospital admissions have also been related to exposure and sensitivity to HDM allergen (17), with continued exposure to high concentrations of HDM associated with an increased risk of readmission.

B. The Importance of Viruses in the Development of Asthma and Allergy

Viral infections are also strongly associated with asthma exacerbations in both adults and children. Respiratory viruses, detected by polymerase chain reaction (PCR) and culture, were identified in 80% to 85% of asthma exacerbations in a cohort of 9- to

11-year-old children who had reported wheeze, cough, or both in a questionnaire. The most frequently identified viruses were RV (2). These studies highlighted that both viruses and allergens were strongly associated with asthma exacerbations, prompting investigators to question whether there was an interaction between viruses and allergens and what the mechanism of such an interaction may be. A case control study in children aged 3 to 17 found that allergen sensitization and exposure in combination with respiratory virus infection substantially increased the risk of hospital admissions in asthmatics (18).

Several viruses have been implicated in interactions with allergens during early life, including respiratory syncytial virus (RSV), influenza viruses, and RV. RSV bronchiolitis requiring hospitalization during infancy has been observed to be highly associated with the development of asthma (43% vs. 8%) and allergic sensitization, determined by skin prick tests to common inhaled allergens (50% vs. 28%; $p = 0.022$) and serum IgE (45% vs. 26%; $p = 0.038$) (19). Similarly, RSV lower respiratory tract infection (LRTI) in early childhood has been associated with the subsequent development of wheeze and lower measurements of forced expiratory volume in children up to the age of 11 years (20). These epidemiological studies suggest that RSV LRTI and bronchiolitis somehow influence the development of asthma and allergy in children. Does RSV LRTI actually cause asthma development or does it simply act as a marker for children who are predisposed to develop asthma? This question of causation versus association between RSV LRTI and development of subsequent asthma and allergy has yet to be definitively answered, though recent studies suggest that both relationships are possible (21,22).

Influenza A LRTI in early childhood has also been implicated in the development of subsequent wheezing episodes. Eriksson et al. examined the incidence of wheeze in the year following hospitalization of children younger than three years with RSV and influenza A (23). Fifty percent of parents reported two or more episodes of wheezing for longer than two weeks; 15% to 20% of these patients were readmitted with wheeze, and the severity of the primary infection correlated with the degree of subsequent wheeze. Results did not differ between the RSV and influenza groups.

RV-induced LRTI are also strongly associated with the development of recurrent wheezing in later childhood. The Childhood Origins of ASThma (COAST) study has demonstrated this association. In children at risk for developing allergic respiratory disease, having at least one parent with one or more positive aeroallergen skin prick tests and/or a history of physician-diagnosed asthma, the most significant risk factor for the development of recurrent wheezing till the age of up to three years was having at least one RV-induced wheezing illness during infancy (OR = 10) (24). The same study identified that the risk was lower with RSV-induced wheezing illness (OR = 3.0) and non-RV/RSV-induced wheezing illness (OR = 3.9) in infancy. Other risk factors for the development of recurrent wheezing in the third year of life identified were passive smoke exposure, allergic sensitization to foods at one year, and any moderate to severe respiratory illness without wheeze during infancy. The same group went on to assess the COAST cohort at six years of age (25). The risk of asthma at six years was again highest among children with RV wheezing illnesses in infancy and early childhood. The mechanisms by which RV infection is associated with the development of asthma are not fully understood.

These studies highlight the finding that viral infections in infancy are associated with increased rates of recurrent wheezing episodes in later childhood. However, there are epidemiological data suggesting that frequent exposure to viral infections in early life may be protective against the development of asthma and recurrent wheeze. Children with older siblings and those who attend day care are at increased risk of infections. Studies examining the effect of day care attendance on the development of asthma and recurrent wheezing have conflicting results. This led investigators to examine this effect in a cohort of children followed prospectively from birth, as part of the Tuscon Children's Respiratory Study (26). The authors concluded that the presence of one or more older sibling at home and attendance at day care during the first six months of life protected against the development of asthma and recurrent wheezing in later childhood. Another longitudinal birth cohort study investigated the association between early childhood infections and the development of asthma, concluding that repeated viral infections, other than LRTI before the age of one, protect against the risk of asthma up to the age of seven (27). The authors proposed that these non-LRT viral infections stimulate the immature immune system toward a T helper 1 (T_h1) phenotype, thereby reducing the risk of subsequent development of asthma. The mechanisms are likely to be more complex as infections may also influence regulatory T-cell function and the development of tolerance to allergens. More work needs to be done in this area to clarify the complex relationships between early-life infection and risk of asthma development.

If there is a causal link between virus infection and development of asthma and allergy, then results of antiviral drug trials may be useful in demonstrating that this relationship is causal and not just associational. An interesting study, carried out by Wenzel et al., evaluated the long-term effects of RSV prophylaxis with high-dose RSV immunoglobulin (RespiGam^{TM}) in children with a high risk of chronic airway disease (28). Children given prophylaxis 7 to 10 years earlier had a significantly better ratio of forced expiratory volume in one second (FEV_1) to forced vital capacity (FVC), were less atopic (determined by skin prick testing to 10 allergens), and had fewer asthma attacks and fewer school absences than the control group. This study was small, nonrandomized, and retrospective; however, similar larger-scale studies could potentially determine if prevention of RSV infection has an effect on the development of allergy and asthma. One such study assessed a cohort of preterm infants, hypothesizing that palivizumab, a human monoclonal antibody against the RSV fusion protein, improves or prevents RSV LRTI, decreasing the occurrence of later recurrent wheezing (22). The incidence of recurrent wheezing, by carer or physician report, was significantly lower in the palivizumab-treated group. This effect remained significant after adjustment for confounding variables, although, as treatment was not randomized, there remains considerable potential for residual confounding. Though the authors acknowledge that the results may not be of relevance in term infants, they concluded that use of palivizumab may have a role in the prevention of recurrent wheeze in premature infants. Prospective randomized placebo-controlled studies will be required to provide definitive evidence to support or refute causation.

C.   Proposed Biological Mechanisms for Viral-Allergy Interactions

What are the likely biological mechanisms for early-life viral-allergy interactions in the development of asthma? The associations are undoubtedly complex and far from fully understood. An early hypothesis was that disruption of the respiratory mucosa by viruses allows allergens to breach the respiratory epithelium, to interact more easily with antigen-presenting cells, and to lead to allergic sensitization. Why should this not lead to tolerance instead of sensitization was not explained, and more recent theories might suggest that simultaneous infection and allergen exposure might result in sensitization, while allergen in the absence of infection might generate tolerance.

CD4$^+$ T cells are functionally divided into T_h1 and T_h2 cells as well as regulatory T cells, T_h17, T_h22, and T_h9 cells. T_h1 cells promote cell-mediated immunity by secreting interferon-γ (IFN-γ). T_h2 cells secrete interleukin-4 (IL-4), IL-5, and IL-13, which are thought to contribute to allergic asthmatic inflammation. There is strong evidence for linkage of total serum IgE concentration and AHR to the T_h2 cytokine cluster on chromosome 5q31 (29). A study examining the in vivo balance between T_h1/T_h2 immune responses of infants infected with natural RSV infection was performed (21). Cytokine levels were determined in nasal lavage fluid by ELISA, and cytokine mRNA was measured from stimulated peripheral blood mononuclear cells (PBMC). The IL-4/IFN-γ ratio was elevated in nasal lavage fluid and stimulated PBMC of infants with acute bronchiolitis compared with infants with upper respiratory tract symptoms only. These excessive T_h2 and deficient T_h1 responses in acute RSV bronchiolitis are consistent with the increased risk of asthma in these patients. An interesting theory has been proposed that suggests a genetic link between atopy and severity of RSV infection (30). In this pilot study of Korean children under two years of age admitted with RSV LRTI, an IL-4 haplotype was found to be overexpressed in the children with severe RSV disease compared with controls (healthy Korean blood donors). Children with this IL-4 haplotype have previously been shown to have increased IL-4 transcription and a predisposition to the development of asthma (30). Severe RSV bronchiolitis has also been associated with polymorphisms in the IL-4 and IL-4 receptor genes (31). These polymorphisms were found more frequently in children hospitalized with RSV than controls. This genetic predisposition to T_h2 responses may help explain the findings that severe RSV bronchiolitis is associated with the development of asthma in later life (19,20).

Other virus-induced cytokines are implicated in the pathogenesis of asthma and recurrent wheeze. IL-10, produced by monocytes, can downregulate T_h1 and T_h2 cytokine production. IL-10 levels were measured in whole-blood cultures stimulated with lipopolysaccharide and IFN-γ in the acute and convalescent phases of RSV bronchiolitis. These IL-10 levels in the acute phase were comparable to that of healthy control subjects but were found to be significantly higher in children who developed recurrent wheeze during the year following the episode of RSV bronchiolitis than that in patients without recurrent wheeze (32). IL-10 levels in stimulated whole blood were also significantly correlated with the number of wheezing episodes. The authors concluded that IL-10 levels in whole blood following stimulation with nonspecific stimuli may have a predictive value for the development of recurrent wheeze after RSV bronchiolitis and that the study indicates that virus-induced changes in monocyte cytokine responses as well as allergen-driven T_h2 cytokine responses can lead to the development of asthma. They propose that the increased IL-10 production could lead to decreased antiviral immunity in the lower airways, resulting in increased inflammation, resulting in wheeze and AHR. This is in contrast to other studies that suggest IL10 is protective against the development of asthma. One such study examines the suppressive responses of allergen-specific CD4$^+$ CD25$^+$ regulatory T cells in a mouse model of airway inflammation and found that the suppressed AHR, eosinophil recruitment, and T_h2 cytokine expression in the lung after allergen challenge were dependent on IL-10 (33). Another study demonstrated that expression of IL-10 by regulatory T cells is essential for the suppression of AHR (34). The differing roles for IL-10 in asthma development need further explanation.

Neutrophilic inflammation is also implicated in asthma pathogenesis. IL-8 is a potent neutrophil chemoattractant. In a study investigating cytokine levels in whole-blood cultures stimulated with nonspecific stimuli in hospitalized, ventilated and non-ventilated RSV bronchiolitis patients, plasma IL-8 levels were significantly higher in ventilated patients than that in nonventilated patients (35). A common variant of the IL-8 gene promoter region, the IL8-251A allele, has been associated with increased IL-8 production in lipopolysaccharide-stimulated whole blood, and the frequency of this allele has been found to be significantly higher in infants with bronchiolitis compared with healthy controls (36). Although these studies investigating cytokine responses in viral infection in infants are interesting, more work is needed to establish which cyto-kines are involved in the development of asthma and atopy.

Viral infections have been shown to alter the individual's response to various stimuli. Nonspecific hyperresponsiveness to both histamine and methacholine is increased with virus infection. Studies also suggest that viral infections alter the response to allergen. Lemanske et al. found that RV infection enhanced airway reactivity and predisposed the allergic patient to develop late asthmatic reactions to ragweed antigen (37). Similarly, Calhoun et al. found that RV-16 augments immediate and late allergic responses in the airways of allergic individuals after antigen challenge (38).

The above work highlights the importance of allergens and viruses in the develop-ment of atopic diseases and asthma. The interaction between viruses and allergens is complex, and more work is needed to define the mechanism of this interaction.

III. Viral-Allergy Interactions in Asthma Exacerbations

Interactions between allergen and virus infection are also important in adults during exacerbations of asthma. RV infection in atopic asthmatics has different clinical man-ifestations from normal, nonasthmatic, nonatopic individuals. Asthmatics do not have increased numbers of RV infections, however, when they do occur, infections are associated with more severe and more prolonged lower respiratory tract symptoms and reductions in lung function (39). A study of experimental RV infection also demon-strated that asthmatics had increased lower respiratory tract symptoms; greater falls in lung function, and increased AHR compared with nonasthmatics (40). There was a strong correlation between symptoms and virus load, suggesting that more severe infections resulted in worse exacerbations. This study emphasizes the importance of RV infections in asthma exacerbations. An interesting feature of the study design was the fact that the asthmatic patients in this study were also atopic and sensitized to a range of common aeroallergens and that they continued to be exposed to these allergens at home, rather than being hospitalized, while experiencing their experimental RV infection. This may be closer to the "real-life" scenario for asthma exacerbations than similar studies in which volunteers were not at home and similar increased illness was not observed.

These studies suggest an interaction between virus infection and allergic processes to induce asthma exacerbations. This is further supported by a case control study of adults admitted with asthma exacerbations to a large district general hospital (41). A synergistic interaction between allergen sensitization, allergen exposure, and virus infection during acute exacerbations was found. The combination of sensitization, high exposure to one or more allergens, and virus detection considerably increased the risk of being admitted with asthma.

An even greater interaction between virus infection and allergic sensitization exists in children. In a study looking at modifiable risk factors for pediatric asthma exacerbations, an increased risk of asthma-related hospital admissions was reported with virus infection and allergen exposure (18). Allergen sensitization and exposure or virus detection alone were not independently associated with hospital admission, but importantly, in combination virus detection, sensitization and high allergen exposure substantially increased the risk of admission to hospital.

These studies illustrate the synergistic effects of virus infection, allergen sensitization, and allergen exposure in increasing risk of asthma exacerbations. The mechanism by which this occurs is not fully understood. Message et al., in a human experimental RV infection model, related airway inflammation to both virus load and clinical symptoms. The authors identified deficient induction of IL-10 and T_h1 cytokines and augmented induction of T_h2 cytokines in asthmatics, supporting a role for RV-induced lower airway inflammation in precipitating asthma exacerbations, perhaps through impaired T_h1/IL-10 and augmented T_h2 responses (40).

To investigate the inflammatory response to combined RV infection and allergen exposure, an intricate study investigated inflammatory responses to allergens in different lung segments (38). Volunteers with allergic rhinitis and normal volunteers were infected with RV and underwent segmental allergen bronchoprovocation and bronchoalveolar lavage (BAL). RV-16 inoculation potentiated airway inflammation after segmental allergen bronchoprovocation in allergic subjects but not in normals. RV inoculation was associated with an enhanced early histamine release after local allergen challenge, persistent histamine release at 48 hours, and a greater recruitment of eosinophils at 48 hours post challenge than that seen in normals. This work suggested that the synergistic effect may be due to an accentuation of allergic responses in the airway contributing to heightened bronchial inflammation. This study was performed in allergic rhinitis patients, but evidence of increased eosinophilic lower airway inflammation has also been reported in experimental RV infection in asthmatics compared with normal subjects, and this was related to virological and clinical outcomes (40).

These two studies support the proposal that viral respiratory tract infections increase the intensity of allergic response, enhancing preexisting inflammation, leading to increased AHR, airway obstruction, and wheeze. How this occurs is not completely understood but may involve damage to epithelium, production of inflammatory mediators or cells recruited as part of the immune response to infection. This may be related to proinflammatory cytokines known to be released during viral infection.

It is also possible that allergic airway inflammation impairs antiviral immunity, leading, at the same time, to greater virus loads and increased virus-induced inflammation. The study by Message et al. was consistent with this hypothesis, as greater virus loads were reported (40), though with the patient numbers studied, these differences were not statistically significant. This hypothesis is also supported by the recent observations of impaired innate immune responses to RV infection in asthma (42,43), which were related to the severity of several clinical an pathological outcomes related to asthma exacerbation severity, as well as to virus load in vivo (43).

Many cytokines have been demonstrated to be raised in nasal secretions during natural and experimental RV infection. These include IL-1, IL-6, IL-8, IL-11, RANTES (regulated on activation, normal T cell expressed and secreted), and many others. There is some evidence linking these cytokines to clinical asthma. IL-8 levels have been shown to be inversely related to PC_{20} in mild atopic asthmatics with confirmed experimental RV infection (44). This placebo-controlled study of 27 asthmatics reported an increase in nasal IL-8 at day 2 with RV infection, suggesting that increase in AHR is associated with chemokines such as IL-8. This group also demonstrated a significant increase in the levels of eosinophil cationic protein (ECP), IL-8, and IL-6 in sputum from these patients, with both IL-6 and IL-8 remaining elevated for up to nine days. Sputum ECP also correlated significantly with the decrease in PC_{20}, suggesting that the enhanced inflammation may be eosinophilic and that this is related to severity of AHR. Notably, the asthmatics in this study did not undergo specific allergen challenge.

In another study of experimental RV infection, virus load in atopic asthmatics was related to lower respiratory symptoms, bronchial hyperreactivity, and reductions in blood total and $CD8^+$ lymphocytes. Virus load and clinical outcomes were strongly related to deficient IFN-γ and IL-10 responses and to augmented IL-4, IL-5, and IL-13 responses, demonstrating relationships between virus load, lower airway inflammation, and asthma exacerbation severity in asthmatics (40). This study suggests that augmented T_h2 or impaired T_h1 or IL-10 immunity may be an important mechanism for this effect. Again, these patients were sensitized and continued to be exposed to aeroallergens but did not undergo specific allergen challenge. Many cytokines have shown an association, although a cause-and-effect relationship has not been demonstrated. It is likely that multiple different cytokines with overlapping effects are involved.

IV. Evidence of Enhanced Inflammation in Animal Models

Given the enhanced respiratory symptoms experienced by asthmatics, there are practical difficulties in investigating combined allergen sensitization, exposure, and virus infection in humans. Although this has been done (45) and suggested that preceding RV infection with allergen exposure did not determine the severity of the resulting exacerbation, most research has been performed in small animal models.

Several rodent models of virus infection and allergen sensitization have been developed. These commonly involve allergen sensitization followed by respiratory viral infection and allergen challenge. Most report that allergen sensitization is associated with eosinophilic airway inflammation and AHR. A number of different models and viruses have been used; however, until recently, RV, the commonest cause of asthma exacerbations, had not been investigated.

A mouse model of RV-induced exacerbations of allergic airway inflammation has now been reported (46). In this model, mice undergo sensitization to ovalbumin (Ova) and are then subjected to Ova challenge in combination with minor-group RV infection (RV-1B). Mice sensitized to and challenged with Ova and then infected with RV demonstrated increased neutrophilic, eosinophilic, and lymphocytic airway inflammation. Significant increases of BAL neutrophils were seen early, whereas the BAL eosinophils were induced later on in the infection. Other significant findings from this model included persistent lymphocytic inflammation, AHR, and mucus secretion. These findings support the hypothesis that the synergistic effect of allergen sensitization, exposure, and virus infection leads to enhanced inflammation. What is not known is if allergic airway inflammation is impairing antiviral responses. Interestingly, both T_h1

and T_h2 cytokines were induced in the RV model with significant early induction of the T_h2 cytokines IL-4 and IL-13, and enhanced induction of virus-specific IFN-γ. Atopic asthma classically produces a T_h2 type of inflammation, whereas virus infection is associated with a T_h1 picture. These can be mutually antagonistic. This model demonstrates that both types of inflammation are enhanced, suggesting a possible augmentation of both responses. The cause and effects of the enhanced inflammation need to be investigated in further studies.

Animal models of allergen sensitization have confirmed that concomitant allergen exposure and viral infection enhance sensitization to the allergen. In a mouse model, concomitant exposure of RSV or influenza A with Ova, as an aeroallergen, led to anaphylactic collapse, with Ova-specific IgG1 and enhanced production of IL-4. This did not occur in the uninfected animals (47). Peebles et al. showed that Ova sensitization prior to RSV infection increased AHR, whereas RSV infection before allergen sensitization led to decreased allergen-induced AHR, supporting the concept that RSV has a greater effect in subjects with underlying allergic disease (48). Interestingly and in contrast to other studies, which demonstrate that RSV infection prior to allergen sensitization in BALB/c mice causes an increase in allergic inflammation (49), this study showed no significant increase in eosinophilia but increases in IFN-γ in mononuclear cells from parabronchial lymph nodes.

A model of RSV-infected mice, subsequently sensitized to aerosolized Ova after resolution of the acute infection, also demonstrated enhanced allergen responses and airway inflammation with both neutrophilic and eosinophilic infiltration (49). Cytokine production was predominantly T_h2 type. AHR was associated with pulmonary eosinophilic inflammation, and treatment with anti-IL-5 antibody abolished AHR. Eosinophilic, but not neutrophilic, inflammation was also abolished in both acutely infected mice and mice sensitized after infection with anti-IL-5 treatment, suggesting T_h2-type inflammation to be important. Interestingly, further investigation in the RSV model identified the importance of T cells in the response. Transfer of T cells, particularly $CD8^+$ cells, from RSV-infected mice to naïve mice resulted in increased lung eosinophils, increased IL-5, and development of AHR following allergen sensitization (50). Dendritic cells, known to be involved in inducing T-cell responses to both viruses and allergens, are also increased in the lung (51). Other models have identified other potentially important inflammatory mediators with IL-4 (52), IL-8 (53), IL-10 (54), and cyteinyl leukotrienes (55) all being implicated.

These interesting studies illustrate that the interaction between virus infections and allergy may not simply be one of additive inflammation. Viruses may actually modify the host response to allergen and vice versa.

V. Conclusions

Although there is good evidence of an interaction between allergen sensitization, exposure, and viral infection, the mechanisms by which they interact are far from understood. Early exposure to aeroallergens increases the risk of allergen sensitization and development of asthma, though at high doses, there may be protection. Also, there is convincing evidence that early-life LRTI, particularly with RVs, RSV, and influenza viruses, is associated with an increased risk of asthma development. Indeed, studies have suggested that prevention of RSV infection may be protective against later development of asthma in preterm infants. Conversely, however, a high overall exposure to infection in early life may also protect against later development of asthma.

The inflammatory response in asthma is characterized by deficient T_h1 and augmented T_h2 immune responses. Severe virus-induced LRTI have been shown to be characterized by excessive T_h2/deficient T_h1 responses, with some evidence implicating the IL-4 and other T_h2 genes. This is consistent with the T_h1/T_h2 imbalance seen in asthma.

Both viral infection and allergen exposure in sensitized individuals stimulate multiple different cytokines that are likely to have overlapping effects. Much further work is needed in animal models to define the functional importance of individual cytokines and other mediators likely to be involved.

As a result of experimental infection studies in asthmatics, several interesting areas for further research have emerged. It will be important to confirm human relevance for findings generated from the mouse studies. It will also be important to repeat these experimental infection studies with nonatopic asthmatics and atopic nonasthmatics to further delineate the roles of atopy and asthma. These studies could potentially shed further light on the synergistic reaction between viral infection and atopy in asthma.

References

1. Nicholson KG, Kent J, Ireland DC. Respiratory viruses and exacerbations of asthma in adults. BMJ 1993; 307(6910):982–986.
2. Johnston SL, Pattemore PK, Sanderson G, et al. Community study of role of viral infections in exacerbations of asthma in 9–11 year old children. BMJ 1995; 310(6989):1225–1229.
3. Pearce N, Pekkanen J, Beasley R. How much asthma is really attributable to atopy? Thorax 1999; 54(3):268–272.
4. Sporik R, Holgate ST, Platts-Mills TA, et al. Exposure to house-dust mite allergen (Der p I) and the development of asthma in childhood. A prospective study. N Engl J Med 1990; 323(8): 502–507.
5. Peat JK, Salome CM, Woolcock AJ. Longitudinal changes in atopy during a 4-year period: relation to bronchial hyperresponsiveness and respiratory symptoms in a population sample of Australian schoolchildren. J Allergy Clin Immunol 1990; 85(1 pt 1):65–74.
6. Ulrik CS, Backer V. Markers of impaired growth of pulmonary function in children and adolescents. Am J Respir Crit Care Med 1999; 160(1):40–44.
7. Platts-Mills TA, Woodfolk JA, Erwin EA, et al. Mechanisms of tolerance to inhalant allergens: the relevance of a modified Th2 response to allergens from domestic animals. Springer Semin Immunopathol 2004; 25(3–4):271–279.
8. Tovey ER, Almqvist C, Li Q, et al. Nonlinear relationship of mite allergen exposure to mite sensitization and asthma in a birth cohort. J Allergy Clin Immunol 2008; 122(1):114–118.
9. Torrent M, Sunyer J, Garcia R, et al. Early-life allergen exposure and atopy, asthma, and wheeze up to 6 years of age. Am J Respir Crit Care Med 2007; 176(5):446–453.
10. Gotzsche PC, Johansen HK. House dust mite control measures for asthma. Cochrane Database Syst Rev 2008; (2):CD001187.
11. von Hertzen L, Haahtela T. Disconnection of man and the soil: reason for the asthma and atopy epidemic? J Allergy Clin Immunol 2006; 117(2):334–344.
12. Takkouche B, Gonzalez-Barcala FJ, Etminan M, et al. Exposure to furry pets and the risk of asthma and allergic rhinitis: a meta-analysis. Allergy 2008; 63(7):857–864.
13. Perzanowski MS, Ronmark E, Platts-Mills TA, et al. Effect of cat and dog ownership on sensitization and development of asthma among preteenage children. Am J Respir Crit Care Med 2002; 166(5):696–702.

14. Custovic A, Hallam CL, Simpson BM, et al. Decreased prevalence of sensitization to cats with high exposure to cat allergen. J Allergy Clin Immunol 2001; 108(4):537–539.
15. Chen CM, Rzehak P, Zutavern A, et al. Longitudinal study on cat allergen exposure and the development of allergy in young children. J Allergy Clin Immunol 2007; 119(5):1148–1155.
16. Rosas I, McCartney HA, Payne RW, et al. Analysis of the relationships between environmental factors (aeroallergens, air pollution, and weather) and asthma emergency admissions to a hospital in Mexico City. Allergy 1998; 53(4):394–401.
17. Sporik R, Platts-Mills TA, Cogswell JJ. Exposure to house dust mite allergen of children admitted to hospital with asthma. Clin Exp Allergy 1993; 23(9):740–746.
18. Murray CS, Poletti G, Kebadze T, et al. Study of modifiable risk factors for asthma exacerbations: virus infection and allergen exposure increase the risk of asthma hospital admissions in children. Thorax 2006; 61(5):376–382.
19. Sigurs N, Gustafsson PM, Bjarnason R, et al. Severe respiratory syncytial virus bronchiolitis in infancy and asthma and allergy at age 13. Am J Respir Crit Care Med 2005; 171(2): 137–141.
20. Stein RT, Sherrill D, Morgan WJ, et al. Respiratory syncytial virus in early life and risk of wheeze and allergy by age 13 years. Lancet 1999; 354(9178):541–545.
21. Legg JP, Hussain IR, Warner JA, et al. Type 1 and type 2 cytokine imbalance in acute respiratory syncytial virus bronchiolitis. Am J Respir Crit Care Med 2003; 168(6):633–639.
22. Simoes EA, Groothuis JR, Carbonell-Estrany X, et al. Palivizumab prophylaxis, respiratory syncytial virus, and subsequent recurrent wheezing. J Pediatr 2007; 151(1):34–42.
23. Eriksson M, Bennet R, Nilsson A. Wheezing following lower respiratory tract infections with respiratory syncytial virus and influenza A in infancy. Pediatr Allergy Immunol 2000; 11(3): 193–197.
24. Lemanske RF Jr., Jackson DJ, Gangnon RE, et al. Rhinovirus illnesses during infancy predict subsequent childhood wheezing. J Allergy Clin Immunol 2005; 116(3):571–577.
25. Jackson DJ, Gangnon RE, Evans MD, et al. Wheezing rhinovirus illnesses in early life predict asthma development in high-risk children. Am J Respir Crit Care Med 2008; 178(7): 667–672.
26. Ball TM, Castro-Rodriguez JA, Griffith KA, et al. Siblings, day-care attendance, and the risk of asthma and wheezing during childhood. N Engl J Med 2000; 343(8):538–543.
27. Illi S, von Mutius E, Lau S, et al. Early childhood infectious diseases and the development of asthma up to school age: a birth cohort study. BMJ 2001; 322(7283):390–395.
28. Wenzel SE, Gibbs RL, Lehr MV, et al. Respiratory outcomes in high-risk children 7 to 10 years after prophylaxis with respiratory syncytial virus immune globulin. Am J Med 2002; 112(8):627–633.
29. Bleecker ER, Amelung PJ, Levitt RC, et al. Evidence for linkage of total serum IgE and bronchial hyperresponsiveness to chromosome 5q: a major regulatory locus important in asthma. Clin Exp Allergy 1995; 25(suppl 2):84–88.
30. Choi EH, Lee HJ, Yoo T, et al. A common haplotype of interleukin-4 gene IL4 is associated with severe respiratory syncytial virus disease in Korean children. J Infect Dis 2002; 186(9): 1207–1211.
31. Hoebee B, Rietveld E, Bont L, et al. Association of severe respiratory syncytial virus bronchiolitis with interleukin-4 and interleukin-4 receptor alpha polymorphisms. J Infect Dis 2003; 187(1):2–11.
32. Bont L, Heijnen CJ, Kavelaars A, et al. Monocyte IL-10 production during respiratory syncytial virus bronchiolitis is associated with recurrent wheezing in a one-year follow-up study. Am J Respir Crit Care Med 2000; 161(5):1518–1523.
33. Kearley J, Barker JE, Robinson DS, et al. Resolution of airway inflammation and hyperreactivity after in vivo transfer of CD4$^+$CD25$^+$ regulatory T cells is interleukin 10 dependent. J Exp Med 2005; 202(11):1539–1547.

34. Presser K, Schwinge D, Wegmann M, et al. Coexpression of TGF-beta1 and IL-10 enables regulatory T cells to completely suppress airway hyperreactivity. J Immunol 2008; 181(11): 7751–7758.

35. Bont L, Heijnen CJ, Kavelaars A, et al. Peripheral blood cytokine responses and disease severity in respiratory syncytial virus bronchiolitis. Eur Respir J 1999; 14(1):144–149.

36. Hull J, Thomson A, Kwiatkowski D. Association of respiratory syncytial virus bronchiolitis with the interleukin 8 gene region in UK families. Thorax 2000; 55(12):1023–1027.

37. Lemanske RF Jr., Dick EC, Swenson CA, et al. Rhinovirus upper respiratory infection increases airway hyperreactivity and late asthmatic reactions. J Clin Invest 1989; 83(1):1–10.

38. Calhoun WJ, Dick EC, Schwartz LB, et al. A common cold virus, rhinovirus 16, potentiates airway inflammation after segmental antigen bronchoprovocation in allergic subjects. J Clin Invest 1994; 94(6):2200–2208.

39. Corne JM, Marshall C, Smith S, et al. Frequency, severity, and duration of rhinovirus infections in asthmatic and non-asthmatic individuals: a longitudinal cohort study. Lancet 2002; 359(9309):831–834.

40. Message SD, Laza-Stanca V, Mallia P, et al. Rhinovirus-induced lower respiratory illness is increased in asthma and related to virus load and Th1/2 cytokine and IL-10 production. Proc Natl Acad Sci U S A 2008; 105(36):13562–13567.

41. Green RM, Custovic A, Sanderson G, et al. Synergism between allergens and viruses and risk of hospital admission with asthma: case-control study. BMJ 2002; 324(7340):763.

42. Wark PA, Johnston SL, Bucchieri F, et al. Asthmatic bronchial epithelial cells have a deficient innate immune response to infection with rhinovirus. J Exp Med 2005; 201(6): 937–947.

43. Contoli M, Message SD, Laza-Stanca V, et al. Role of deficient type III interferon-lambda production in asthma exacerbations. Nat Med 2006; 12(9):1023–1026.

44. Grunberg K, Timmers MC, Smits HH, et al. Effect of experimental rhinovirus 16 colds on airway hyperresponsiveness to histamine and interleukin-8 in nasal lavage in asthmatic subjects in vivo. Clin Exp Allergy 1997; 27(1):36–45.

45. de Kluijver J, Evertse CE, Sont JK, et al. Are rhinovirus-induced airway responses in asthma aggravated by chronic allergen exposure? Am J Respir Crit Care Med 2003; 168(10): 1174–1180.

46. Bartlett NW, Walton RP, Edwards MR, et al. Mouse models of rhinovirus-induced disease and exacerbation of allergic airway inflammation. Nat Med 2008; 14(2):199–204.

47. O'Donnell DR, Openshaw PJ. Anaphylactic sensitization to aeroantigen during respiratory virus infection. Clin Exp Allergy 1998; 28(12):1501–1508.

48. Peebles RS Jr., Hashimoto K, Collins RD, et al. Immune interaction between respiratory syncytial virus infection and allergen sensitization critically depends on timing of challenges. J Infect Dis 2001; 184(11):1374–1379.

49. Schwarze J, Hamelmann E, Bradley KL, et al. Respiratory syncytial virus infection results in airway hyperresponsiveness and enhanced airway sensitization to allergen. J Clin Invest 1997; 100(1):226–233.

50. Schwarze J, Makela M, Cieslewicz G, et al. Transfer of the enhancing effect of respiratory syncytial virus infection on subsequent allergic airway sensitization by T lymphocytes. J Immunol 1999; 163(10):5729–5734.

51. Beyer M, Bartz H, Horner K, et al. Sustained increases in numbers of pulmonary dendritic cells after respiratory syncytial virus infection. J Allergy Clin Immunol 2004; 113(1): 127–133.

52. Barends M, Van Oosten M, De Rond CG, et al. Timing of infection and prior immunization with respiratory syncytial virus (RSV) in RSV-enhanced allergic inflammation. J Infect Dis 2004; 189(10):1866–1872.

53. Bossios A, Gourgiotis D, Skevaki CL, et al. Rhinovirus infection and house dust mite exposure synergize in inducing bronchial epithelial cell interleukin-8 release. Clin Exp Allergy 2008; 38(10):1615–1626.
54. Makela MJ, Kanehiro A, Borish L, et al. IL-10 is necessary for the expression of airway hyperresponsiveness but not pulmonary inflammation after allergic sensitization. Proc Natl Acad Sci U S A 2000; 97(11):6007–6012.
55. Volovitz B, Welliver RC, De Castro G, et al. The release of leukotrienes in the respiratory tract during infection with respiratory syncytial virus: role in obstructive airway disease. Pediatr Res 1988; 24(4):504–507.

7
Viral Respiratory Infections in Infancy and Chronic Asthma

JAMES E. GERN
University of Wisconsin Medical School, Madison, Wisconsin, U.S.A.

I. Introduction

Many children with asthma begin wheezing in infancy, and these illnesses are predominantly caused by respiratory viruses. This relationship has led to speculation that respiratory infections in early life can, in fact, cause asthma. Although proof of this theory is lacking, there is experimental evidence to support this concept from a variety of different sources and study designs including animal models, studies of isolated cells and tissues, case control and birth cohort studies, and epidemiologic studies. Of course, asthma is multifactorial in nature, and a variety of host, lifestyle, and environmental factors, together with respiratory viral infections, collectively determine the risk of developing asthma. In this review, evidence linking viral respiratory infections to the onset of asthma will be reviewed, and potential interactions between viral illnesses and other factors known to promote asthma will be explored.

II. Viral Infections and Infantile Wheezing

Viral respiratory infections, although seasonal, are ubiquitous in infancy, and it is estimated that up to 50% of infants develop virus-induced wheezing. Bronchiolitis is the most common wheezing illness in infancy and can be caused by a number of different respiratory viruses that vary in frequency with the season of the year. In the Northern Hemisphere, respiratory syncytial virus (RSV), metapneumovirus, and coronaviruses are most often found in winter, while human rhinovirus (HRV) and parainfluenza viruses account for most wheezing illnesses at other times of the year (1–3). Influenza viruses, bocavirus, adenoviruses, polyomaviruses, and bacterial pathogens are less common causes of wheezing in children (4–6). In the Southern Hemisphere, these patterns are offset by six months (7). There is relatively little data to describe seasonal patterns of virus-induced wheezing in equatorial regions. Mixed viral infections (e.g., RSV and HRV) can also occur and tend to cause more severe illnesses (8). Most viral respiratory illnesses are one to two weeks in duration, although adenovirus can be shed for several weeks or months (9). Prolonged illnesses can occur and are most often caused by a series of respiratory viruses rather than prolonged infection with a single pathogen (9). Despite major differences in viral structure and viral replication cycles, the clinical manifestations of infections with diverse respiratory viruses are quite similar.

A. RSV Bronchiolitis

RSV infects all children by two to three years of age. The season for RSV infections generally extends from December through March, but there is considerable variability from year to year. There are two serotypes of RSV, although reinfections are common because low titers of antibody, including that acquired transplacentally, are incompletely protective (10,11). The initial RSV infection is typically the most severe and causes bronchiolitis in 20% to 30% of infants. Over 120,000 children are hospitalized with bronchiolitis each year in the United States, and RSV causes up to 80,000 of these hospitalizations (12). For reasons that are unclear, the number of infants hospitalized for bronchiolitis is increasing (13). In older children and adults, RSV can cause common cold symptoms. These illnesses do not cause serious morbidity but can serve to spread the virus to more susceptible individuals.

RSV has a number of characteristics that promote lower respiratory illnesses. First, RSV nonstructural proteins 1 and 2 inhibit type I interferon (IFN) responses, thereby slowing innate immune responses to the infection (14). In addition, RSV can infect both airway cells and types 1 and 2 alveolar pneumocytes (15) and frequently causes pneumonia in addition to bronchiolitis. Finally, RSV infection can induce intense secretion of mucus (16), which, together with necrotic cells, can severely obstruct airways (15).

B. HRV as a Lower Airway Pathogen

Recent studies have demonstrated that HRV, once considered to be limited to the upper airway, is an important cause of lower respiratory infections (17). HRV consist of 99 canonical serotypes divided into groups A and B initially on the basis of patterns of inhibition with certain antiviral compounds. More recently, partial and complete genetic sequencing of viruses detected using molecular techniques have revealed that the number of HRV strains has been severely underestimated, and in fact, evidence is growing for a third group of HRV ("HRV C") that appears to be as different from HRV groups A and B as it is from other enteroviruses (18–26). These newly discovered viruses are quite common and comprise up to 50% of HRV detected in some clinical studies (21). Clinical manifestations are similar to other HRV and range from asymptomatic infection to common colds to severe wheezing illnesses in infants and in children with asthma. The frequency of detection appears to be consistently high in studies conducted in the United States, Europe, Asia, and Australia.

It was long assumed that infections were limited to the upper airway because HRV replicate best at relatively cool temperatures (33–35°C) and were closely associated with common colds. In fact, temperatures in large and medium-sized airways are ideal for HRV replication (27), and HRV has been present in lower airway fluids and cells of experimentally inoculated adult volunteers (28–30), and secretions obtained by suctioning the lower airways of children with tracheostomies (31). Furthermore, HRV is often the only pathogen detected in young children with wheezing illnesses and those hospitalized for pneumonia (1,3,17,26,32,33). A recent year-long population-based study found that HRV was detected in 26% of children <5 years of age hospitalized for respiratory symptoms or fever (32).

HRV infections are an important cause of wheezing illnesses, and yet HRV are also frequently detected in asymptomatic infants and children (1,34,35). This observation raises the question as to whether there are more virulent HRV strains that are more likely to cause wheezing illnesses. This is certainly the case for other respiratory viruses (e.g., influenza), and with 150 strains identified to date, it is likely that this is also true for HRV. Identifying more virulent strains, together with the molecular mechanisms that determine this characteristic, will be important in developing new therapeutic strategies to reduce the severity of HRV illnesses.

C. Risk Factors for Virus-Induced Wheezing

Risk factors for bronchiolitis and viral lower respiratory infection (LRI) include young age, small lung size, male gender, season of birth, and exposure to tobacco smoke (36). The peak age for hospitalization with RSV is two to four months of life, and this probably coincides with a nadir in transplacentally acquired neutralizing antibody along with immaturity of innate antiviral immune responses. Lung-specific factors such as preexisting limitation to airflow also increase the risk of viral LRI (37). In addition, several genetic factors modify the risk of RSV-induced wheezing, including polymorphisms in genes encoding surfactant proteins, cytokines, chemokines, and innate immune receptors (38). Although data are more limited for HRV infections, polymorphisms in IL-10 may influence the severity of illnesses with this virus (39). Finally, vitamin D deficiency is common in colder climates in wintertime and may be associated with an increased risk for recurrent wheezing illnesses (40).

III. Do Viral Respiratory Infections Cause Asthma?

The coughing, wheezing, and tachypnea associated with viral respiratory illnesses closely resemble exacerbations of asthma in older children, and 30% to 50% of children with recurrent virus-induced wheezing in infancy go on to develop asthma. This progression suggests that viral respiratory infections might damage the airways and initiate asthma. It is also possible that the relationship is not causal and that virus-induced wheezing episodes, instead, reveal a preexisting tendency for asthma secondary to impaired lung physiology or antiviral responses. A third possibility, which combines elements of the first two, is a "two-hit hypothesis," in which viral infections promote asthma mainly in predisposed children (41,42). Understanding the host-pathogen interactions that determine the severity of respiratory illnesses and long-term sequelae would be of great help in identifying at-risk individuals and in designing new and more effective treatments and preventive strategies.

A. Risk Factors for Asthma Following Viral Infection

Long-term studies have demonstrated that infants hospitalized with RSV bronchiolitis have a two- to threefold increase in the risk of developing asthma later in childhood (43). This risk is further increased by a strong family history of atopy, or the development of atopic features, particularly if this occurs during early childhood (42). The relationship between virus-induced wheezing in infancy and subsequent asthma was recently evaluated in a large Tennessee Medicaid database (44). As noted in previous studies, infants born approximately 120 days before the peak of RSV season had the highest rate of hospitalization for bronchiolitis or other wheezing illnesses. Follow-up of these children revealed that timing of birth date with respect to the peak of the winter bronchiolitis season also tracked with the risk of developing asthma. These findings suggest that children who are four months old during the peak of the viral bronchiolitis season are most likely to go on to develop asthma, suggesting a causative relationship. In a second report analyzing the same population, children born four months before the fall HRV season were at even greater risk for developing asthma, although fewer infants wheezed in the fall season compared with that in winter (45).

The type of virus-induced wheezing episode also appears to influence the risk of subsequent asthma. Wheezing illnesses caused by RSV, parainfluenza viruses, or influenza A appear to have similar long-term prognosis. In contrast, a case control study conducted in Finland demonstrated that infants hospitalized with HRV-induced wheezing were found to have a particularly high risk for subsequent asthma, and this relationship persisted at least through the late teen years (46,47). This finding is supported by findings from two birth cohort studies. The Childhood Origins of Asthma (COAST) study is a high-risk birth cohort study in which families with at least one parent with allergies or asthma were enrolled prenatally and both immune development and respiratory illnesses were prospectively evaluated (41). Through the use of polymerase chain reaction (PCR) technology, viral etiologies were identified in 90% of wheezing illnesses. Notably, moderate to severe HRV infections (with and without wheezing) during infancy were a significant risk factor [odds ratio (OR) = 10] for persistent wheezing at age three years (1). Moreover, RV wheezing illnesses in the first three years of life were significantly associated with the development of asthma at age six years (48). The combination of allergic sensitization and HRV induced by age three years was associated with the highest risk of developing asthma. Similarly, in high-risk infants who were followed prospectively in Australia, Kusel and colleagues prospectively evaluated 198 Australian children and compared respiratory illnesses in the first year of life with respiratory outcomes at age five years (49). Wheezing illnesses with either HRV or RSV were associated with asthma at age five years. Interestingly, these associations were only significant in the children with early-onset (by age two years) allergic sensitization. Both of these studies highlight the role of virus-induced wheezing in infancy, HRV in particular, in determining the risk for subsequent asthma. Children who develop allergic sensitization at an early age and also wheeze with HRV are at high risk for developing asthma.

B. Respiratory Viral Infections and the Hygiene Hypothesis

The "hygiene hypothesis" proposes that certain viral or bacterial infections might actually *protect* against the subsequent development of allergies and asthma (50,51). However, there is no evidence that viral infections of the respiratory tract protect against either allergies or asthma, and in fact, bronchiolitis and pneumonias in infancy signal an increased risk of subsequent asthma. This has led to speculation that the site of infection might also be an important factor related to asthma risk, and it is possible that the gastrointestinal infections are protective. Other epidemiologic and biologic factors that have been associated with reduced rates of allergic diseases include early exposure to pets, a farming lifestyle, alterations in bacterial flora of the gut, and increased use of antibiotics (52). Collectively, these studies suggest that exposure to microbes may have a greater effect than actual infections on immune development and the risk of atopy and asthma.

IV. Mechanisms for Long-Term Effects of Acute Viral Respiratory Infections

A. Viral Infections and Postnatal Lung Development

Lung development begins at about four weeks of gestation and continues after birth (53). The differentiation of the respiratory airways and respiratory gas exchange (acinar) units is largely completed by 40 weeks of gestation. Postnatally, there is continued formation of new alveoli for at least two to three years. Lung growth is maximal at this time, and early childhood can be considered a period of continuous airway and lung structural "remodeling." Murine models of gene deletion and overexpression have been used to identify factors that regulate lung growth and alveolarization, including epidermal growth factor (EGF), vascular endothelial growth factor (VEGF), transforming growth factor β (TGF-β), and platelet-derived growth factor (PDGF).

This period of rapid lung growth and development is coincident with frequent viral respiratory illnesses, raising the possibility that these illnesses could disrupt normal development and lead to abnormalities of lung structure and function. In the Tucson Children's Respiratory Study, children with persistent wheezing have normal lung function soon after birth but show signs of airway obstruction by six years of age (54). These findings raise the possibility that viral respiratory infections contribute to the reduction in lung function in "persistent wheezers" during the first few years of life.

B. Interactions with Allergy

Atopic features such as atopic dermatitis, elevated total IgE, allergic sensitization, and food allergy are strong predictors of recurrent wheezing and asthma in infants with a history of virus-induced wheezing (42). Sensitization to foods, particularly egg, or aeroallergens indicates an increased risk for persistent wheezing and lower lung function in childhood (37,49,55). Sensitization in early life, persistent sensitization, multiple positive skin tests, and high levels of antigen-specific IgE all predict recurrent wheezing and/or increased asthma risk (48,49,55–57). Eosinophils or eosinophil degranulation products, together with the detection of a respiratory virus, most commonly HRV, synergistically increased the risk of wheezing in a study conducted in a pediatric emergency department (35). Finally, atopic, but not nonatopic, eczema in infancy is a risk factor for subsequent asthma (58).

These observations have led to the development of predictive scoring systems, which attempt to synthesize multiple risk factors into a clinically useful prognostic tool for asthma (59). These indices have good predictive value for transient wheezing but are less able to identify infants with early stages of asthma. Improving the ability to classify infants at an early age would have benefits related to clinical decisions regarding therapy and follow-up, as well as clinical research studies of asthma prevention.

C. Influence of Host Immune Responses

The outcome of respiratory viral infections depends on a kinetic race between viral replication and antiviral responses of the host. Innate immunity is likely the most important factor during the acute phase of the infection, since these responses are rapidly induced by early events of viral life cycles. Virus-induced inflammation limits viral replication and transmission to other cells, but for viruses such as HRV, which infect relatively few cells in the airway (30,60,61), inflammation also contributes to respiratory symptoms. Upon infection, viral RNA activates innate immune responses by binding to molecules such as toll-like receptor (TLR)-3, TLR-7, the dsRNA-dependent protein kinase (PKR), retinoic acid inducible gene-I (RIG-I), and melanoma differentiation-associated gene-5 (MDA-5) (62–64). In addition, RSV is known to interact with TLR-4. These mechanisms activate a host of antiviral effector mechanisms, including the secretion of chemokines to recruit additional inflammatory cells into the airway (65). Once replication is under way, mononuclear cells strengthen the antiviral response through the secretion of IFN, proinflammatory cytokines, and chemokines (66,67). Viral infections can also indirectly activate and cause degranulation of eosinophils through a lymphocyte-dependent mechanism (42,68). This effect could contribute to the enhanced risk of virus-induced wheeze in children with allergic sensitization (35).

Necrotic epithelial and inflammatory cells together with mucus production and airway edema can cause airway obstruction and wheezing.

There is clinical evidence that innate immune responses in early life are clinically important. For example, babies with low ex vivo IFN responses in early life are more likely to have frequent viral respiratory illnesses, including those associated with wheezing (8,69,70). These experimental findings suggest that an impaired IFN response could increase the risk of more severe viral respiratory infections in infancy and perhaps promote long-term damage to airway structures. Interestingly, reduced IFN-γ responses in infancy are also observed in children with atopic features (71,72), which could help to explain why atopy is a risk factor for virus-induced wheezing and the progression to asthma. In addition, it has been proposed that asthma may be associated with an inherent defect in antiviral responses. For example, airway epithelial cells cultured from adults with asthma were reported to produce reduced amounts of IFN-β, IFN-γ, and IFN-λ in response to HRV and support enhanced viral replication (73–75). Collectively, these findings suggest that infants who have persistently low innate antiviral responses could develop more severe viral respiratory infections and that repeated lower respiratory infections damage the airways and/or disturb lung development to promote airway obstruction and asthma (Fig. 1).

D. Effects of Viral Infections on Lung Growth Factors

Respiratory viruses can induce the synthesis of cytokines and growth factors that regulate airway remodeling and alveolar development, including VEGF (76,77), NO (78), TGF-β (79), amphiregulin (77), activin A (77), and fibroblast growth factor (FGF) (80). In addition, viral infections can induce neurotrophins that can direct remodeling of the airway neural network and possibly promote airway hyperresponsiveness (81). How the repeated induction of these regulatory factors affects lung development and remodeling is unknown, but is of interest regarding the long-term effects on lung function and asthma. These questions can be studied in animal models, and recently, two different models for HRV infections in the mouse (82,83) as well as methods for serial passage of mouse epithelial cells for propagation of HRV have been published (84).

E. Intervention Studies

Interventional studies utilizing effective antiviral therapies are needed to definitively test the role of viral respiratory infections in the pathogenesis of asthma. Although definitive studies are not yet available, there are some encouraging early results. Results of a recent

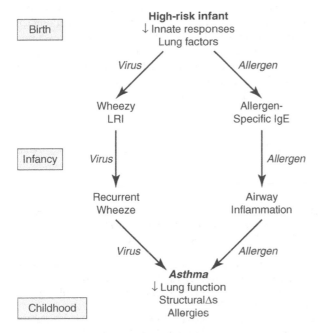

Figure 1 Risk factors for virus-induced wheezing and asthma. Infants with impaired innate antiviral responses are prone to more severe viral respiratory infections and also to allergic sensitization. In children with persistent impairment, repeated infections and allergic airway inflammation could lead to airway remodeling, airway hyperresponsiveness, and the development of asthma.

nonrandomized clinical trial of palivizumab suggest that preventing or moderating the severity of RSV infections in infancy also reduces subsequent asthma (85). Clinical trials have also been conducted to determine whether early treatment of children with virus-induced wheezing with asthma control medications might lessen the risk of asthma. Unfortunately, neither montelukast nor inhaled corticosteroids modify the risk of recurrent wheezing or asthma in high-risk children (86,87). Furthermore, treatment of children with bronchiolitis with systemic steroid has little or no effect on either the acute illness or the risk of recurrent wheeze. One possible exception is the case of HRV bronchiolitis. In a single study, treatment of infants with systemic corticosteroid during acute wheezing illnesses caused by HRV, but not RSV, reduces the subsequent risk of recurrent wheeze (88). Collectively, these findings provide hope that prevention or early treatment of viral LRI in early childhood could reduce long-term morbidity related to asthma.

V. Conclusions

There is no doubt that viral respiratory infections cause nearly all wheezing illnesses in infancy and are usually detected in episodes of recurrent wheezing and in children with acute asthma exacerbations. Although circumstantial evidence is mounting, it is still uncertain as to whether viral infections actually cause asthma. Prospective randomized interventional trials to prevent viral infections and assess effects on asthma prevention are needed to test this hypothesis. Passive immunization to prevent RSV is available, although not yet economically practical for widespread use. Preventive treatments for HRV and other common causes of wheezing illnesses in infancy are not yet available and represent a major unmet need for the health of infants and young children.

Acknowledgement

NIH NIAID U19 AI070503-01, RFP/contract NIH-NIAID-DAIT-02-11, and NIH-NHLBI P01 HL070831.

References

1. Lemanske RF Jr., Jackson DJ, Gangnon RE, et al. Rhinovirus illnesses during infancy predict subsequent childhood wheezing. J Allergy Clin Immunol 2005; 116:571–577.
2. Jartti T, van den HB, Garofalo RP, et al. Metapneumovirus and acute wheezing in children. Lancet 2002; 360:1393–1394.
3. Legg JP, Warner JA, Johnston SL, et al. Frequency of detection of picornaviruses and seven other respiratory pathogens in infants. Pediatr Infect Dis J 2005; 24:611–616.
4. Chung JY, Han TH, Kim SW, et al. Detection of viruses identified recently in children with acute wheezing. J Med Virol 2007; 79:1238–1243.
5. Ren L, Gonzalez R, Xie Z, et al. WU and KI polyomavirus present in the respiratory tract of children, but not in immunocompetent adults. J Clin Virol 2008; 43:330–333.
6. Bosis S, Esposito S, Niesters HG, et al. Role of respiratory pathogens in infants hospitalized for a first episode of wheezing and their impact on recurrences. Clin Microbiol Infect 2008; 14:677–684.
7. Kusel MM, de Klerk N, Holt PG, et al. Occurrence and management of acute respiratory illnesses in early childhood. J Paediatr Child Health 2007; 43:139–146.
8. Gern JE, Brooks GD, Meyer P, et al. Bidirectional interactions between viral respiratory illnesses and cytokine responses in the first year of life. J Allergy Clin Immunol 2006; 117:72–78.
9. Jartti T, Lee WM, Pappas T, et al. Serial viral infections in infants with recurrent respiratory illnesses. Eur Respir J 2008; 32:314–320.
10. Englund JA. Prevention strategies for respiratory syncytial virus: passive and active immunization. J Pediatr 1999; 135:38–44.
11. Lamprecht CL, Krause HE, Mufson MA. Role of maternal antibody in pneumonia and bronchiolitis due to respiratory syncytial virus. J Infect Dis 1976; 134:211–217.
12. Shay DK, Holman RC, Roosevelt GE, et al. Bronchiolitis-associated mortality and estimates of respiratory syncytial virus-associated deaths among US children, 1979–1997. J Infect Dis 2001; 183:16–22.
13. Shay DK, Holman RC, Newman RD, et al. Bronchiolitis-associated hospitalizations among US children, 1980–1996. JAMA 1999; 282:1440–1446.
14. Spann KM, Tran KC, Collins PL. Effects of nonstructural proteins NS1 and NS2 of human respiratory syncytial virus on interferon regulatory factor 3, NF-kappaB, and proinflammatory cytokines. J Virol 2005; 79:5353–5362.
15. Johnson JE, Gonzales RA, Olson SJ, et al. The histopathology of fatal untreated human respiratory syncytial virus infection. Mod Pathol 2007; 20:108–119.
16. Moore ML, Chi MH, Luongo C, et al. A chimeric A2 strain respiratory syncytial virus (RSV) with the fusion protein of RSV strain line 19 exhibits enhanced viral load, mucus, and airway dysfunction. J Virol 2009; 83(9):4185–4194.

17. Turner RB. Rhinovirus: more than just a common cold virus. J Infect Dis 2007; 195:765–766.
18. Kiang D, Kalra I, Yagi S, et al. An assay for 5' noncoding region analysis of all human rhinovirus prototype strains. J Clin Microbiol 2008; 46(11):3736–3745.
19. McErlean P, Shackelton LA, Andrews E, et al. Distinguishing molecular features and clinical characteristics of a putative new rhinovirus species, human rhinovirus C (HRV C). PLoS ONE 2008; 3:e1847.
20. Renwick N, Schweiger B, Kapoor V, et al. A recently identified rhinovirus genotype is associated with severe respiratory-tract infection in children in Germany. J Infect Dis 2007; 196:1754–1760.
21. Lee WM, Kiesner C, Pappas T, et al. A diverse group of previously unrecognized human rhinoviruses are common causes of respiratory illnesses in infants. PLoS ONE 2007; 2:e966.
22. Lau SK, Yip CC, Tsoi HW, et al. Clinical features and complete genome characterization of a distinct human rhinovirus (HRV) genetic cluster, probably representing a previously undetected HRV species, HRV-C, associated with acute respiratory illness in children. J Clin Microbiol 2007; 45:3655–3664.
23. Kistler A, Avila PC, Rouskin S, et al. Pan-viral screening of respiratory tract infections in adults with and without asthma reveals unexpected human coronavirus and human rhinovirus diversity. J Infect Dis 2007; 196:817–825.
24. Lamson D, Renwick N, Kapoor V, et al. MassTag polymerase chain-reaction detection of respiratory pathogens, including a new rhinovirus genotype, that caused influenza-like illness in New York State during 2004–2005. J Infect Dis 2006; 194:1398–1402.
25. Palmenberg AC, Spiro D, Kuzmickas R, et al. Sequencing and analyses of all known human rhinovirus genomes reveals structure and evolution. Science 2009; 324(5923):55–59.
26. Miller EK, Edwards KM, Weinberg GA, et al. A novel group of rhinoviruses is associated with asthma hospitalizations. J Allergy Clin Immunol 2009; 123:98–104.
27. McFadden ER Jr., Pichurko BM, Bowman HF, et al. Thermal mapping of the airways in humans. J Appl Physiol 1985; 58:564–570.
28. Gern JE, Galagan DM, Jarjour NN, et al. Detection of rhinovirus RNA in lower airway cells during experimentally-induced infection. Am J Respir Crit Care Med 1997; 155:1159–1161.
29. Papadopoulos NG, Bates PJ, Bardin PG, et al. Rhinoviruses infect the lower airways. J Infect Dis 2000; 181:1875–1884.
30. Mosser AG, Vrtis R, Burchell L, et al. Quantitative and qualitative analysis of rhinovirus infection in bronchial tissues. Am J Respir Crit Care Med 2005; 171:645–651.
31. Simons E, Schroth MK, Gern JE. Analysis of tracheal secretions for rhinovirus during natural colds. Pediatr Allergy Immunol 2005; 16:276–278.
32. Miller EK, Lu X, Erdman DD, et al. Rhinovirus-associated hospitalizations in young children. J Infect Dis 2007; 195:773–781.
33. Kusel MM, de Klerk NH, Holt PG, et al. Role of respiratory viruses in acute upper and lower respiratory tract illness in the first year of life: a birth cohort study. Pediatr Infect Dis J 2006; 25:680–686.
34. Johnston SL, Sanderson G, Pattemore PK, et al. Use of polymerase chain reaction for diagnosis of picornavirus infection in subjects with and without respiratory symptoms. J Clin Microbiol 1993; 31:111–117.
35. Rakes GP, Arruda E, Ingram JM, et al. Rhinovirus and respiratory syncytial virus in wheezing children requiring emergency care. IgE and eosinophil analyses. Am J Respir Crit Care Med 1999; 159:785–790.
36. Simoes EA. RSV disease in the pediatric population: epidemiology, seasonal variability, and long-term outcomes. Manag Care 2008; 17:3–6, discussion 18–19.
37. Martinez FD, Wright AL, Taussig LM, et al. Group Health Medical Associates: asthma and wheezing in the first six years of life. N Engl J Med 1995; 332:133–138.

38. Singh AM, Moore PE, Gern JE, et al. Bronchiolitis to asthma: a review and call for studies of gene-virus interactions in asthma causation. Am J Respir Crit Care Med 2007; 175:108–119.
39. Helminen M, Nuolivirta K, Virta M, et al. IL-10 gene polymorphism at -1082 A/G is associated with severe rhinovirus bronchiolitis in infants. Pediatr Pulmonol 2008; 43:391–395.
40. Camargo CA Jr., Rifas-Shiman SL, Litonjua AA, et al. Maternal intake of vitamin D during pregnancy and risk of recurrent wheeze in children at 3 y of age. Am J Clin Nutr 2007; 85:788–795.
41. Lemanske RF Jr. The childhood origins of asthma (COAST) study. Pediatr Allergy Immunol 2002; 13(suppl 15):38–43.
42. Sly PD, Boner AL, Bjorksten B, et al. Early identification of atopy in the prediction of persistent asthma in children. Lancet 2008; 372:1100–1106.
43. Stein RT, Sherrill D, Morgan WJ, et al. Respiratory syncytial virus in early life and risk of wheeze and allergy by age 13 years. Lancet 1999; 354:541–545.
44. Wu P, Dupont WD, Griffin MR, et al. Evidence of a causal role of winter virus infection during infancy in early childhood asthma. Am J Respir Crit Care Med 2008; 178:1123–1129.
45. Carroll KN, Wu P, Gebretsadik T, et al. Season of infant bronchiolitis and estimates of subsequent risk and burden of early childhood asthma. J Allergy Clin Immunol 2009; 123(4): 964–966.
46. Kotaniemi-Syrjanen A, Vainionpaa R, Reijonen TM, et al. Rhinovirus-induced wheezing in infancy–the first sign of childhood asthma? J Allergy Clin Immunol 2003; 111:66–71.
47. Hyvarinen MK, Kotaniemi-Syrjanen A, Reijonen TM, et al. Teenage asthma after severe early childhood wheezing: an 11-year prospective follow-up. Pediatr Pulmonol 2005; 40:316–323.
48. Jackson DJ, Gangnon RE, Evans MD, et al. Wheezing rhinovirus illnesses in early life predict asthma development in high-risk children. Am J Respir Crit Care Med 2008; 178:667–672.
49. Kusel MM, de Klerk NH, Kebadze T, et al. Early-life respiratory viral infections, atopic sensitization, and risk of subsequent development of persistent asthma. J Allergy Clin Immunol 2007; 119:1105–1110.
50. Strachan DP. Hay fever, hygiene, and household size. BMJ 1989; 299:1259–1260.
51. Bufford JD, Gern JE. The hygiene hypothesis revisited. Immunol Allergy Clin North Am 2005; 25:247–262.
52. Schaub B, Lauener R, von Mutius E. The many faces of the hygiene hypothesis. J Allergy Clin Immunol 2006; 117:969–977.
53. Gern JE, Rosenthal LA, Sorkness RL, et al. Effects of viral respiratory infections on lung development and childhood asthma. J Allergy Clin Immunol 2005; 115:668–674.
54. Taussig LM, Wright AL, Holberg CJ, et al. Tucson children's respiratory study: 1980 to present. J Allergy Clin Immunol 2003; 111:661–675.
55. Illi S, von ME, Lau S, Niggemann B, et al. Perennial allergen sensitisation early in life and chronic asthma in children: a birth cohort study. Lancet 2006; 368:763–770.
56. Kulig M, Bergmann R, Tacke U, et al. Long-lasting sensitization to food during the first two years precedes allergic airway disease. The MAS Study Group, Germany. Pediatr Allergy Immunol 1998; 9:61–67.
57. Guilbert TW, Morgan WJ, Zeiger RS, et al. Atopic characteristics of children with recurrent wheezing at high risk for the development of childhood asthma. J Allergy Clin Immunol 2004; 114:1282–1287.
58. Lowe AJ, Hosking CS, Bennett CM, et al. Skin prick test can identify eczematous infants at risk of asthma and allergic rhinitis. Clin Exp Allergy 2007; 37:1624–1631.
59. Castro-Rodriguez JA, Holberg CJ, Wright AL, et al. A clinical index to define risk of asthma in young children with recurrent wheezing. Am J Respir Crit Care Med 2000; 162:1403–1406.
60. Mosser AG, Brockman-Schneider RA, Amineva SP, et al. Similar frequency of rhinovirus-infectable cells in upper and lower airway epithelium. J Infect Dis 2002; 185:734–743.

61. Arruda E, Boyle TR, Winther B, et al. Localization of human rhinovirus replication in the upper respiratory tract by in situ hybridization. J Infect Dis 1995; 171:1329–1333.
62. Edwards MR, Slater L, Johnston SL. Signalling pathways mediating type I interferon gene expression. Microbes Infect 2007; 9:1245–1251.
63. Edwards MR, Hewson CA, Laza-Stanca V, et al. Protein kinase R, IkappaB kinase-beta and NF-kappaB are required for human rhinovirus induced pro-inflammatory cytokine production in bronchial epithelial cells. Mol Immunol 2007; 44:1587–1597.
64. Alexopoulou L, Holt AC, Medzhitov R, et al. Recognition of double-stranded RNA and activation of NF-kappaB by toll-like receptor 3. Nature 2001; 413:732–738.
65. Gern JE, French DA, Grindle KA, et al. Double-stranded RNA induces the synthesis of specific chemokines by bronchial epithelial cells. Am J Respir Cell Mol Biol 2003; 28:731–737.
66. Hall DJ, Bates ME, Guar L, et al. The role of p38 MAPK in rhinovirus-induced monocyte chemoattractant protein-1 production by monocytic-lineage cells. J Immunol 2005; 174: 8056–8063.
67. Korpi-Steiner NL, Bates ME, Lee WM, et al. Human rhinovirus induces robust IP-10 release by monocytic cells, which is independent of viral replication but linked to type I interferon receptor ligation and STAT1 activation. J Leukoc Biol 2006; 80:1364–1374.
68. Davoine F, Cao M, Wu Y, et al. Virus-induced eosinophil mediator release requires antigen-presenting and CD4+ T cells. J Allergy Clin Immunol 2008; 122:69–77.
69. Copenhaver CC, Gern JE, Li Z, et al. Cytokine response patterns, exposure to viruses, and respiratory infections in the first year of life. Am J Respir Crit Care Med 2004; 170:175–180.
70. Stern DA, Guerra S, Halonen M, et al. Low IFN-gamma production in the first year of life as a predictor of wheeze during childhood. J Allergy Clin Immunol 2007; 120:835–841.
71. Tang MLK, Kemp AS, Thorburn J, et al. Reduced interferon-g production in neonates and subsequent atopy. Lancet 1994; 344:983–985.
72. Holt PG, Sly PD. Interactions between respiratory tract infections and atopy in the aetiology of asthma. Eur Respir J 2002; 19:538–545.
73. Papadopoulos NG, Stanciu LA, Papi A, et al. A defective type 1 response to rhinovirus in atopic asthma. Thorax 2002; 57:328–332.
74. Contoli M, Message SD, Laza-Stanca V, et al. Role of deficient type III interferon-lambda production in asthma exacerbations. Nat Med 2006; 12:1023–1026.
75. Wark PA, Johnston SL, Bucchieri F, et al. Asthmatic bronchial epithelial cells have a deficient innate immune response to infection with rhinovirus. J Exp Med 2005; 201:937–947.
76. Lee CG, Yoon HJ, Zhu Z, et al. Respiratory syncytial virus stimulation of vascular endothelial cell growth Factor/Vascular permeability factor. Am J Respir Cell Mol Biol 2000; 23:662–669.
77. Leigh R, Oyelusi W, Wiehler S, et al. Human rhinovirus infection enhances airway epithelial cell production of growth factors involved in airway remodeling. J Allergy Clin Immunol 2008; 121:1238–1245.
78. Sanders SP. Asthma, viruses, and nitric oxide. Proc Soc Exp Biol Med 1999; 220:123–132.
79. Dosanjh A. Transforming growth factor-beta expression induced by rhinovirus infection in respiratory epithelial cells. Acta Biochim Biophys Sin (Shanghai) 2006; 38:911–914.
80. Dosanjh A, Rednam S, Martin M. Respiratory syncytial virus augments production of fibroblast growth factor basic in vitro: implications for a possible mechanism of prolonged wheezing after infection. Pediatr Allergy Immunol 2003; 14:437–440.
81. Tortorolo L, Langer A, Polidori G, et al. Neurotrophin overexpression in lower airways of infants with respiratory syncytial virus infection. Am J Respir Crit Care Med 2005; 172:233–237.
82. Bartlett NW, Walton RP, Edwards MR, et al. Mouse models of rhinovirus-induced disease and exacerbation of allergic airway inflammation. Nat Med 2008; 14:199–204.
83. Newcomb DC, Sajjan US, Nagarkar DR, et al. Human rhinovirus 1B exposure induces phosphatidylinositol 3-kinase-dependent airway inflammation in mice. Am J Respir Crit Care Med 2008; 177:1111–1121.

84. Brockman-Schneider RA, Amineva SP, Bulat MV, et al. Serial culture of murine primary airway epithelial cells and ex vivo replication of human rhinoviruses. J Immunol Methods 2008; 339(2):264–269.
85. Simoes EA, Groothuis JR, Carbonell-Estrany X, et al. Palivizumab prophylaxis, respiratory syncytial virus, and subsequent recurrent wheezing. J Pediatr 2007; 151:34–42.
86. Guilbert TW, Morgan WJ, Zeiger RS, et al. Long-term inhaled corticosteroids in preschool children at high risk for asthma. N Engl J Med 2006; 354:1985–1997.
87. Bisgaard H, Flores-Nunez A, Goh A, et al. Study of montelukast for the treatment of respiratory symptoms of post-respiratory syncytial virus bronchiolitis in children. Am J Respir Crit Care Med 2008; 178:854–860.
88. Lehtinen P, Ruohola A, Vanto T, et al. Prednisolone reduces recurrent wheezing after a first wheezing episode associated with rhinovirus infection or eczema. J Allergy Clin Immunol 2007; 119:570–575.

8

Bacterial Respiratory Infections and Asthma

E. RAND SUTHERLAND
National Jewish Health and University of Colorado Health Sciences Center, Denver, Colorado, U.S.A.

I. Introduction

There is a growing body of literature to suggest that *Mycoplasma pneumoniae* and *Chlamydophila pneumoniae* (formerly *Chlamydia pneumoniae*), two "atypical" bacteria, are important cofactors in patients with asthma, potentially with regard both to asthma onset and asthma phenotype (1). Additionally, more "typical" bacterial pathogens, such as *Streptococcus pneumoniae*, *Moraxella catarrhalis*, and *Haemophilus influenzae* may be implicated in elevating asthma risk in young children as well. This chapter will discuss the data and the challenges faced in elucidating the relationship between bacterial infection and asthma with regard to issues such as animal models, methods of detection, and controversies surrounding the importance of infectious agents relative to other risk factors in the pathogenesis and prognosis of asthma.

II. Respiratory Tract Infection and Asthma Pathogenesis

The exact role of respiratory tract infections in asthma pathogenesis is controversial, but basic scientific, epidemiologic, and clinical research support the conclusion that there is an association between early childhood respiratory infection and asthma. Two distinct observations have been made at the clinical level: (*i*) early childhood respiratory tract infections, especially those occurring before six months of age, are associated with wheezing during active infection (2), and (*ii*) patients with recurrent wheezing and diminished lung function often have a history of respiratory tract infections in early life (3). These observations have led to the conclusion that childhood respiratory tract infections may predispose to subsequent asthma, although ongoing research is evaluating whether viral or bacterial infections are associated with differential risk in this regard.

Although evidence suggests that early-life respiratory tract infection elevates subsequent asthma risk, other studies have indicated that these infections may actually protect against the subsequent development of asthma (4). These investigators postulate that bacterial and viral infections occurring during the first six months of life provide important signals to the developing immune system, deviating the immunologic phenotype to a predominantly T_h1 or a more balanced $T_h1:T_h2$ phenotype in response to intracellular bacteria and viruses, resulting in reduced immunoglobulin E (IgE) synthesis and a less prominent "allergic" response (5,6).

Longitudinal studies such as the Tucson Children's Respiratory Study have contributed importantly to our understanding with regard to the relationship between infection and wheeze or asthma, particularly with regard to a potential protective effect of infection. For example, Martinez and colleagues reported that a history of recurrent nonwheezing respiratory tract infections was associated with decreased levels of serum IgE and skin test reactivity (7), and similar conclusions were drawn by Ball and colleagues from their questionnaire study of asthma incidence and wheezing prevalence in children participating in the Tucson cohort (8). They found that the presence of one or more older siblings at home (which presumably increases the exposure of the youngest child to infectious agents) appeared to protect against the development of asthma (on the basis of a parent-reported doctor's diagnosis of asthma or a reported exacerbation within the previous year), with an adjusted relative risk of 0.8 per older sibling [95% confidence interval (CI), 0.7–1.0; $p = 0.04$]. Attendance at day care within the first six months of life was also associated with a reduction in the risk of subsequent asthma, with an adjusted relative risk of 0.4 (95% CI, 0.2–1.0; $p = 0.04$). Serum IgE levels were reported as being lower in children with two or more older siblings or day care exposure, with a relative risk of high IgE (serum levels above the 95th percentile) of 0.8 (relative risk 0.8; 95% CI, 0.6–1.0; $p = 0.03$).

While the authors concluded that their results confirmed the observation that early-life infectious exposure protects against the later development of asthma, they also reported the conflicting observation that children with increased exposure to others at home or day care were more likely to demonstrate frequent (parent-reported) wheezing at age two years than children with little or no exposure (adjusted relative risk 1.4; 95% CI, 1.1–1.8; $p = 0.01$), although this wheezing was less likely to persist in these children from ages six through thirteen years (8). These observations bring forth the potentially important interaction between infection and allergy in modifying clinical expression of asthma and wheezing. This interaction appears to be a key in the development of the asthma phenotype, although much work remains to be done to further clarify this relationship.

In attempts to delineate the relative importance of infection and allergic sensitization, a significant body of research has focused on the role of viral pathogens in inducing both acute and chronic airway inflammation and airway responsiveness, and this topic is addressed extensively elsewhere in this volume. The relative importance of typical and atypical bacterial pathogens in chronic asthma is less well established but is an area of active interest by multiple investigators, and one which is being enhanced by the development of novel molecular methods to detect bacteria in the lower airways.

III. Studies of Typical Bacteria and Asthma

A recent example of prospective cohort studies suggesting that bacterial infection may play a role in the onset of asthma in children comes from the Copenhagen Prospective Study on Asthma in Childhood (9), in which investigators evaluated the relationship between early-life colonization with bacteria such as *H. influenzae*, *M. catarrhalis*, *Staphylococcus aureus*, *S. pneumoniae*, and *S. pyogenes* and the risk of developing recurrent wheeze or asthma in the first five years of life (10). In this study, hypopharyngeal sampling was performed in 321 asymptomatic infants in the first month of life and at age 12 months, and the samples were then cultured for the organisms noted above. The investigators, blinded to the results of the respiratory cultures, then assessed the development of clinical end points such as persistent wheeze or other respiratory symptoms over the course of the study and the development of asthma at age five years (defined by the presence of typical symptoms and treatment with both an inhaled cor-ticosteroid and a rescue bronchodilator).

Rates of bacterial colonization at one month of age ranged from <1% for *S. pyogenes* to 61% with *Staphylococcus aureus*, and 21% of the participants were colonized with one or more of *H. influenzae, M. catarrhalis*, or *S. pneumoniae*. Although there were no clinically significant differences between infants who were and were not colonized with these three organisms at birth, the risk of wheeze was found to be increased in infants colonized with one or more of *H. influenzae, M. catarrhalis*, or *S. pneumoniae*, with an adjusted hazard ratio of developing persistent wheeze of 2.01 (95% CI, 1.13–3.57). Colonization with these organisms also significantly increased the risk of being hospitalized with wheeze, with an adjusted hazard ratio of 3.57 (1.55–8.23). At five years of age, the prevalence of asthma was 33% in colonized children and 14% in culture-negative children, with an odds ratio of 4.57 (2.18–9.57). Significant differences in lung function (airway resistance) were not demonstrated, while elevations of total IgE and blood eosinophil counts (both measured at four years) were observed in colonized infants. Finally, the relationship between colonization and asthma-related phenotypes was time dependent, as similar outcomes were not able to be demonstrated with regard to culture positivity at 12 months of age (10).

The investigators suggested that their findings appeared to be relevant in the context of prior observations that young children with severe recurrent wheeze are more likely to manifest a neutrophil-predominant airway inflammatory phenotype (11,12) and that children with early-onset wheezing have an airway inflammatory phenotype that appears to differ from that of patients with asthma that begins later in life (12). Although the phenotypic characterization study of Krawiec and colleagues, which demonstrated that young children with wheeze demonstrate a relative increase in macrophages and neutrophils in the lavage fluid, excluded acute lower airway bacterial infection, as defined by culture of bronchoalveolar lavage (BAL), the cellular com-position of BAL fluid was similar to that observed in the inflammatory phenotype characterization study of Marguet and colleagues (13), in which the majority of patients with infantile wheeze demonstrated BAL culture positivity for one or more bacteria. Therefore, the findings of Bisgaard and colleagues appear to support prior assertions (14) that bacterial colonization of the upper airway is associated with the initiation of inflammatory events, which lead to the development of wheeze and, ultimately, asthma.

Little is known, however, about how bacterial colonization might interact with host processes to increase the likelihood of developing asthma, although von Mutius has proposed that bacterial colonization in the first month of life may be reflective of a defective innate immune response (15). Specifically, alterations in the development of T_h1-associated immune responses could either increase risk of infection with bacteria or viruses or reduce the ability to clear these infections, perhaps mediated by genetic variation in toll-like receptor 2 (TLR2) (16).

A. *Mycoplasma pneumoniae*: Biology and Relevance to Asthma

M. pneumoniae, a common cause of atypical pneumonia and tracheobronchitis (17), attaches to ciliated airway epithelial cells by means of a terminal organelle, infecting the cell and causing epithelial damage and ciliary dysfunction (18). Evidence linking

M. pneumoniae to new-onset wheezing, exacerbations of prevalent asthma, and long-term decrements in lung function suggest that this organism can play an important role in asthma.

Reports in the late 1930s (19) and early 1940s (20) noted that some cases of acute pneumonitis in young adults were atypical in both their clinical course and lack of response to antibiotics. In 1944, Eaton and colleagues demonstrated the infectious nature of an agent of atypical pneumonia (21), which was later observed by Marmion and Goodburn to be similar to that of *M. mycoides*, the agent that causes contagious bovine pleuropneumonia (22). In 1961, Koch's postulates were satisfied after laboratory-isolated *M. pneumoniae* were used to infect human volunteers, resulting in atypical pneumonia (23). *M. pneumoniae* is now known as an important cause of pneumonia, tracheo-bronchitis, and pharyngitis (24) and has been associated with a variety of extrapulmonary manifestations, including articular, hepatopancreatic, exanthematic, cardiovascular, and central nervous system syndromes (24,25).

Mycoplasmas have a filamentous shape with specialized polar tip organelles, which facilitate attachment to host target cells by means of adhesion proteins called adhesins (25). Cell adherence is the initial step in mycoplasma infection, which is followed by the potential for induction of a wide range of immunomodulatory events, including lymphocyte activation and cytokine production (17). Adhesins share signifi-cant sequence homology with mammalian structural proteins, which may trigger an "anti-self" response to structural proteins such as myosin, keratin, and fibrinogen (25) and form the basis for bacterially mediated autoimmune disease.

Mycoplasmas are fastidious organisms, which are highly dependent on the sur-rounding host or culture microenvironment for growth. Mycoplasmas appear to be capable of fusing with host cells because of characteristics of their cholesterol-containing cell membranes, and their intracellular location allows them to survive long courses of appropriate antibiotic treatment (17). Intact mycoplasmas have been demonstrated in the cytoplasm and perinuclear regions of human cells both in vitro and in vivo (24).

The absence of an acute antibody response to *M. pneumoniae* has been reported both in acute infections and in more chronic infections/colonization (26,27). In adults and children with community-acquired pneumonia, up to 6% of subjects will demon-strate evidence of infection by polymerase chain reaction (PCR) analysis or culture while remaining seronegative (28). In 1999, Dorigo-Zetsma and colleagues reported the results of a study in which they prospectively compared the utility of PCR, culture, and serology for the diagnosis of *M. pneumoniae* respiratory tract infection in children (29). In the setting of active respiratory tract infection and using a "gold standard" for active *M. pneumoniae* infection of positive culture and/or positive complement fixation, they demonstrated a sensitivity of PCR of 78%, with specificity and positive predictive values of 100%. IgM immunofluorescence antibody (IFA) testing demonstrated a sen-sitivity equal to that of PCR, but it had a specificity of 92% and a positive predictive value of only 57%. The authors concluded that the IgM IFA should not be utilized as a single assay to make the diagnosis of acute mycoplasma infection and that the sensitivity of PCR is increased when used in concert with complement fixation assays (29).

The test characteristics described above have been determined in the setting of acute infection, where the organism load is presumably higher than that seen in states of chronic mycoplasma colonization. The diagnosis of active *M. pneumoniae* infection becomes more challenging in states where chronic carriage, with lower total organism burdens, is the case. This is particularly important in asthma, where *M. pneumoniae* has been reported to be present in the airways of approximately 55% of subjects with persistent stable asthma (27). Detection of *M. pneumoniae* in these subjects was by PCR; the organism was unable to be cultured from lower respiratory specimens of any subjects, reflecting the observation that culture of *M. pneumoniae* from the airways of chronic asthmatics has been an ineffective means of detecting the pathogen. In fact, culture was the least sensitive of the methods used to detect mycoplasma in the cohort of Kraft and colleagues (27). This is likely due to a combination of factors, including the organism's extreme fastidiousness and dependence on an intracellular environment for growth, as well as the low level of organisms present in the airways of subjects without acute infection. Although culture methods are now well standardized, the low burden of organisms in the setting of chronic infection further complicates the diagnosis of this infection by culture alone. Similar findings in asthma were reported in 2001, when Martin and colleagues (30) published their systematic evaluation of mycoplasma and chlamydophila infection in the upper and lower airways of adults with persistent stable asthma. The investigators evaluated 55 stable asthmatics and 11 normal controls for the presence of *M. pneumoniae* and *C. pneumoniae*, performing serology, culture, and PCR for these organisms on specimens obtained from the naso- and oropharynx, BAL, and endobronchial biopsy. *M. pneumoniae* or *C. pneumoniae* was detected by PCR in 56.4% of asthmatic subjects compared with 9% of controls ($p = 0.02$), but cultures for both organisms were negative in all subjects.

Important questions have been raised about the importance of *M. pneumoniae* in asthma, particularly with regard to what role it plays in modifying the clinical and/or inflammatory phenotypes in human subjects with asthma. *M. pneumoniae* is known to bind to TLR2 on airway epithelial cells, initiating an inflammatory response and increased expression of MUC5AC (31), the major mucin protein in the asthmatic airway (32). Kraft and colleagues cultured primary human airway epithelial cells obtained via bronchoscopy from patients with asthma and healthy control subjects and demonstrated that coculture of these cells with *M. pneumoniae* increased MUC5AC mRNA and protein expression in asthmatic, but not healthy, airway epithelial cells. This effect was attenuated by the addition of a nuclear factor–kappa B (NF-κB) inhibitor and a TLR2 inhibitor, suggesting that the mechanism of this upregulation of MUC5AC expression involves both TLR2 and NF-κB activation (32) and suggesting that *M. pneumoniae*, like other bacterial and viral respiratory pathogens (33,34), is an important inducer of airway mucin expression in asthma.

Although sporadic case reports have suggested that antecedent mycoplasma infection can be associated with subsequent development of asthma (35), a stronger and perhaps more clinically relevant association is the importance of *M. pneumoniae* as a precipitant of exacerbations in asthmatics. One example of this is the report by Lieberman and colleagues of a prospective study of atypical bacterial infections in patients hospitalized with acute asthma exacerbation, which demonstrated serologic evidence of acute *M. pneumoniae* infection in 18% of patients with an asthma exacerbation, compared with a prevalence of 3% in a matched control group ($p = 0.0006$) (36). In an earlier series of children with preexisting asthma, *M. pneumoniae* infection was similarly seen in 7 of 40 (18%) episodes of acute exacerbation (37).

In addition to causing a decrement in pulmonary function during acute infection, *M. pneumoniae* might also be associated with long-term impairment of pulmonary function in both asthmatics and nonasthmatics. In a series of 108 children with lower respiratory tract infection caused by *M. pneumoniae* (detected by increased complement fixation titers), 40% of subjects presented with wheezing as an initial clinical finding, and at both three months and three years of age, there were decrements in forced vital capacity (FVC) (93.1% vs. 100.8% of predicted, $p < 0.01$) and forced expiratory volume in one second (FEV_1) (94.5% vs. 100.6% of predicted, $p < 0.02$) in infected nonasthmatic subjects compared with controls (38). The reported strength of this association is variable; however, as a separate series of 50 children evaluated 1.5 to 9.5 years after clinical and radiographic recovery from *M. pneumoniae* pneumonia did not demonstrate persistent reductions in FVC or FEV_1 (39). A report by Kim and colleagues suggested a potential anatomic substrate for impaired lung function after acute *M. pneumoniae* pneumonia, in that high-resolution chest CT scanning performed in 37 children at a mean interval of 1.5 years after the episode of pneumonia demonstrated findings such as bronchial wall thickening, mosaic perfusion, and air trapping, features that were not seen in a control population of 17 children with mycoplasma upper airway infection (40).

B. *Chlamydophila pneumoniae*: Biology and Relevance to Asthma

The first clinical isolate of *C. pneumoniae* to cause respiratory disease AR-39 was isolated in 1983. *C. pneumoniae* was first thought to be a strain of *C. psittaci*, but subsequent investigation revealed it to be a separate species; there is <10% sequence homology between *C. pneumoniae* and other chlamydophilae, and its morphology differs as well.

Chlamydophilae are obligate intracellular pathogens, which survive in the host cell within the confines of a membrane-bound inclusion. Host cell invasion is affected by the elementary body of *C. pneumoniae*, which then differentiates to a more metabolically active reticulate body. This reticulate body then replicates by binary fission and ultimately returns to the elementary body form, which is then released from infected host cells to continue the cycle of infection and replication (41). Respiratory epithelium appears to be the primary target of *C. pneumoniae* infection, but other host cells including smooth muscle cells, vascular endothelium, and mononuclear cells can be infected by the organism in vitro (42).

Diagnostic techniques for *C. pneumoniae* vary somewhat from those utilized for *M. pneumoniae*. In the setting of acute respiratory tract infection, Gaydos and colleagues (43) evaluated PCR–enzyme immunoassay (PCR-EIA) and serology in 56 subjects with respiratory symptoms and 80 control subjects. Using a gold standard for diagnosis of either positive broth culture or positive direct fluorescent antibody (DFA), they reported a sensitivity of 74.2% and a specificity of 96.2% for PCR-EIA. Serology testing with microimmunofluorescence, using the criteria of Grayston and colleagues (IgM $\geq 1:16$ or IgG $\geq 1:512$) (44), did not perform as well. 75% of asymptomatic subjects had some level of antibody response to *C. pneumoniae*, and 18.8% of asymptomatic subjects had antibody levels considered to be diagnostic of acute infection with *C. pneumoniae*. The authors concluded that PCR-EIA was more reliable than serology for the diagnosis of acute *C. pneumoniae* infection (43). More recently, Verkooyen and colleagues, on the basis of the results of their prospective study of 156 subjects with community-acquired pneumonia, reported that recombinant lipopolysaccharide enzyme-linked immunosorbent assay may be the test of choice for diagnosis of acute *C. pneumoniae* infection and that microimmunofluorescence was the test of choice for the diagnosis of *C. pneumoniae* infection in the community (45).

Less information is available about the utility of these tests in individuals who are chronically infected. In the study of chronic stable asthmatics by Kraft and colleagues, a high prevalence (33%) of serologic response to *C. pneumoniae* was seen, whereas the prevalence of positive PCR and culture was lower or zero, respectively, perhaps because of a lower organism load than that seen in acute infection (27).

A number of potential explanations for these findings exist. In the general population, overall seropositivity for *C. pneumoniae* increases over each decade of life, with a peak prevalence of 50% to 60% seropositivity (46). This serves to reduce the sensitivity and specificity of serologic criteria for the diagnosis of acute infection in adults. The criteria that have been proposed for the serologic diagnosis of *C. pneumoniae* infection (particularly those using a single Ig titer) are arbitrary and may, in fact, lead to the overdiagnosis of acute *C. pneumoniae* infection in population-based studies, as described above. The serologic assays utilized for *C. pneumoniae* have also been complicated by cross-reactivity of antibodies to bacterial lipopolysaccharide antigens of a variety of different *Chlamydophila* species (47), making accurate identification of *C. pneumoniae* more difficult. In a recent study, Routes and colleagues reported a lack of correlation between *C. pneumoniae* antibody titers and adult-onset asthma, providing further indication that serology alone is an inadequate means of strengthening the evidence for a relationship between *C. pneumoniae* and asthma (48). Further studies are required to determine the most reliable means of detecting chronic infection with *C. pneumoniae* in subjects with asthma.

C. pneumoniae may result in chronic infections (49), and like *M. pneumoniae*, has been associated with subsequent wheezing illness. *C. pneumoniae* also causes exacerbations of preexisting asthma, as reported in case series such as that of Allegra and colleagues, where in a cohort of seventy adults presenting with asthma exacerbation, 10% were shown by serology to be acutely infected with *C. pneumoniae* (50). In a community-based cohort of 365 patients with lower respiratory tract illness, 47% of patients with acute *C. pneumoniae* infection were found to wheeze during the course of the infection, with a statistically significant dose-response relationship between the level of *C. pneumoniae* IgG titer and prevalence of wheezing in the cohort. There was also an association of *C. pneumoniae* antibody titers and subsequent development of "asthmatic bronchitis" after the acute illness, which was seen in 32% of cases (odds ratio = 7.2; 95% CI, 2.2–23.4) (51).

In the 2001 study of Martin and colleagues (30), 18 asthmatic subjects and one normal control had positive serologic results for *C. pneumoniae*. Of the 18, 10 had positive results by IgG, and 5 by IgM criteria, with 3 of the subjects demonstrating both positive IgG and positive IgM. However, only seven subjects had positive PCR results for *C. pneumoniae*, and of these, only three had positive serologic results. On the basis of these data, the authors concluded that a majority of adults with chronic, stable asthma are chronically infected with *M. pneumoniae* with a significantly greater frequency than nonasthmatic subjects and that serologic evaluation does not reliably indicate lower airway PCR status (30). At this time, more study is needed to evaluate whether chlamydophila infection is a pathogenic factor in asthma or merely an epiphenomenon somehow related to the enhanced airway inflammation seen in chronic asthma.

IV. Relevant Animal Models of Atypical Bacterial Infection

Although the topic of animal models of infection and asthma is reviewed in great detail in this volume, brief commentary on the relevance of certain animal experiments to human asthma is warranted. Although *M. pneumoniae* is not a natural mouse pathogen, Wubbel and colleagues demonstrated that intranasal introduction of *M. pneumoniae* into BALB/c mice results in acute respiratory tract infection on the basis of positive broth culture data from BAL specimens performed up to 15 days following infection (52). Murine infection with *M. pneumoniae* also results in an active immunologic response, with 62% of animals demonstrating ELISA evidence of *M. pneumoniae*–specific IgM production and 97% of animals demonstrating positive immunoblots for *M. pneumoniae*. Many animals also demonstrated histologic evidence of airway epithelial disruption following *M. pneumoniae* infection (52).

Pietsch and colleagues studied the inflammatory response of BALB/c mice during acute primary and secondary infection with *M. pneumoniae*. Following infection, the investigators evaluated in vivo cytokine gene expression in the spleens and lungs of these animals (53). During the acute phase of infection, the authors found elevated expression of tumor necrosis factor α (TNF-α), interleukin-1 (IL-1), IL-6, and interferon-γ (IFN-γ). IL-2 and IL-2 receptor gene expression was seen only during reinfection. Expression of cytokines also varied over the course of infection; IL-2 mRNA levels fell over the first 24 hours of infection and were not detectable after 24 hours, and IL-10 mRNA levels rose over this same period. Furthermore, during reinfection with *M. pneumoniae*, mRNA levels of IL-6 and TNF-α were 10-fold higher than those seen during acute infection. IFN-γ mRNA levels were 50-fold higher following reinfection than that following acute infection (53).

To investigate the relationship between timing of mycoplasma infection, allergic sensitization, and subsequent pulmonary physiologic and immune response, Chu and colleagues investigated the effect of experimental *M. pneumoniae* infection both before and after ovalbumin sensitization and challenge on airway hyperresponsiveness (AHR), lung inflammation, and protein levels of T_h1 and T_h2 cytokines in BALB/c mice. When experimental mycoplasma infection was instituted three days prior to ovalbumin sensitization and challenge, this sequence resulted in reduced AHR and reduction in lung inflammatory cell influx, and induced a predominantly T_h1 response with increases in the ratio of IFN-γ to the T_h2 cytokine IL-4 in the BAL fluid. Inoculation and infection with *M. pneumoniae* 48 hours after ovalbumin challenge initially caused a temporary reduction in AHR, followed by augmented AHR, lung inflammation score, and BAL IL-4 concentration with a concomitant reduction in BAL IFN-γ concentration. The authors concluded that mycoplasma infection can modulate physiologic and inflammatory responses to allergic airway inflammation and that their findings with regard to timing of infection versus allergic sensitization supported the "hygiene hypothesis" of asthma, in which protection against asthma and/or allergic diseases occurs in those experiencing infections early in life (i.e., prior to allergen sensitization) (54).

Although the data cited above suggest that mycoplasma could modulate events occurring early in the development of asthma, questions remain about what effect chronic infection might have on the airways over a long term. In a series of mouse experiments in which animals with experimental *M. pneumoniae* infections were followed for up to 56 days, Chu and colleagues investigated whether infection could lead to alterations in airway collagen deposition. In mice in whom infection was preceded by allergic sensitization and challenge, an increase in airway wall collagen deposition was observed at 42, but not 14, days post infection, a finding accompanied by increased lung expression of transforming growth factor (TGF)-β1 mRNA and protein (as evaluated by immunohistochemistry). In allergen-naive mice, mycoplasma infection did not alter airway wall collagen. Although these findings require further investigation, this study suggests that mycoplasma infection could, over a long term, modulate airway collagen deposition and thereby possibly airway fibrosis and remodeling (55).

Although no animal reservoir has been implicated in the transmission of *C. pneumoniae* (56), animal models of *C. pneumoniae* have been successfully established in mice, rabbits, and monkeys. Kishimoto and colleagues have demonstrated homogenous infection in mice following nasal inoculation with *C. pneumoniae*, with interstitial pneumonitis on the third day after inoculation, pneumonia on the fifth day, and a strong antibody response peaking three to four weeks following intranasal inoculation. These pathologic changes were observed for several weeks after the acute infection (57). Furthermore, *C. pneumoniae* DNA can be detected in lungs by PCR and in situ DNA hybridization, even after the organism can no longer be cultured from the lungs (58). *C. pneumonia* also appears to establish chronic latent infection in mice; if immunosuppressive medications such as corticosteroids are administered after recovery from primary infection, *C. pneumoniae* can once again be cultured from lung tissue within 14 days following immunosuppression with corticosteroids (59).

V. Antibiotics in the Treatment of Chronic Asthma

Antibiotics do not currently play a major role in the treatment of persistent stable asthma. There is emerging evidence, however, that symptoms and markers of airway inflammation may improve when patients who have atypical bacterial infection as a cofactor in their asthma are treated with macrolide antibiotics. In a double-blind protocol, Kraft and colleagues treated 55 asthmatics with chronic, stable asthma with clarithromycin (500 mg po b.i.d.) for six weeks. At the end of the treatment course, there was a significant improvement in FEV_1 in those who were PCR positive on endobronchial biopsy for either *M. pneumoniae* or *C. pneumoniae*, a clinical finding accompanied by reduction of TNF-α, IL-5, and IL-12 mRNA expression in BAL and of TNF-α mRNA expression in airway epithelial cells in these subjects (60). However, the observation that PCR positivity appeared to predict response to macrolide antibiotic therapy was a post hoc one, and the Asthma Clinical Research Network is conducting a PCR-stratified, prospective study (the Macrolides in Asthma trial, Clinicaltrials.gov identifier NCT00318708) to explore further the importance of PCR positivity in determining response to macrolide antibiotic therapy.

Pilot studies focusing on macrolide antibiotic treatment of subjects with chronic asthma who have positive serology for *C. pneumoniae* have been performed. In an open-label trial of 48 adults with stable persistent asthma published in 1995, Hahn and colleagues reported significant clinical improvement or complete remission of asthma symptoms after three to nine weeks of antibiotic therapy. In this study, the majority of subjects received azithromycin, although other antibiotics were used as well (61). In a follow-up study, these investigators conducted a community-based, randomized, placebo-controlled trial of azithromycin (600 mg po for three days, followed by 600 mg each week for five weeks) in subjects with persistent asthma. Macrolide antibiotic therapy did not result in a significant improvement by the Asthma Quality of Life Questionnaire, but there was a treatment-related improvement in asthma symptoms (62). As noted previously, the diagnosis of *C. pneumoniae* in study participants was based on serology alone, and only baseline serum IgA was associated with a positive treatment response. A similarly modest effect was observed in a six-week treatment trial of roxithromycin in 232 subjects with chronic asthma and serologic (IgG titer $\geq$1:64 or IgA titer $\geq$1:16) evidence of *C. pneumoniae* infection. Although numerically small, statistically significant increases in morning and evening peak flow rates were observed; these findings were not sustained at three and six months following the end of treatment (63).

VI. Summary

Mounting evidence from both animal and human studies suggests that bacterial infections are an important acquired factor in the pathogenesis and clinical expression of asthma. Ongoing research into the relationship between bacterial infection and asthma will elucidate questions about whether these infections are important in disease development and/or whether their prevalence is increased in asthmatics because of yet poorly understood mechanisms. Current studies will further define the role of macrolide antibiotics in the treatment of stable asthma, ultimately determining whether these therapeutic agents have a place in the management of stable asthma.

References

1. Sutherland ER, Martin RJ. Asthma and atypical bacterial infection. Chest 2007; 132:1962–1966.
2. Wright AL, Taussig LM, Ray CG, et al. The Tucson Children's Respiratory Study. II. Lower respiratory tract illness in the first year of life. Am J Epidemiol 1989; 129:1232–1246.
3. Castro-Rodriguez JA, Holberg CJ, Wright AL, et al. Association of radiologically ascertained pneumonia before age 3 yr with asthmalike symptoms and pulmonary function during childhood: a prospective study. Am J Respir Crit Care Med 1999; 159:1891–1897.
4. Shaheen SO, Aaby P, Hall AJ, et al. Measles and atopy in guinea-bissau. Lancet 1996; 347:1792–1796.
5. Holt PG. Environmental factors and primary t-cell sensitisation to inhalant allergens in infancy: reappraisal of the role of infections and air pollution. Pediatr Allergy Immunol 1995; 6:1–10.
6. Romagnani S. Human th1 and th2 subsets: regulation of differentiation and role in protection and immunopathology. Int Arch Allergy Immunol 1992; 98:279–285.
7. Martinez FD, Wright AL, Taussig LM, et al. Asthma and wheezing in the first six years of life. The group health medical associates. N Engl J Med 1995; 332:133–138.
8. Ball TM, Castro-Rodriguez JA, Griffith KA, et al. Siblings, day-care attendance, and the risk of asthma and wheezing during childhood. N Engl J Med 2000; 343:538–543.
9. Bisgaard H. The Copenhagen prospective study on asthma in childhood (copsac): design, rationale, and baseline data from a longitudinal birth cohort study. Ann Allergy Asthma Immunol 2004; 93:381–389.
10. Bisgaard H, Hermansen MN, Buchvald F, et al. Childhood asthma after bacterial colonization of the airway in neonates. N Engl J Med 2007; 357:1487–1495.
11. Saglani S, Malmstrom K, Pelkonen AS, et al. Airway remodeling and inflammation in symptomatic infants with reversible airflow obstruction. Am J Respir Crit Care Med 2005; 171:722–727.
12. Krawiec ME, Westcott JY, Chu HW, et al. Persistent wheezing in very young children is associated with lower respiratory inflammation. Am J Respir Crit Care Med 2001; 163:1338–1343.
13. Marguet C, Jouen-Boedes F, Dean TP, et al. Bronchoalveolar cell profiles in children with asthma, infantile wheeze, chronic cough, or cystic fibrosis. Am J Respir Crit Care Med 1999; 159:1533–1540.

14. Bisgaard H. Persistent wheezing in very young preschool children reflects lower respiratory inflammation. Am J Respir Crit Care Med 2001; 163:1290–1291.

15. von Mutius E. Of attraction and rejection—asthma and the microbial world. N Engl J Med 2007; 357:1545–1547.

16. Eder W, Klimecki W, Yu L, et al. Toll-like receptor 2 as a major gene for asthma in children of European farmers. J Allergy Clin Immunol 2004; 113:482–488.

17. Baseman JB, Tully JG. Mycoplasmas: sophisticated, reemerging, and burdened by their notoriety. Emerg Infect Dis 1997; 3:21–32.

18. Andersen P. Pathogenesis of lower respiratory tract infections due to Chlamydia, Mycoplasma, Legionella and viruses. Thorax 1998; 53:302–307.

19. Reimann HA. An acute infection of the respiratory tract with atypical pneumonia. JAMA 1938; 111:2377–2384.

20. Gallagher RJ. Acute pneumonitis: a report of 87 cases among adolescents. Yale J Biol Med 1941; 13:663–678.

21. Eaton M, Meiklejohn G, van Herick W. Studies on the etiology of primary atypical pneumonia: a filterable agent transmissible to cotton rats, hamsters, and chick embryos. J Exp Med 1944; 79:649–668.

22. Marmion B, Goodburn G. Effect of an organic gold salt on Eaton's primary atypical pneumonia agent and other observations. Nature 1961; 189:247–248.

23. Chanock R, Hayflick L, Barile M. Growth on artificial medium of an agent associated with atypical pneumonia and its identification as a PPLO. Proc Nat Acad of Sci U S A 1962; 48:41–49.

24. Baseman JB, Reddy SP, Dallo SF. Interplay between Mycoplasma surface proteins, airway cells, and the protean manifestations of Mycoplasma-mediated human infections. Am J Respir Crit Care Med 1996; 154:S137–S144.

25. Waites KB, Talkington DF. Mycoplasma pneumoniae and its role as a human pathogen. Clin Microbiol Rev 2004; 17:697–728.

26. Block S, Hedrick J, Hammerschlag MR, et al. Mycoplasma pneumoniae and Chlamydia pneumoniae in pediatric community-acquired pneumonia: comparative efficacy and safety of clarithromycin versus erythromycin ethylsuccinate. Pediatr Infect Dis J 1995; 14:471–477.

27. Kraft M, Cassell GH, Henson JE, et al. Detection of Mycoplasma pneumoniae in the airways of adults with chronic asthma. Am J Respir Crit Care Med 1998; 158:998–1001.

28. Marmion BP, Williamson J, Worswick PA, et al. Experience with newer techniques for the laboratory detection of Mycoplasma pneumoniae infection: Adelaide, 1978–1991. Clin Infect Dis 1993; 17:S90–S99.

29. Dorigo-Zetsma J, Zaat S, Wertheim-van Dillen P, et al. Comparison of PCR, culture, and serological tests for diagnosis of Mycoplasma pneumoniae respiratory tract infection in children. J Clin Microbiol 1999; 37:14–17.

30. Martin RJ, Kraft M, Chu HW, et al. A link between chronic asthma and chronic infection. J Allergy Clin Immunol 2001; 107:595–601.

31. Chu HW, Jeyaseelan S, Rino JG, et al. Tlr2 signaling is critical for Mycoplasma pneumoniae-induced airway mucin expression. J Immunol 2005; 174:5713–5719.

32. Kraft M, Adler KB, Ingram JL, et al. Mycoplasma pneumoniae induces airway epithelial cell expression of muc5ac in asthma. Eur Respir J 2008; 31:43–46.

33. Hashimoto K, Graham BS, Ho SB, et al. Respiratory syncytial virus in allergic lung inflammation increases muc5ac and gob-5. Am J Respir Crit Care Med 2004; 170:306–312.

34. Inoue D, Yamaya M, Kubo H, et al. Mechanisms of mucin production by rhinovirus infection in cultured human airway epithelial cells. Respir Physiol Neurobiol 2006; 154:484–499.

35. Yano T, Ichikawa Y, Komatu S, et al. Association of Mycoplasma pneumoniae antigen with initial onset of bronchial asthma. Am J Respir Crit Care Med 1994; 149:1348–1353.

36. Lieberman D, Printz S, Ben-Yaakov M, et al. Atypical pathogen infection in adults with acute exacerbation of bronchial asthma. Am J Respir Crit Care Med 2003; 167:406–410.

37. Berkovich S, Millian SJ, Snyder RD. The association of viral and Mycoplasma infections with recurrence of wheezing in the asthmatic child. Ann Allergy 1970; 28:43–49.
38. Sabato AR, Martin AJ, Marmion BP, et al. Mycoplasma pneumoniae: acute illness, antibiotics, and subsequent pulmonary function. Arch Dis Child 1984; 59:1034–1037.
39. Mok JY, Waugh PR, Simpson H. Mycoplasma pneumonia infection. A follow-up study of 50 children with respiratory illness. Arch Dis Child 1979; 54:506–511.
40. Kim CK, Chung CY, Kim JS, et al. Late abnormal findings on high-resolution computed tomography after Mycoplasma pneumonia. Pediatrics 2000; 105:372–378.
41. LaVerda D, Kalayoglu MV, Byrne GI. Chlamydial heat shock proteins and disease pathology: new paradigms for old problems? Infect Dis Obstet Gynecol 1999; 7:64–71.
42. Redecke V, Dalhoff K, Bohnet S, et al. Interaction of Chlamydia pneumoniae and human alveolar macrophages: infection and inflammatory response. Am J Respir Cell Mol Biol 1998; 19:721–727.
43. Gaydos CA, Roablin PM, Hammerschlag MR, et al. Diagnostic utility of PCR-enzyme immunoassay, culture and serology for detection of Chlamydia pneumoniae in symptomatic and asymptomatic patients. J Clin Microbiol 1994; 32:903–905.
44. Grayston JT, Campbell LA, Kuo CC, et al. A new respiratory tract pathogen: Chlamydia pneumoniae strain TWAR. J Infect Dis 1990; 161:618–625.
45. Verkooyen RP, Willemse D, Hiep-van Casteren SC, et al. Evaluation of PCR, culture, and serology for diagnosis of Chlamydia pneumoniae respiratory infections. J Clin Microbiol 1998; 36:2301–2307.
46. Grayston JT. Infections caused by Chlamydia pneumoniae strain TWAR. Clin Infect Dis 1992; 15:757–761.
47. Kern DG, Neill MA, Schachter J. A seroepidemiologic study of Chlamydia pneumoniae in Rhode Island: evidence of serologic cross-reactivity. Chest 1993; 104:208–213.
48. Routes JM, Nelson HS, Noda JA, et al. Lack of correlation between Chlamydia pneumoniae antibody titers and adult-onset asthma. J Allergy Clin Immunol 2000; 105:391–392.
49. Grayston JT, Kuo CC, Wang SP, et al. A new Chlamydia psittaci strain, TWAR, isolated in acute respiratory tract infections. N Engl J Med 1986; 315:161–168.
50. Allegra L, Blasi F, Centanni S, et al. Acute exacerbations of asthma in adults: role of Chlamydia pneumoniae infection. Eur Respir J 1994; 7:2165–2168.
51. Hahn DL, Dodge RW, Golubjatnikov R. Association of Chlamydia pneumoniae (strain TWAR) infection with wheezing, asthmatic bronchitis, and adult-onset asthma. JAMA 1991; 266:225–230.
52. Wubbel L, Jafri HS, Olsen K, et al. Mycoplasma pneumoniae pneumonia in a mouse model. J Infect Dis 1998; 178:1526–1529.
53. Pietsch K, Ehlers S, Jacobs E. Cytokine gene expression in the lungs of BALB/c mice during primary and secondary intranasal infection with Mycoplasma pneumoniae. Microbiology 1994; 140 (pt 8):2043–2048.
54. Chu HW, Honour JM, Rawlinson CA, et al. Effects of respiratory Mycoplasma pneumoniae infection on allergen-induced bronchial hyperresponsiveness and lung inflammation in mice. Infect Immun 2003; 71:1520–1526.
55. Chu HW, Rino JG, Wexler RB, et al. Mycoplasma pneumoniae infection increases airway collagen deposition in a murine model of allergic airway inflammation. Am J Physiol Lung Cell Mol Physiol 2005; 289:L125–L133.
56. Kuo CC, Jackson LA, Campbell LA, et al. Chlamydia pneumoniae (TWAR). Clin Microbiol Rev 1995; 8:451–461.
57. Kishimoto T. [Studies on Chlamydia pneumoniae, strain TWAR, infection. I. Experimental infection of C. pneumoniae in mice and serum antibodies against TWAR by MFA]. Kansen-shogaku Zasshi 1990; 64:124–131.

58. Kaukoranta-Tolvanen SE, Laurila AL, Saikku P, et al. Experimental Chlamydia pneumoniae infection in mice: effect of reinfection and passive immunization. Microb Pathog 1995; 18:279–288.
59. Malinverni R, Kuo CC, Campbell LA, et al. Reactivation of Chlamydia pneumoniae lung infection in mice by cortisone. J Infect Dis 1995; 172:593–594.
60. Kraft M, Cassell GH, Pak J, et al. Mycoplasma pneumoniae and Chlamydia pneumoniae in asthma: effect of clarithromycin. Chest 2002; 121:1782–1788.
61. Hahn DL. Treatment of Chlamydia pneumoniae infection in adult asthma: a before-after trial. J Fam Pract 1995; 41:345–351.
62. Hahn DL, Plane MB, Mahdi OS, et al. Secondary outcomes of a pilot randomized trial of azithromycin treatment for asthma. PLoS Clin Trials 2006; 1:e11.
63. Black PN, Blasi F, Jenkins CR, et al. Trial of roxithromycin in subjects with asthma and serological evidence of infection with Chlamydia pneumoniae. Am J Respir Crit Care Med 2001; 164:536–541.

9
Increased Susceptibility to Viral Infection at the Origins of Asthma

FERNANDO D. MARTINEZ
Arizona Respiratory Center, The University of Arizona, Tucson, Arizona, U.S.A.

I. Introduction

The association between viral infection and asthma has been the matter of great scrutiny and scientific and clinical interest. As will be reviewed below, it is now clearly established that infants who will go on to develop asthma later in life are more likely to have lower respiratory illnesses (LRI) triggered by infections with the respiratory syncytial virus (RSV) (1) and rhinoviruses (RV) (2). However, it has not yet been clearly established if this association is causal or if the LRI are an indication of a preexisting susceptibility to asthma and allergies. In older children and adults with asthma, viral infections, especially those due to RV, are also involved in most acute exacerbations of the disease (3), suggesting that subjects with asthma may have inappropriate inflammatory responses to RV and other viruses, but the nature of these alterations has not been elucidated.

The main objective of this review is to summarize our current knowledge about the potential determinants of the peculiar susceptibility of subjects with asthma to acute viral infections. The author has recently and extensively analyzed the association between viral infection in early life and subsequent development of asthma (4).

II. Morbidity Associated with Acute Asthma Exacerbations

The recent third version of the Guidelines for the Treatment of Asthma by the National Asthma Education and Prevention Panel (NAEPP) (5) introduced for the first time the concept that there are two dimensions to the clinical expression of the disease: impairment and risk. Whereas impairment considers the continuous day-to-day expression of the disease, risk includes mainly the development of acute worsening of symptoms beyond the more usual and less pronounced periodic variation, which is characteristic of asthma. These exacerbations are a prominent contributor to morbidity in both children and adults (6,7) and often require the use of oral corticosteroids, with their associated potential for long- and short-term side effects (8).

Studies of the natural history of asthma have shown that most cases of the disease begin during the first years of life (9). It is of great interest that, during the preschool school years, the most frequent expression of the disease is acute episodes of airway obstruction that mimic in duration and symptoms those occurring in older children and adults. These episodes account for the bulk of the morbidity and health care costs in this age group (10,11), and it is not possible to distinguish clinically between those occurring in children who will go on to develop asthma (so-called "persistent wheezers") and those affecting children with transient wheezing, who will grow out of their symptoms by the early school years (12). In both these phenotypes, however, periods between episodes are usually symptom-free, and in fact, the presence of more persistent respiratory morbidity (so-called "atypical wheezing") is indication for further diagnostic assessments (13). In this sense, the pattern of disease expression in this age group is very different from that of older children and adults.

Two recent longitudinal studies, one performed in Madison, Wisconsin, and the other one in Perth, Australia, have contributed important new information regarding the etiology of these acute episodes. In the Madison study, Lemanske et al. (2,14) observed that viruses could be recovered from nasal washes in 78% of infants with severe LRI and parental history of allergies, as compared with 31% of infants with no respiratory symptoms. More relevantly, viruses were recovered from 90% of all wheezing illnesses during the first three years of life (14). Thus, the proportion of wheezing episodes attributable to viral infection was approximately 60%. Similarly, in the Perth Study, Kusel and colleagues (15) assessed the potential viral etiology of acute respiratory illnesses in infants also at high risk for asthma and allergies. They could detect viruses (mainly RV and RSV) in nasopharyngeal aspirates of 68% to 70% of children with wheezing LRI, nonwheezing LRI, and upper respiratory illnesses (URI), and also in one-fourth of these same children at times when they had had no apparent respiratory illness for at least four weeks. These two studies thus confirmed and extended our findings from the early 1980s (16) and, by using much more sophisticated molecular diagnostics, stressed for the first time the major role of RV in acute episodes of airway obstruction in young children. Nevertheless, there was no difference in the viral etiology of LRI and URI in these children, suggesting that it is not the virus itself but the nature of the response to the virus that is of importance.

III. Early-Life Wheezing and Subsequent Asthma: Common Susceptibility to Viruses?

Until recently, little was known about the alterations that determined increased susceptibility to viral infections in children with recurrent wheezing episodes in early life. Some clues were provided by the same two studies in Madison and Perth quoted earlier. Both of these studies confirmed our own previous report that RSV infection during the first years of life is associated with a three- to fourfold risk of recurrent wheezing at the age of six years (1). Of note, our own studies followed these children with RSV infections in early life up to age 13 and showed that this risk decreased significantly with age, whereas data from the Madison and Perth studies are only available up to the age of six years. However, both these latter studies also showed that wheezing illnesses associated with RV infection were also strongly associated with increased risk of subsequent asthma. Of note, investigators in the Madison study used novel genomic technologies and identified rhinoviral subspecies not previously recognized as potential triggers of wheezing LRI (17). As a consequence, these investigators were able to determine that, when compared with children who did not have wheezing episodes in early life, those with RV wheezing were up to 10 times more likely to have asthma by the age of six years. Since the main cause of acute exacerbations of asthma after the age of three years is RV infections (18,19), these studies clearly suggested that a common, perhaps congenital susceptibility to RV infection could explain, at least in part, the connection between wheezing in early life and the subsequent development of asthma.

Recent longitudinal and cross-sectional studies have shed important new light into the nature of this shared susceptibility. Guerra et al. (20) showed that, when compared with children with no wheezing in the first year of life, those who had recurrent episodes of wheezing had lower interferon-γ responses by peripheral blood mononuclear cells stimulated nonspecifically during the first months of life. Moreover, Macaubas et al. (21) reported that detectable cord blood concentrations of IL-4 and interferon-γ were each associated with significantly lower risk of physician-diagnosed asthma, current asthma, and current wheeze at the age of six years. More recently, we showed that interferon-γ responses to nonspecific stimuli at a mean age of nine months were inversely related to the likelihood of having frequent wheezing episodes between the ages of 2 and 13 years (22). Taken together, these results suggested that either diminished interferon-γ responses themselves were responsible for the increased susceptibility to viral infection present in both wheezing young children and older children with asthma or they were a marker for other potential alterations in immune responses that explain the association.

Strong support for the latter conclusion has come from studies in which responses by type I interferons [i.e., interferon-α and interferon-β (23)] and type III interferon [i.e., interferon-λ also called IL-28a, IL-28b, IL-29 (24,25)] were assessed. Wark et al. examined virus replication and innate responses to RV-16 infection of primary bronchial epithelial cells from asthmatic and healthy controlled subjects (26). Viral RNA expression and late viral release into supernatance were increased 50 and 7 fold, respectively, in asthmatic cells compared with healthy controls. Examination of early innate immune responses revealed profound impairment of virus-induced interferon-β and mRNA expression in asthmatic cultures, which produced more than 2.5 times less interferon-β protein than normal cells. Contoli et al. (27), from the same laboratory, performed similar experiments and showed that bronchial epithelial cells from asthmatics had significantly diminished type III interferon responses as compared with cells from normal controls. Bufe et al. (28) assessed induced interferon-α production in blood cultures and showed that children with allergic asthma produced significantly lower amounts of interferon-α than healthy children and patients with nonallergic asthma. Subsequently, Gehlhar et al. (29) extended those analyses to adults. They found that virus-induced interferon-$\alpha2$ release from blood cells of allergic asthmatic patients was significantly lower than that observed with healthy controls, both when the cells were stimulated with New Castle disease virus and with RSV. In neither of these studies, however, were cells directly exposed to RV. No studies are available in which cells obtained in younger children were exposed to virus to determine responsiveness to type I or type III interferon. However and taken together with studies of interferon-γ responsiveness in younger children, these results strongly suggest that a common factor that could explain the association between viral wheezing respiratory illness in early life and subsequent asthma could be an alteration in viral responsiveness that predisposes both groups of children to the development of lower respiratory symptoms during viral infections.

IV. Natural Course of Asthma: From Episodic to Persistent

Although the studies reviewed above showing altered interferon responses could explain why young children with recurrent wheezing could become the older child with acute asthma episodes triggered by the same viruses (e.g., RV), many other aspects of the natural history of asthma remain unexplained. Specifically, children with persistent asthma not only have acute virus-induced exacerbations but often have weekly or even daily symptoms associated with bronchial obstruction that are unrelated to any evidence of a viral infection. Moreover, persistent asthma is associated with chronic airway inflammation, bronchial hyperresponsiveness, and mean levels of airway function that are lower than those present in children without asthma (30,31). Although a study from a birth cohort in Norway suggested that some deficits in airway function may be already present in the neonatal period in children who subsequently developed asthma (32), our own studies suggest that deficits in lung function present in children who have persistent wheezing are much more pronounced at the age of six years than shortly after birth (33), strongly indicating that these deficits may be acquired to the greatest extent during this age interval. Recent studies by Saglani et al. (34,35) provide strong anatomical support for this assumption. These authors performed bronchial biopsies in infants with recurrent wheezing and reversible airway obstruction in preschoolers with recurrent wheezing and in older children with asthma. They found no signs of reticular basement membrane thickening in the infant wheezers, but a certain degree of thickening was already present in the preschoolers and became much more pronounced and similar to that observed in adults with asthma in school-age children with the disease. Although these studies were not performed repeatedly in the same children, they mirror the changes in airway function that our group had previously reported in persistent wheezers as compared with children who did not wheeze during the first six years of life.

Particularly revealing from a clinical point of view was the Prevention of Early Asthma in Kids (PEAK) trial (36). In this study, two- to three-year-old children with recurrent wheezing and a positive asthma predictive index (37) were randomized to either twice-daily fluticasone proprionate inhaler or placebo treatment for two years. At the end of the second year, treatment was discontinued and children were followed for a third year to determine if the frequency of symptoms during the third year of treatment differed between the two groups. Interestingly, children treated with placebo showed a steady decrease in the number of episode-free days, that is, days during which there were no asthma-like symptoms and no use of asthma medications between the beginning of treatment and the end of the trial three years late. Specifically, children treated with placebo had only 5% of days in which they had symptoms or needed treatment at the beginning of follow-up compared with 15% of such days at the end of follow-up. These results thus mirror from a clinical point of view both those of our own studies of deficits in lung function growth during this same period and those obtained from bronchial biopsies by Saglani et al. (35): asthma starts in early life as an episodic disease and, with time, becomes a more persistent chronic disease that involves not only acute, virally triggered events but also such events that are associated with cough, wheezing, and other respiratory symptoms not related to infection.

V. Interaction Between Viruses and Allergies at the Beginnings of Asthma

Several lines of research suggest that skin test reactivity to local aeroallergens by age six is a strong determinant of the long-term outcome of children with recurrent viral wheezing during the preschool years (14,38). Specifically, we reported that most preschool wheezers who remained symptomatic during the school years were atopic and vice versa, and wheezing remitted in a very high proportion of nonatopics (39). These findings were confirmed and extended by Illi et al. using data from the German Multicenter Asthma and Allergy Study (MAAS) (38). They found that children who were sensitized were not only more unlikely to remit if they wheezed as preschoolers but were also more likely to have bronchial hyperresponsiveness at age seven. Murray et al. (40), analyzing data for specific airway conductance in the Manchester Asthma Study (MAS), showed that the effect of allergic sensitization on airway function could be detected as early as at age three. We further explored in the Tucson study the characteristics that, when present in early life, predispose viral wheezers for persistent asthma later in life (37). We identified parental asthma and atopic dermatitis in the child as major factors, whereas rhinitis, wheezing without colds, and peripheral blood eosinophilia were minor factors: preschool wheezers with either one of the former or two of the latter had 75% chance of having asthma during the school years. A careful analysis of these factors reveals that they are markers of either an allergic predisposition, a genetic susceptibility to asthma, or the premature development of persistent, nonvirally triggered wheezing. Very recently, Jackson et al. (14) showed that having had a confirmed RV wheezing illness at ages one or three and being sensitized to aeroallergens at either of these ages were both independent risk factors for asthma at age six, defined by the presence of one of several clinical criteria, and there was no significant interaction between these two factors. However, a thorough analysis of their data suggests that the incidence of asthma at age six was 86% (6/7) among children with RV wheezing and allergic sensitization by age one, compared with 39% to 45% among children who had either RV wheezing or sensitization, but not both, by that age. It is thus possible that small numbers may have precluded attainment of sufficient power in these studies. By contrast, Kusel et al. (15) showed that the association between RV viral infection in infancy and asthma at the age of five years was only observed among children who had become atopic by the age of two years and not among those who did not become atopic during the preschool years or among those who became sensitized after that age. The authors thus suggested that RV wheezing and allergy sensitization interact to determine asthma risk by six years of age. It is important to consider here that Stein et al. (39) and Illi et al. (38) have shown that a large proportion of nonatopic wheezers remit after the age of six. It will be thus of great interest to determine what is the relative importance of early RV wheezing, allergic sensitization, and their interaction on asthma later during the school years.

In all these studies, two main elements thus seem essential: viral infection and allergens/allergic conditions. Viruses, especially RV, are by far the main triggers of recurrent episodes of airway obstruction in early life, and this propensity persists in children who will go on to develop asthma, but only if concomitantly they are exposed and susceptible to becoming sensitized to allergens. Why nonatopic children lose this propensity to virus-induced airway obstruction is not understood, but it is likely that maturation of airways and inflammatory responses makes the growing child less susceptible to becoming symptomatic during viral respiratory infection.

It is currently unknown whether the susceptibility to viral infection is due to common genetic and developmental factors in atopic and nonatopic wheezers. We showed that, among the future persistent wheezers, serum total IgE was significantly higher at the time of the first ascertained episode of viral wheezing than that away from this illness, whereas no significant increase in total serum IgE was observed among transient wheezers (41). These findings suggested to us that a predisposition to IgE-mediated responses was already present at the time of the first LRI in persistent wheezers. However, we could not determine from these studies if it was the IgE-mediated response that caused the wheezing episode or if it was simply a marker for the atopic predisposition present in these children. Most likely, different factors contribute to the development of altered responses to RV and to the development of virus-induced airway obstruction in early life. Nevertheless, the fact that aeroallergen sensitization is a major predictor of school-age asthma among preschool wheezers strongly suggests that the development of allergen-triggered mechanisms can perpetuate the "infantile" pattern of response to viral infection. There is a strong association between aeroallergen sensitization and bronchial hyperresponsiveness as early as at age six (42), and it is thus plausible to surmise that the chronic allergic inflammation during the vulnerable preschool years may predispose to the functional and anatomic changes in the airways that appear to develop during this period in future asthmatics. In strong support of this contention, Illi et al. (38) showed that children who were exposed to the same perennial aeroallergens (house-dust mites and cats) to which they were sensitized had significant evidence of airway obstruction by the school years as compared with children who were sensitized but not exposed, exposed but not sensitized, or neither exposed nor sensitized. When this process first develops is still not clear. However, at least for schoolchildren with persistent asthma in developed countries, aeroallergy is most often an essential risk factor for their disease. What is relevant here, however, is that, in most children with persistent asthma, allergy is not the only predisposing factor implicated in the pathogenesis of the disease: most children and adults with persistent asthma are both atopic and susceptible to viruses. In fact, in most schoolchildren with asthma, symptoms started before they develop clear evidence of aeroallergen responsiveness, suggesting that the predisposition to virus-related bronchial obstruction is not originally caused by aeroallergies. The requirement of the concomitant presence of these two susceptibilities in most children with asthma is the most important and most novel clue derived from recent studies of the natural history of the disease.

VI. Conclusions

The evidence discussed in the above sections identifies a specific asthma phenotype that usually begins in early childhood and is associated with an early [and often severe (43)] susceptibility to viruses, which carries on into childhood and even adulthood, with early aeroallergen sensitization. This phenotype is a major risk factor for persistent disease into adult life. However, I do not intend to surmise that this is the only form of asthma present in schoolchildren. It is well recognized, for example, that asthma can first emerge in children and adults with allergic rhinitis (44) who are usually sensitized to seasonal allergens and whose symptoms often appear when they are exposed to these allergens. Similarly, we have described a form of nonatopic asthma that begins in the preadolescent years in girls who become overweight during those years (45). In developing countries, atopy is not an important risk factor for a frequent and severe form of childhood asthma that strongly resembles that of younger children in developed countries, in that it is mainly triggered by infection (46). However, there is strong evidence to suggest that the phenotype that we first branded as persistent wheezers identifies a group of virus-susceptible children at risk for lifetime chronic asthma. In these children, susceptibility to viral infection seems to appear concomitantly with evidence of an allergic diathesis and both seem to contribute separately to the development of severe obstructive episodes (47) and of chronic changes in airway function and structure that predispose to continuous asthma symptoms up to the early adult years (48).

Acknowledgment

Dr. Martinez was funded with grants HL056177, HL080083, and HL064307 from the National Heart, Lung, and Blood Institute.

Disclaimer: F.D.M. has served on the Merck Advisory Board and participated in one MedImmune Advisory Board meeting. He also served as a consultant for GlaxoSmithKline, Pfizer, Genentech, and MedImmune. In the last three years he has also received lecture fees for events sponsored by Merck and Genentech. No additional relationships exist between Dr. Martinez and these (or any other) commercial entities.

References

1. Stein RT, Sherrill D, Morgan WJ, et al. Respiratory syncytial virus in early life and risk of wheeze and allergy by age 13 years. Lancet 1999; 353:541–545.
2. Lemanske RF Jr., Jackson DJ, Gangnon RE, et al. Rhinovirus illnesses during infancy predict subsequent childhood wheezing. J Allergy Clin Immunol 2005; 116:571–577.
3. Message SD, Johnston SL. Viruses in asthma. Br Med Bull 2002; 61:29–43.
4. Martinez FD. Respiratory syncytial virus bronchiolitis and the pathogenesis of childhood asthma. Pediatr Infect Dis J 2003; 22:S76–S82.
5. National Asthma Education Prevention Program Coordinating Committee. Expert Panel. Guidelines for the diagnosis and management of asthma. Bethesda, M.D.: National Institutes of Health, 2008.
6. Lane S, Molina J, Plusa T. An international observational prospective study to determine the cost of asthma exacerbations (COAX). Respir Med 2006; 100:434–450.
7. Martinez FD. Managing childhood asthma: challenge of preventing exacerbations. Pediatrics 2009; 123(suppl 3):S146–S150.
8. Hanania NA, Chapman KR, Kesten S. Adverse effects of inhaled corticosteroids. Am J Med 1995; 98:196–208.
9. Yunginger J, Reed CE, O'Connell EJ, et al. A community-based study of the epidemiology of asthma. Incidence rates, 1964–1983. Am Rev Respir Dis 1992; 146:888–894.
10. Juniper EF, Guyatt GH, Epstein RS, et al. Evaluation of impairment of health related quality of life in asthma: development of a questionnaire for use in clinical trials. Thorax 1992; 47: 76–83.
11. Hoskins G, McCowan C, Neville RG, et al. Risk factors and costs associated with an asthma attack. Thorax 2000; 55:19–24.
12. Martinez FD, Wright AL, Taussig LM, et al. Asthma and wheezing in the first six years of life. N Engl J Med 1995; 332:133–138.
13. Martinez FD, Godfrey S. Wheezing Disorders in the Preschool Child. New York: Martin Dunitz, Taylor & Francis Group, 2003.
14. Jackson DJ, Gangnon RE, Evans MD, et al. Wheezing rhinovirus illnesses in early life predict asthma development in high risk children. Am J Respir Crit Care Med 2008; 178(7): 667–672.

15. Kusel MM, de Klerk NH, Kebadze T, et al. Early-life respiratory viral infections, atopic sensitization, and risk of subsequent development of persistent asthma. J Allergy Clin Immunol 2007; 119:1105–1110.

16. Wright AL, Taussig LM, Ray CG, et al. The Tucson Children's Respiratory Study. II. Lower respiratory tract illness in the first year of life. Am J Epidemiol 1989; 129:1232–1246.

17. Lee WM, Kiesner C, Pappas T, et al. A diverse group of previously unrecognized human rhinoviruses are common causes of respiratory illnesses in infants. PLoS ONE 2007; 2:e966.

18. Rakes GP, Arruda E, Ingram JM, et al. Rhinovirus and respiratory syncytial virus in wheezing children requiring emergency care. IgE and eosinophil analyses. Am J Respir Crit Care Med 1999; 159:785–790.

19. Johnston SL, Pattemore PK, Sanderson G, et al. The relationship between upper respiratory infections and hospital admissions for asthma: a time-trend analysis. Am J Respir Crit Care Med 1996; 154:654–660.

20. Guerra S, Lohman IC, Halonen M, et al. Reduced interferon gamma production and soluble CD14 levels in early life predict recurrent wheezing by 1 year of age. Am J Respir Crit Care Med 2004; 169:70–76.

21. Macaubas C, de Klerk NH, Holt BJ, et al. Association between antenatal cytokine production and the development of atopy and asthma at age 6 years. Lancet 2003; 362:1192–1197.

22. Stern DA, Guerra S, Halonen M, et al. Low IFN-gamma production in the first year of life as a predictor of wheeze during childhood. J Allergy Clin Immunol 2007; 120:835–841.

23. Zhang SY, Boisson-Dupuis S, Chapgier A, et al. Inborn errors of interferon (IFN)-mediated immunity in humans: insights into the respective roles of IFN-alpha/beta, IFN-gamma, and IFN-lambda in host defense. Immunol Rev 2008; 226:29–40.

24. Sheppard P, Kindsvogel W, Xu W, et al. IL-28, IL-29 and their class II cytokine receptor IL-28R. Nat Immunol 2003; 4:63–68.

25. Kotenko SV, Gallagher G, Baurin VV, et al. IFN-lambdas mediate antiviral protection through a distinct class II cytokine receptor complex. Nat Immunol 2003; 4:69–77.

26. Wark PA, Johnston SL, Bucchieri F, et al. Asthmatic bronchial epithelial cells have a deficient innate immune response to infection with rhinovirus. J Exp Med 2005; 201:937–947.

27. Contoli M, Message SD, Laza-Stanca V, et al. Role of deficient type III interferon-lambda production in asthma exacerbations. Nat Med 2006; 12:1023–1026.

28. Bufe A, Gehlhar K, Grage-Griebenow E, et al. Atopic phenotype in children is associated with decreased virus-induced interferon-alpha release. Int Arch Allergy Immunol 2002; 127:82–88.

29. Gehlhar K, Bilitewski C, Reinitz-Rademacher K, et al. Impaired virus-induced interferon-alpha2 release in adult asthmatic patients. Clin Exp Allergy 2006; 36:331–337.

30. Tantisira KG, Colvin R, Tonascia J, et al. Airway responsiveness in mild to moderate childhood asthma: sex influences on the natural history. Am J Respir Crit Care Med 2008; 178:325–331.

31. Strunk RC, Weiss ST, Yates KP, et al. Mild to moderate asthma affects lung growth in children and adolescents. J Allergy Clin Immunol 2006; 118:1040–1047.

32. Haland G, Carlsen KC, Sandvik L, et al. Reduced lung function at birth and the risk of asthma at 10 years of age. N Engl J Med 2006; 355:1682–1689.

33. Morgan WJ, Stern DA, Sherrill DL, et al. Outcome of asthma and wheezing in the first 6 years of life: follow-up through adolescence. Am J Respir Crit Care Med 2005; 172:1253–1258.

34. Saglani S, Malmstrom K, Pelkonen AS, et al. Airway remodeling and inflammation in symptomatic infants with reversible airflow obstruction. Am J Respir Crit Care Med 2005; 171:722–727.

35. Saglani S, Payne DN, Zhu J, et al. Early detection of airway wall remodeling and eosinophilic inflammation in preschool wheezers. Am J Respir Crit Care Med 2007; 176:858–864.

36. Guilbert TW, Morgan WJ, Zeiger RS, et al. Long-term inhaled corticosteroids in preschool children at high risk for asthma. N Engl J Med 2006; 354:1985–1997.
37. Castro-Rodriguez JA, Holberg CJ, Wright AL, et al. A clinical index to define risk of asthma in young children with recurrent wheezing. Am J Respir Crit Care Med 2000; 162:1403–1406.
38. Illi S, von Mutius E, Lau S, et al. Perennial allergen sensitisation early in life and chronic asthma in children: a birth cohort study. Lancet 2006; 368:763–770.
39. Stein RT, Holberg CJ, Morgan WJ, et al. Peak flow variability, methacholine responsiveness and atopy as markers for detecting different wheezing phenotypes in childhood. Thorax 1997; 52:946–952.
40. Lowe LA, Woodcock A, Murray CS, et al. Lung function at age 3 years: effect of pet ownership and exposure to indoor allergens. Arch Pediatr Adolesc Med 2004; 158:996–1001.
41. Martinez FD, Stern DA, Wright AL, et al. Differential immune responses to acute lower respiratory illness in early life by subsequent development of persistent wheezing and asthma. J Allergy Clin Immunol 1998; 102:915–920.
42. Lombardi E, Morgan WJ, Wright AL, et al. Cold air challenge at age 6 and subsequent incidence of asthma. A longitudinal study. Am J Respir Crit Care Med 1997; 156:1863–1869.
43. Devulapalli CS, Carlsen KC, Haland G, et al. Severity of obstructive airways disease by age 2 years predicts asthma at 10 years of age. Thorax 2008; 63:8–13.
44. Guerra S, Sherrill DL, Martinez FD, et al. Rhinitis as an independent risk factor for adult-onset asthma. J Allergy Clin Immunol 2002; 109:419–425.
45. Castro-Rodriguez JA, Holberg CJ, Morgan WJ, et al. Increased incidence of asthma-like symptoms in girls who become overweight or obese during the school years. Am J Respir Crit Care Med 2001; 163:1344–1349.
46. Mallol J, Castro-Rodriguez JA, Cortez E, et al. Heightened bronchial hyperresponsiveness in the absence of heightened atopy in children with current wheezing and low income status. Thorax 2008; 63:167–171.
47. Murray CS, Poletti G, Kebadze T, et al. Study of modifiable risk factors for asthma exacerbations: virus infection and allergen exposure increase the risk of asthma hospital admissions in children. Thorax 2006; 61:376–382.
48. Stern DA, Morgan WJ, Halonen M, et al. Wheezing and bronchial hyper-responsiveness in early childhood as predictors of newly diagnosed asthma in early adulthood: a longitudinal birth-cohort study. Lancet 2008; 372:1058–1064.

10

Pulmonary Surfactant, Innate Immunity, and Asthma

MARI NUMATA and DENNIS R. VOELKER
National Jewish Health, Denver, Colorado, U.S.A.

I. Introduction

Pulmonary surfactant is a phospholipid-rich, protein-containing secretion present at the air-liquid interface of the alveolar compartment that functions both to reduce surface tension and to regulate innate immune functions within the lung (1). Although primarily produced in the alveolar compartment and the small conducting airways, the constituents of pulmonary surfactant can also be found in larger airways. Increasing evidence demonstrates that pulmonary surfactant lipids and proteins play important roles in the pathogenesis of bronchial asthma through direct interactions with microbes, allergens, epithelial cells, and cells of the immune system. The components of the pulmonary surfactant system can function to both facilitate the recognition and phagocytosis of microbes and suppress inflammatory responses of the lung elicited by environmental stimuli. These interactions suggest that pulmonary surfactant components may have significant and untapped potential for use in the treatment of chronic lung diseases including asthma.

II. Fundamentals of Pulmonary Surfactant

A. The Composition of Alveolar Pulmonary Surfactant in the Lung

Pulmonary surfactant was initially identified as a lipoprotein complex consisting of approximately 90% lipid and 10% protein (Fig. 1). The major lipid components of pulmonary surfactant are phospholipids, with a small amount of neutral lipids (5–10 wt%) such as cholesterol. The levels of phospholipid in the pulmonary surfactant layer that resides above the alveolar epithelium are extraordinarily high, with estimates ranging from 15 to 30 mg/mL (2). The most abundant phospholipids in this surfactant layer belong to the phosphatidylcholine (PC) class, with dipalmitoylphosphatidylcholine (DPPC) as the major molecular species, accounting for approximately 50 wt% of the total surfactant lipid. Biophysical studies demonstrate that interfacial films of DPPC play an essential role in reducing alveolar surface tension, thereby preventing alveolar collapse at the end of the expiratory phase of the respiratory cycle (3). DPPC is unusual because it contains two saturated fatty acids, whereas most phospholipids found in mammalian systems contain at least one unsaturated fatty acid. The presence of two saturated fatty acids in DPPC imparts high surface activity to surface films of the lipid, thus enabling the reduction of surface tension. Although DPPC is the dominant lipid in surfactant, lesser amounts of unsaturated PC are also present in the secretion, but these are believed to be selectively removed from surface films as they are compressed at

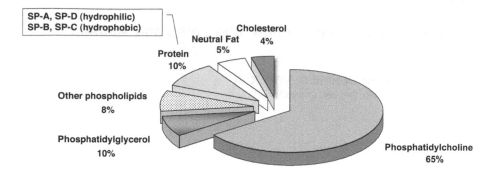

Figure 1 The composition of human pulmonary surfactant in bronchoalveolar lavage fluid. Pulmonary surfactant is mainly composed of phospholipids, with phosphatidylcholine and phosphatidylglycerol as the major molecular classes. About 10% of surfactant is protein and contains the hydrophilic proteins, SP-A and SP-D, as well as hydrophobic SPs, SP-B and SP-C. *Abbreviation*: SP, surfactant protein.

reduced alveolar diameters (3,4). In addition to the PC class, surfactant also contains significant amounts ($\sim 10\%$ of total lipid) of the phosphatidylglycerol (PG) class of phospholipids, which, in humans, is predominately composed of unsaturated molecular species. The presence of PG is also highly unusual, as this lipid typically occurs in only trace amounts in mammalian cells, and has not been identified in other tissue secretions. Lesser quantities of other classes of phospholipids, including phosphatidylinositols, phosphatidylethanolamines, and sphingomyelins, which, in aggregate, constitute about 8% of the total lipid, are also present (4).

The surfactant proteins (SPs) SP-A, SP-B, SP-C, and SP-D are associated with extracellular surfactant lipids in the lung (1). SP-A and SP-D are hydrophilic, whereas SP-B and SP-C are extraordinarily hydrophobic. The association of SP-A and SP-D with surfactant lipids is Ca^{2+} dependent. SP-A and SP-D are structurally related and belong to the collectin family of proteins, characterized by the presence of collagen-like domains and Ca^{2+}-dependent carbohydrate binding (C-type lectin) domains (5). The monomeric molecular size of SP-A is 24 kDa, and that of SP-D is 36 kDa, and variable levels of glycosylation contribute another 2 to 12 kDa to the size of the mature secreted proteins present in surfactant. Both SP-A and SP-D undergo covalent (disulfide-dependent) and noncovalent (collagen domain–dependent and coiled coil domain–dependent) oligomerization such that mature SP-A forms 18-mers and mature SP-D forms 12-mers. The overall organization of SP-A oligomers is arranged in a bouquet motif comprised of six trimeric subunits, whereas the organization of SP-D is arranged in a cruciform motif comprised of four trimeric subunits (1,5). The trimerization of the SP-A and SP-D occurs via noncovalent interactions of the collagen and coiled coil domains. Further oligomerization of the proteins occurs upon disulfide cross-linking of the trimers. The high degree of oligomerization of the pulmonary collectins promotes high-affinity reactions with cognate ligands present on host cell surfaces, and foreign microbial surfaces, which play important roles in the regulation of innate immunity in the lung (1,5–7). The hydrophobic SP-B and SP-C are initially synthesized as larger hydrophilic proteins that undergo extensive intracellular posttranslational processing before secretion as mature forms, which appear as dimeric SP-B (17 kDa) and monomeric, fatty acid–modified SP-C (4.2 kDa). SP-B and SP-C participate in intracellular phospholipid packaging in lamellar bodies (LBs) (8) and promote the highly efficient adsorption of extracellular surfactant lipid to the air-liquid interface, which is essential for reduction of alveolar surface tension (4).

Alveolar type II cells are the primary source of the surfactant lipids and proteins, which are stored in a unique secretory organelle known as the LB (Fig. 2). The LB contains high concentrations of SP-B, SP-C, and the surfactant lipids and is released

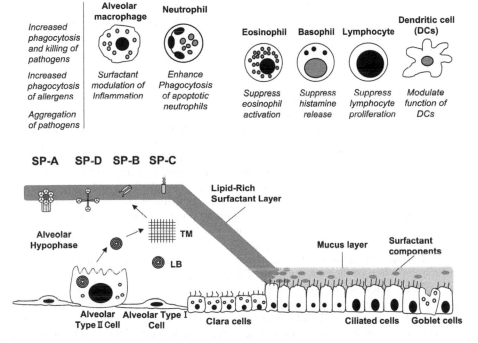

Figure 2 Fundamentals of pulmonary surfactant. Pulmonary surfactant is synthesized, stored, and secreted by alveolar type II cells. Intracellular surfactant is stored in specialized organelles known as LBs. Upon secretion, LBs transform into TM before absorption of the lipids and hydrophobic proteins to the air-liquid interface. The surfactant layer contains the peripherally associated hydrophilic proteins, SP-A and SP-D, which associate with the lipid in a Ca^{2+}-dependent manner. The hydrophobic proteins, SP-B and SP-C, are insoluble in the aqueous compartment and behave as integral components of the lipid layer. Pulmonary surfactant components are partially extruded into the mucus layer of conducting airways and larger airways by mechanical processes and mucociliary escalator function. SP-A and SP-D mainly mediate host defense function and interact with multiple species of pathogens and complex allergens. These proteins also interact with multiple cells of the immune system including macrophages, neutrophils, eosinophils, basophils, lymphocytes, and dendritic cells and regulate innate immune responses in the lung. Selected surfactant components including SP-A, SP-D, and phospholipids are also found interspersed within the mucus layer of large airways. *Abbreviations*: SP, surfactant protein; LB, lamellar body; TM, tubular myelin.

from the cell by regulated exocytosis (9). In contrast to the hydrophobic proteins, most of the SP-A and SP-D is delivered to the extracellular compartment via constitutive secretion, although recycling pools of surfactant may deliver SP-A and SP-D to the LB (10). Surfactant secretion can be elicited by subjecting alveolar type 2 cells to stretch stimuli in vitro, which approximates the cyclical expansion and contraction of the alveolar compartment during respiration (11). The stretch stimuli transduce intracellular signals through a Ca^{2+}/calmodulin-dependent protein kinase pathway (10). In addition, β-adrenergic agonists acting through cyclic adenosine monophosphate (AMP) signaling cascades and agonists activating protein kinase C pathways also elicit surfactant secretion (10). SP-A, SP-B, and SP-D are also synthesized by airway cells, including Clara cells and submucosal gland cells (12–16). SP-A is encoded by two genes located on chromosome 10 in humans. Adjacent to the SP-A locus, the single human gene encoding SP-D is also found on chromosome 10. The human gene encoding for SP-B is located on chromosome 2, and the human gene encoding for human SP-C is present on chromosome 8.

B. Airway Pulmonary Surfactant

Although the alveoli are the principal synthetic center for the production of pulmonary surfactant, the airways are supplied with surfactant components via the sweeping action of the mucociliary escalator, as the surfactant film at the alveolar air-liquid interface is partly extruded into adjacent conducting airways during expiration. Current findings estimate that 7% of alveolar surfactant reaches the bronchial tree by this mechanism (13,17). SP synthesis has been described in Clara cells (12,15,16) and more proximal parts of the respiratory tract (14), but quantitative estimates of the contributions of distinct regions of the lung to the resident airway pools are lacking. Biophysical considerations have been put forward to argue that the presence of surfactant in small airways plays an important role in promoting and maintaining their patency (13,17,18). Currently, accurate sampling of small-airway surfactant pools is technically challenging, and the definition of the constituents remains unresolved.

Examination of the constituents of large-airway secretions obtained by tracheal washings of porcine lungs demonstrated some similarities in phospholipid composition of this material compared with alveolar surfactant (19). Subfractionation of the cell-free tracheal secretions by density gradient centrifugation revealed lipoprotein complexes, which contained lipids, nearly identical to purified surfactant, and SP-A. However, these subfractions were devoid of SP-B and SP-C. The synthesis of surfactant components by airway cells and its regulation by specific environmental factors, including micro-particulates, xenobiotics, and infectious microorganisms, remains poorly understood.

III. The Functions of Pulmonary Surfactant
A. Biophysical Functions of Surfactant

Pulmonary surfactant was initially identified as a lipoprotein complex that acts to reduce surface tension at the air-liquid interface of the lung (20). Biophysical studies demonstrate that surfactant prevents collapse of the alveoli and fluid occlusion of small conducting airways during expiration (3,18). The biophysical properties of surfactant also facilitate inspiratory opening of the lungs (1,4,13,17). The location of surfactant at the air-liquid interface makes it the first biological material encountered by airborne microorganisms that are deposited in the alveolar compartment. The surfactant film also has the ability to trap microparticulate material and promote its physical removal from the alveoli and small airways, and integrate these compartments with the mucociliary transport system (13).

B. Immunological Functions of Surfactant Proteins

Multiple host defense functions of surfactant are now recognized to be mediated by SP-A and SP-D (1,5,7). These pulmonary collectins interact with glycoconjugates, lipids, and proteins present on the surface of a variety of microorganisms and allergens. In addition, the interactions with multiple host cell proteins enable SP-A and SP-D to potently regulate pulmonary innate immunity. SP-A and SP-D exhibit high-affinity binding interactions to multiple species of bacteria, fungi, viruses, and complex allergens (1,21,22). The majority of specific interactions of the proteins with microorganisms occur through the carbohydrate recognition domains (CRDs) of the collectins, but the N-linked oligosaccharide of SP-A also participates in specific interactions (23,24). The consequences of SP-A and SP-D ligation to viruses, bacteria, and fungi are multiple, resulting in (*i*) aggregation of pathogens (25–28), (*ii*) opsonization of microorganisms and enhancement of their phagocytosis by leukocytes (29–31), (*iii*) amplification of microbial killing via oxidative mechanisms (32–34), (*iv*) growth inhibition by direct bacteriostatic and fungistatic effects (35–37), (*v*) viral neutralization (38–40), and (*vi*) modulation of cytokine and chemokine secretion at the site of infection (7). The enhancement of phagocytosis by the collectins also extends to increased removal of apoptotic cells, especially neutrophils, from the lungs, as part of the resolution phase of inflammatory processes (41).

SP-A and SP-D can modulate cellular inflammatory responses by their direct interaction with pattern recognition receptors. Specifically, SP-A interacts with CD14 on alveolar macrophages and inhibits the binding of smooth lipopolysaccharide (LPS) to CD14 and thereby reduces TNF-α expression induced by LPS (42). SP-A can also directly bind to toll-like receptor (TLR)2 and TLR4 and prevent the interactions of these proteins with ligands (43,44). SP-D also directly binds to TLR2 and interferes with ligand recognition by the receptor (45). In the absence of external challenges by microbes or their proinflammatory substituents, the lectin domains of SP-A and SP-D can bind signal regulatory phosphatase binding protein-1α (SIRP-1α) and maintain a quiescent state with respect to inflammation (46). However, displacement of the lectin domains from SIRP1α by ligation of the collectins to microbial surfaces releases the suppression of inflammation. Concomitantly, the aggregation of SP-A and SP-D effected by pathogen recognition and direct interaction with the lectin domains induces aggregation of the collagen domains of these molecules and recognition by cell surface calreticulin, resulting in the triggering of proinflammatory responses (46).

SP-A and SP-D also modulate the functions of dendritic cells (DCs) and T cells (1,6,13). SP-A suppresses the maturation of DCs and their ability to respond to chemotactic stimuli and phagocytose particles (47). In contrast, SP-D promotes antigen uptake and processing and surface presentation by DCs (48). SP-A and SP-D have also been shown to mediate a number of anti-allergic effects, including inhibition of IgE binding to allergens, suppression of histamine release from basophils, and inhibition of lymphocyte proliferation in the late phase of inflammation (1,6,13). SP-A binds to pollen grains, and both SP-A and SP-D interact with mite allergens in a carbohydrate-specific and calcium-dependent manner (49). There is now compelling evidence that

SP-A and SP-D play an important role in regulating the transition between innate and adaptive immunity in the lung.

Although much of the work examining surfactant and innate immunity in the lung has focused on SP-A and SP-D, there is also evidence demonstrating that mature SP-C can directly interact with CD14 (50) and LPS. These latter studies raise the possibility that this hydrophobic protein may also play a significant role in pulmonary immunology both during acute lung injury and chronic lung disease (8,51).

The most abundant constituents of surfactant are phospholipids, but their roles in the regulation of pulmonary innate immunity have not been studied in detail. Changes in surfactant phospholipids correlate with the pathogenesis of pulmonary diseases [e.g., acute respiratory distress syndrome (ARDS) (52), interstitial lung disease (ILD) (53), and bronchial asthma (54)]. Especially noteworthy is the minor surfactant phospholipid class PG, which is comprised primarily of the molecular species harboring one or two oleic acid moieties. The PG levels of surfactant strongly correlate with the prognosis of patients with pulmonary fibrosis (IPF) (53,55). The phospholipid components of surfactant can inhibit both T-lymphocyte activation and the neutrophil respiratory burst oxidase response (13,56). Surfactant phospholipids, especially PI and PG can also regulate inflammatory cell function in the lungs (57,58). Additional studies will be required to elucidate the role of surfactant lipids in regulating immune response in the lung and whether these components have therapeutic potential for suppressing chronic inflammation.

C.   Alterations in Pulmonary Surfactant in Lung Disease

Historically, surfactant deficiency was first characterized in premature newborns as a developmental disease resulting from insufficient maturation of alveolar type II cells and inadequate expression of the genes encoding the surfactant components. Now, a variety of pathological processes and intrinsic genetic mutations are recognized that modify surfactant abundance, structure, and function and thereby contribute to lung diseases at various stages of life by disrupting the homeostatic role of the surfactant components. Significant changes in SPs and phospholipids recovered from bronchoalveolar lavage fluid (BALF) have been reported for several lung diseases (17). The alteration of SP levels correlates with susceptibility, severity, and prognosis of selected lung diseases. Quantitative changes in surfactant components have been described in obstructive lung diseases including asthma, allergic bronchopulmonary aspergillosis (ABPA), bronchiolitis, and chronic obstructive pulmonary disease (COPD) (7,17). Alterations in surfactant have been described following lung transplantation and in ARDS, pulmonary edema, diseases specific to infants (chronic lung disease of prematurity and SP-B deficiency), ILD (sarcoidosis, idiopathic IPF, and hypersensitive pneumonitis), pulmonary alveolar proteinosis, and infection suppurative lung disease (cystic fibrosis, pneumonia, and HIV) (17).

SP-A and SP-D are primarily confined to the environmental surfaces of the lung but compromise of epithelial integrity in disease processes can promote access of the proteins to the vasculature. Smokers and patients with COPD exhibit higher serum levels of SP-D compared with normal control subjects (59). Significant changes in both lavage and serum levels of SP-A and SP-D have been described for both ARDS and subacute lung disease (60,61). Serum SP-A and SP-D levels can be used as important biomarkers for predicting the course of IPF (62). McCormack et al. also found that BAL fluid levels of phospholipids and SP-A, and SP-A/PL ratio could be used to predict outcome of patients with IPF (53).

Pulmonary collectin deficiency has been detected in BALF from cystic fibrosis (CF) subjects, and the levels of these proteins are inversely correlated with inflammation in patient airways (63,64). SP-A and SP-D bind directly to *Pseudomonas aeruginosa*, which is the predominate pathogen associated with CF. The pulmonary collectins facilitate phagocytosis of the bacteria (65,66). In a reciprocally antagonistic process, *P. aeruginosa* proteases degrade SP-A and SP-D, and in CF this depletion of the pulmonary collectins may play an important mechanistic role in establishing chronic bacterial infection (67). Glasser et al. reported that SP-C-deficient mice were more susceptible to *P. aeruginosa* infection and thus, SP-C may also play a role in maintaining the integrity of the innate immune system within the lung (68).

Changes in surfactant lipids also correlate with disease processes. BALF from patients with pneumonia has reduced PC and PG content, and alterations in fatty acid composition (52,69,70). The quantitative changes in surfactant lipids associated with microbial infection are similar to those observed in patients with ARDS (52).

Polymorphisms in genes encoding pulmonary SPs have been reported in association with a number of different pulmonary diseases. Such polymorphisms may alter the level of protein expression and/or functional activity and stability of the gene products and thus contribute to disease processes. The human SP-A locus consists of one pseudogene and two functional genes, SP-A1 and SP-A2. Within the SP-A1 gene, single-nucleotide polymorphisms (SNPs) that characterize the 6A4 allele were found with higher frequency in IPF (71). An SNP present in SP-B genetic variants was also associated with IPF (71). Risk factors for high-altitude pulmonary edema are associated with multiple polymorphisms in both the SP-A1 and SP-A2 (72) genes. Additional polymorphisms within the SP-A2 gene were associated with severe RSV-induced bronchiolitis (73). Polymorphisms in SP-D specifying amino acid Met or Thr at position 11 of the mature protein are differentially associated with diseases. The heterozygous Met/Thr 11 is protective against RSV infection, whereas the homozygous Met 11 is associated with RSV bronchiolitis (74). In contrast, the homozygous Thr11 is associated with increased susceptibility to *Mycobacterium tuberculosis* infections (75). Homozygous inactivating mutations to SP-B cause infantile respiratory distress and respiratory failure in newborns (76). Individuals heterozygous for inactivating mutations exhibit partial defects in SP-B function that are associated with chronic ILD with childhood onset (77). Mutations in SP-C exert a dominant effect and are associated with respiratory distress and ILD in both newborns and older individuals (51,78).

IV. Pulmonary Surfactant and Asthma
A. Surfactant Protein Modulation of Allergic Inflammation and Hypersensitivity

Increasing evidence demonstrates that surfactant components play an important role in regulating host responses to inflammatory and allergic stimuli. The insufficiency or inactivation of surfactant components may result in the loss of anti-inflammatory checkpoints controlling the activation of lymphocytes, eosinophils, macrophages, and DCs (1,6,7). The roles of SPs in asthma, especially SP-A and SP-D, are multifactorial, involving both the recognition and processing of allergens and immunogens and the regulation of cellular responses to these agents. SP-D levels are significantly increased during the acute asthmatic response in animal models and clinical human studies (79). SP-A and SP-D are also increased in BALF in patients with asthma (80). The serum levels of SP-D were also significantly elevated in allergic asthmatic patients both before and following allergen challenge (79). The increased levels of SP-A and SP-D may exert a protective role during allergic inflammation in asthma. These data suggest that SPs, especially SP-A and SP-D, appear to be quite important in resisting allergic challenge and hypersensitivity reactions in the lung and pathogenesis in asthma. The alterations in SPs in asthma are not restricted to the collectins. Reduction in SP-C levels occurs in BALF after segmental allergen challenge in patients with asthma (81). SP-C maintains a stable association of surfactant with the interface and permits resistance to surface inhibition by invading plasma protein (4,8). The protective role of SP-C in asthma may be a consequence of the maintenance of biophysical surfactant function in terminal airways.

Several important allergens directly interact with the pulmonary collectins. SP-A and SP-D bind to dust mite allergens (Der p1 and Der f1) (82), grass pollen allergens (83,84), conidia, and various glycoprotein allergens (gp55, gp45) from *Aspergillus fumigatus* (gp55, gp45) (85–87). SP-D also binds to pollen starch granules (84). These physical interactions appear to primarily involve the CRD regions of the proteins. The consequences of these physical binding interactions have important implications for asthma. The binding of SP-A and SP-D to glycoprotein allergens derived from *Aspergillus* inhibits the binding of IgE to these same allergens, thereby blocking the activation of basophils and the release of histamine (88). The interaction of SP-D with pollen starch granules suppresses their induction of mast cell degranulation (89). SP-D also enhances the binding and phagocytosis of starch granules by alveolar macrophages (84).

The pulmonary collectins also directly interact with multiple cells of the immune system and modulate their responses to mitogens, allergens, pyrogens, and immunogens. These interactions are complex and depend on the nature of the activating ligand, or organism that interacts with the SPs and the responding cell. In addition, the response of a particular cell can be influenced by whether it is naive or has been previously exposed to cytokines or inflammatory mediators. With lymphocytes, SP-A and SP-D inhibit proliferation and IL-2 production induced by mitogen (e.g., phytohemagglutinin) stimulation (90). In addition, lymphocyte proliferation induced by dust mite allergen is also suppressed by the pulmonary collectins (85). Although these suppressive interactions between the pulmonary collectins and lymphocytes are partially defined, pharmaceutical preparations of pulmonary surfactants devoid of SP-A and SP-D have also been reported to suppress lymphocyte proliferation (91,92). The general suppression of lymphocyte proliferation by surfactant components within the lung is expected to afford protection from allergic immune responses. However, lymphocytes from asthmatic children were largely refractory to the anti-proliferative effects of pulmonary collectins (85), and preactivation of lymphocytes in vitro with mitogens or IL-2 within an appropriate time frame can also bypass the suppressive effects of SP-D on proliferation (93). Thus, issues of collectin concentrations and pre-activation states of lymphocytes are important parameters to consider with regard to the utility of SP-A and SP-D in suppressing cell proliferation.

Eosinophils play important roles in asthma by secreting inflammatory mediators, which damage tissue and promote long-term remodeling changes to airways. The pulmonary collectins alter eosinophil function and turnover. SP-A suppresses the production and release of IL-8 by eosinophils stimulated with ionomycin (94). Resting eosinophils appear to be unaffected by SP-D, but eosinophils exposed to IL-5 show increased apoptosis when treated with a recombinant truncated form of SP-D (95). Likewise, esosinophils from asthmatics respond to a truncated recombinant SP-D treatment with increased rates of apoptosis. Apoptotic eosinophils show increased binding to SP-D, which facilitates their clearance by macrophages. Consistent with these findings, pretreatment of ovalbumin-sensitized mice with SP-D suppresses the recovery of eosinophils from the lungs upon ovalbumin challenge (96). Eosinophil-dependent inflammation is also suppressed by recombinant SP-D in *Aspergillus*- and dust mite (Der p)-sensitized mice (87,97). Thus, the pulmonary collectins act dually to suppress the activation of eosinophils and facilitate their removal.

DCs play a critical function in bridging innate and adaptive immunity (98). Resting DCs within the lung have an immature, phagocytic phenotype. Under the appropriate stimulation by microbial ligands and cytokines, lung DCs undergo differentiation to a mature antigen-presenting and T cell–stimulatory phenotype (99). SP-D suppresses antigen presentation by lung DCs (100). In contrast to lung DCs, bone marrow DCs are induced to mature and present antigen by SP-D (48). Conversely, SP-A inhibits maturation of bone marrow DCs (47). Thus, DCs undergo critical changes within the pulmonary environment that alter their responsiveness to pulmonary collectins. In the context of the lung, the collectins act to suppress the processing of antigens for the development of adaptive immunity.

B. Surfactant Phospholipids in Asthma

In addition to the actions of the SPs, surfactant phospholipids may also play an important role in the pathogenesis of asthma. After segmental allergen challenge of asthmatic patients, changes in surfactant phospholipid composition and inhibition of surface tension–lowering activity have been observed (54,101). Hite et al. reported that antigen challenge significantly altered the partitioning of surfactant phospholipids between the large surfactant aggregates (LAs), which exhibit high surface activity, and small surfactant aggregates (SAs) with reduced surface activity (54). The LA/SA ratio is thought to reflect the dynamic flux of surfactant between its surface-active and surface-inactive forms. The reduction in surface activity could adversely affect the patency of small airways. The minor anionic surfactant phospholipids PG and PI were also significantly reduced in the LA of the asthmatic BALF after antigen challenge. PG is thought to have a key function in interacting with SP-B to maintain alveolar surfactant layer by enhancing the adsorption of DPPC and re-spreading the monolayer after maximum compression (102,103). Depletion of PG was also reported in other lung diseases (53,55,70,104). PG and PI also act as regulators of inflammatory cell function in the lungs (57,58). Surfactant lipids also suppress lymphocyte function and proliferation, inhibit the activation of neutrophils, and decrease the production of superoxide anions, and the release of proinflammatory mediators (13,58).

C. Dysfunction of Pulmonary Surfactant in Asthma

Surfactant impairment occurs in many lung diseases (17,105). Environmental agents, serum components, enzymes produced by tissue injury, and microbes have been identified as factors that physically inhibit or chemically alter pulmonary surfactant and

reduce its surface activity (4,106). Inhibitors of the biophysical activity of lung surfactant include plasma proteins (e.g., albumin, hemoglobin, fibrinogen), unsaturated cell
membrane phospholipids, lysophospholipids, cholesterol, free fatty acid, and meconium.
Inhibition of pulmonary surfactant function can also be caused by degradation of surfactant lipids by phospholipases, lysophospholipases, proteases, and reactive oxygen and
nitrogen derivatives including superoxide and nitroxide radicals. Extrinsic agents that
inactivate pulmonary surfactant can be in the form of gases, dusts, and microparticulates.
The intrinsic agents can be produced during infection and/or as a consequence of chronic
pulmonary inflammation. Surfactant dysfunction in asthma has been well documented
(13,60,107). Multiple studies have identified pulmonary surfactant impairment as a
consequence of leakage of plasma proteins into the airway (13,101,108). Additional
studies identify the hydrolytic activities of secretory phospholipases (sPLA2s) as another
class of important factors that can degrade and inactivate surfactant lipids (109).

Low molecular weight phospholipases of the sPLA2 family are released by human
airway epithelial cells, neutrophils, eosinophils, and probably other cell types and
hydrolyze phospholipids at the 2-acyl ester position, generating lysophospholipids and
free fatty acids (109,110). Both of these degradation products have detergent activity
capable of diminishing the surface tension–lowering properties of native surfactant and
altering the interaction of the hydrophobic SPs with lipids. Circulating levels of sPLA2s
increase in several illnesses including sepsis, ARDS, shock, traumatic injury, and
pancreatitis (111,112). The accumulation of eosinophils in the lung is one important
feature of the pathogenesis of asthma. sPLA2s can promote arachidonic acid (AA)
release and eosinophil activation. AA functions as an essential precursor for prosta-
glandins and leukotrienes. After antigen challenge, sPLA2 activity was increased in the
BALF of patients with asthma (113) and generated lysophospholipids at levels sufficient
to cause surfactant dysfunction (54). The sPLA2 activation produced significant
reduction in the PC and PG classes of phospholipid (113). The eosinophil release of
sPLA2s catalyzes the hydrolysis of PC and LPC and has been linked to small-airway
obstruction (114,115). Eosinophils exhibit more sPLA2 and LPLase activity than neutrophils and mononuclear leukocytes (116). Recent examination of mice lacking group
X sPLA2 in the context of an ovalbumin-induced model of asthma revealed that sPLA2
contributes to lymphocyte and eosinophil infiltration, goblet cell metaplasia, tissue
remodeling, and the production of T_h2 cytokines and eicosanoids (117).

V.   Microbes, Asthma Exacerbations, and Surfactant
A.   Asthma Exacerbation and Microbes

Asthma exacerbations can occur in response to multiple factors, but microbial infection is
typically the most common inducer of these episodes. The leading cause of asthma
exacerbation in all age groups is respiratory virus infection (118,119). The most
important viruses implicated in exacerbation of asthma are rhinovirus (RV), respiratory
syncytial virus (RSV), influenza A virus (IAV), influenza B virus, parainfluenza virus,
corona virus, and adenovirus (120–122). RV is numerically the most important virus in
asthma exacerbations (118) and is especially problematic in childhood asthma. RV
increases airway responsiveness in allergic individuals compared with nonallergic individuals and enhances both the immediate and the late-phase responses to allergen (123).
However, RSV and influenza virus have a greater propensity to trigger acute asthma

symptoms. RSV infection also alters SP-A and SP-D levels in human lung (124–126). Levine et al. reported that SP-A levels were increased in the BALF of patients with RSV infection (126), but there are variations in clinical studies (125), which may be related to individual responsiveness and the timing of sampling relative to the progress of the viral infection. Significantly, upon in vitro challenge, RSV causes increased expression of SP-A mRNA in human alveolar type II cells (127). SP-A and SP-D are also implicated in the prevention and attenuation of RSV infection in vivo. RSV expresses two major surface proteins that function in viral attachment (G protein) and fusion (F protein) (128). Both F and G proteins are important for entry of RSV into host cells. SP-A binds to F protein (38) and enhances clearance of RSV in vivo. SP-A null mice are markedly defective in clearing RSV infections and show elevated levels of inflammation. Reconstitution of SP-A null mice with exogenous human SP-A significantly reduced RSV infection and its accompanying pathology (129). Decreased RSV clearance is also observed in SP-D null mice, and deficiency of the protein is associated with elevated inflammatory responses induced by the virus (130). SP-D plays a role in innate defense to RSV infection by directly binding viral F and G glycoproteins, which interact with the CRD, thereby enhancing phagocytosis of the virus by alveolar macrophages.

SP-A and SP-D also play important roles in the innate immune response to IAV infection. SP-A binds IAV and neutralizes the virus by directly occupying the hemagglutinin (HA) cell attachment site via the terminal sialic acid of the N-linked oligosaccharide located in the CRD of SP-A (24). SP-A enhances influenza clearance from the lung and decreases lung inflammation in vivo (131). Both SP-A and SP-D agglutinate influenza virus (132), enhance virus uptake by neutrophils, and potentiate the reactive oxygen production by these cells (133). Interestingly, the protective effects of SP-D against IAV infection are bypassed in viral strains lacking glycosylation, at the N165 site of the H3N2 subtype HA protein and at the N104 site of H1N1 subtype HA protein (134,135). However, current work also reveals that the susceptibility or resistance of IAV is also dependent on other glycosylation sites on HA whose alteration over time can induce sensitivity in resistant strains and resistance in sensitive strains. SP-D can also bind to oligosaccharides on the viral HA and neuraminidase (NA) (136), and this protective role of SP-D against IAV infection strongly depends on the state of glycosylation of HA protein. Reconstitution of SP-D–/– mice with recombinant SP-D attenuates the severity of IAV infection (137). Acute respiratory viral infections are often accompanied by robust neutrophil influx into the upper and lower respiratory secretions. There is evidence that activated neutrophils, through the release of elastase, can markedly upregulate goblet cell secretion of mucus (138), which leads to significant aggravation of asthma. SP-A and SP-D are also susceptible to proteolysis catalyzed by neutrophil elastase, which could reduce the beneficial effects of the proteins as regulators of lymphocyte proliferation, and eosinophil and macrophage activation in asthmatics; thereby compounding the effects of the viral infection. Thus, the antiviral properties of SP-A and SP-D make them important intrinsic agents for counteracting the effects of viruses as exacerbants of asthma.

The atypical bacteria *Mycoplasma pneumoniae* (Mp) and *Chlamydia pneumoniae* (Cp) also play a role in severe asthma exacerbation and asthma pathogenesis (121,139) (see chap. 6). Mp has also been implicated in the long-term impairment of pulmonary function in both asthmatic subjects and nonasthmatic subjects (140,141). Both SP-A and SP-D can bind to Mp (36,142) with high affinity. SP-A binding to Mp markedly attenuates the growth of the organism (36). In mouse experimental systems, SP-A potentiates host cell–dependent killing of *Mycoplasma pulmonis* by enhancing in vivo production of peroxinitrite by alveolar macrophages (32), and SP-A null mice exhibit reduced clearance of the bacteria (143). The robust interactions between the human pulmonary collectins and Mp are predicted to protect individuals from the bacteria, but it is uncertain why some asthmatics appear to be colonized by the bacteria and not effectively protected by either SP-A or SP-D.

VI. Pulmonary Surfactant Therapy for Asthma

Increasing evidence suggests that pulmonary surfactant can play an important role in the pathogenesis of asthma. The therapeutic use of exogenous surfactant treatment is well established in premature infants with respiratory distress syndrome (144,145). There are several commercially available surfactants that are either animal derived or synthetic (146). Animal and in vitro experiments demonstrate the potential protective effects of surfactant in models of asthma (81,87,96,147) and experimental suppression of allergic reactions (84,89,148). Currently, the results of clinical trials with therapeutic application of pulmonary surfactant for asthma have produced variable results. In one pilot study, exogenous synthetic surfactant, composed of phospholipids, significantly improved lung function in patients during an asthmatic attack (149). Another study showed beneficial effects from synthetic surfactant phospholipids (Pumacutant) in antigen-challenged asthmatic patients. In this latter study, exogenous surfactant treatment only inhibited the early asthmatic response (150). In contrast, the nebulization of Bovactant (which is an animal-derived surfactant) in children with asthma did not change airflow obstruction or bronchial hyperresponsiveness to histamine (151). Finally, the application of natural porcine surfactant (Curosurf) augmented the eosinophilic inflammation after local allergen challenge in patients with asthma (152).

There are numerous issues that need to be addressed to effectively examine the efficacy of surfactant for treatment of asthma, including the source of the surfactant, mode, dose, timing, and frequency of administration. Despite the successes of surfactant therapy in treating premature newborns, the utility of surfactant treatment for asthma may require a different frame of reference. Under conditions of newborn respiratory distress, the greatest need appears to be for the biophysical properties of surfactant. Conversely, in asthmatics the anti-inflammatory and immunoregulatory functions of surfactant may need to be supplemented. Although pulmonary surfactants devoid of SP-A and SP-D are effective for treatment of respiratory distress of the newborn, it is likely that these missing proteins are important, if not essential, for successful treatment of asthma. In addition to SP-A and SP-D, more specific attention should also be given to the lipid components of surfactant and their potential role in regulating inflammation and innate immunity.

References

1. Wright JR. Immunoregulatory functions of surfactant proteins. Nat Rev Immunol 2005; 5:58–68.
2. Lewis JF, Jobe AH. Surfactant and the adult respiratory distress syndrome. Am Rev Respir Dis 1993; 147:218–233.

3. Nieman GF, Bredenberg CE, Clark WR, et al. Alveolar function following surfactant deactivation. J Appl Physiol 1981; 51:895–904.
4. Zuo YY, Veldhuizen RA, Neumann AW, et al. Current perspectives in pulmonary surfactant—inhibition, enhancement and evaluation. Biochim Biophys Acta 2008; 1778:1947–1977.
5. Sano H, Kuroki Y. The lung collectins, SP-A and SP-D, modulate pulmonary innate immunity. Mol Immunol 2005; 42:279–287.
6. Pastva AM, Wright JR, Williams KL. Immunomodulatory roles of surfactant proteins A and D: implications in lung disease. Proc Am Thorac Soc 2007; 4:252–257.
7. Kishore U, Greenhough TJ, Waters P, et al. Surfactant proteins SP-A and SP-D: structure, function and receptors. Mol Immunol 2006; 43:1293–1315.
8. Mulugeta S, Beers MF. Surfactant protein C: its unique properties and emerging immunomodulatory role in the lung. Microbes Infect 2006; 8:2317–2323.
9. Dietl P, Haller T. Exocytosis of lung surfactant: from the secretory vesicle to the air-liquid interface. Annu Rev Physiol 2005; 67:595–621.
10. Andreeva AV, Kutuzov MA, Voyno-Yasenetskaya TA. Regulation of surfactant secretion in alveolar type II cells. Am J Physiol Lung Cell Mol Physiol 2007; 293:L259–L271.
11. Wirtz HR, Dobbs LG. Calcium mobilization and exocytosis after one mechanical stretch of lung epithelial cells. Science 1990; 250:1266–1269.
12. Auten RL, Watkins RH, Shapiro DL, et al. Surfactant apoprotein A (SP-A) is synthesized in airway cells. Am J Respir Cell Mol Biol 1990; 3:491–496.
13. Hohlfeld JM. The role of surfactant in asthma. Respir Res 2002; 3:4.
14. Madsen J, Kliem A, Tornoe I, et al. Localization of lung surfactant protein D on mucosal surfaces in human tissues. J Immunol 2000; 164:5866–5870.
15. Mason RJ. Surfactant synthesis, secretion, and function in alveoli and small airways. Review of the physiologic basis for pharmacologic intervention. Respiration 1987; 51(suppl 1):3–9.
16. Voorhout WF, Veenendaal T, Kuroki Y, et al. Immunocytochemical localization of surfactant protein D (SP-D) in type II cells, Clara cells, and alveolar macrophages of rat lung. J Histochem Cytochem 1992; 40:1589–1597.
17. Griese M. Pulmonary surfactant in health and human lung diseases: state of the art. Eur Respir J 1999; 13:1455–1476.
18. Enhorning G, Holm BA. Disruption of pulmonary surfactant's ability to maintain openness of a narrow tube. J Appl Physiol 1993; 74:2922–2927.
19. Bernhard W, Haagsman HP, Tschernig T, et al. Conductive airway surfactant: surface-tension function, biochemical composition, and possible alveolar origin. Am J Respir Cell Mol Biol 1997; 17:41–50.
20. Pattle RE. Properties, function and origin of the alveolar lining layer. Nature 1955; 175:1125–1126.
21. Lawson PR, Reid KB. The roles of surfactant proteins A and D in innate immunity. Immunol Rev 2000; 173:66–78.
22. van de Wetering JK, van Golde LM, Batenburg JJ. Collectins: players of the innate immune system. Eur J Biochem 2004; 271:1229–1249.
23. van Iwaarden JF, van Strijp JA, Visser H, et al. Binding of surfactant protein A (SP-A) to herpes simplex virus type 1-infected cells is mediated by the carbohydrate moiety of SP-A. J Biol Chem 1992; 267:25039–25043.
24. Benne CA, Benaissa-Trouw B, van Strijp JA, et al. Surfactant protein A, but not surfactant protein D, is an opsonin for influenza A virus phagocytosis by rat alveolar macrophages. Eur J Immunol 1997; 27:886–890.
25. Ferguson JS, Voelker DR, McCormack FX, et al. Surfactant protein D binds to Mycobacterium tuberculosis bacilli and lipoarabinomannan via carbohydrate-lectin interactions resulting in reduced phagocytosis of the bacteria by macrophages. J Immunol 1999; 163:312–321.

26. Hartshorn KL, Crouch E, White MR, et al. Pulmonary surfactant proteins A and D enhance neutrophil uptake of bacteria. Am J Physiol 1998; 274:L958–L969.
27. Hartshorn KL, White MR, Shepherd V, et al. Mechanisms of anti-influenza activity of surfactant proteins A and D: comparison with serum collectins. Am J Physiol 1997; 273: L1156–L1166.
28. Schelenz S, Malhotra R, Sim RB, et al. Binding of host collectins to the pathogenic yeast Cryptococcus neoformans: human surfactant protein D acts as an agglutinin for acapsular yeast cells. Infect Immun 1995; 63:3360–3366.
29. Kabha K, Schmegner J, Keisari Y, et al. SP-A enhances phagocytosis of Klebsiella by interaction with capsular polysaccharides and alveolar macrophages. Am J Physiol 1997; 272:L344–L352.
30. McNeely TB, Coonrod JD. Aggregation and opsonization of type A but not type B Hemophilus influenzae by surfactant protein A. Am J Respir Cell Mol Biol 1994; 11: 114–122.
31. O'Riordan DM, Standing JE, Kwon KY, et al. Surfactant protein D interacts with Pneumocystis carinii and mediates organism adherence to alveolar macrophages. J Clin Invest 1995; 95:2699–2710.
32. Hickman-Davis J, Gibbs-Erwin J, Lindsey JR, et al. Surfactant protein A mediates mycoplasmacidal activity of alveolar macrophages by production of peroxynitrite. Proc Natl Acad Sci U S A 1999; 96:4953–4958.
33. van Rozendaal BA, van Spriel AB, van De Winkel JG, et al. Role of pulmonary surfactant protein D in innate defense against Candida albicans. J Infect Dis 2000; 182:917–922.
34. Weikert LF, Lopez JP, Abdolrasulnia R, et al. Surfactant protein A enhances mycobacterial killing by rat macrophages through a nitric oxide-dependent pathway. Am J Physiol Lung Cell Mol Physiol 2000; 279:L216–L223.
35. McCormack FX, Gibbons R, Ward SR, et al. Macrophage-independent fungicidal action of the pulmonary collectins. J Biol Chem 2003; 278:36250–36256.
36. Piboonpocanun S, Chiba H, Mitsuzawa H, et al. Surfactant protein A binds Mycoplasma pneumoniae with high affinity and attenuates its growth by recognition of disaturated phosphatidylglycerols. J Biol Chem 2005; 280:9–17.
37. Wu H, Kuzmenko A, Wan S, et al. Surfactant proteins A and D inhibit the growth of Gram-negative bacteria by increasing membrane permeability. J Clin Invest 2003; 111: 1589–1602.
38. Ghildyal R, Hartley C, Varrasso A, et al. Surfactant protein A binds to the fusion glycoprotein of respiratory syncytial virus and neutralizes virion infectivity. J Infect Dis 1999; 180:2009–2013.
39. Hartshorn KL, White MR, Mogues T, et al. Lung and salivary scavenger receptor glycoprotein-340 contribute to the host defense against influenza A viruses. Am J Physiol Lung Cell Mol Physiol 2003; 285:L1066–L1076.
40. Hickling TP, Bright H, Wing K, et al. A recombinant trimeric surfactant protein D carbohydrate recognition domain inhibits respiratory syncytial virus infection in vitro and in vivo. Eur J Immunol 1999; 29:3478–3484.
41. Vandivier RW, Ogden CA, Fadok VA, et al. Role of surfactant proteins A, D, and C1q in the clearance of apoptotic cells in vivo and in vitro: calreticulin and CD91 as a common collectin receptor complex. J Immunol 2002; 169:3978–3986.
42. Sano H, Sohma H, Muta T, et al. Pulmonary surfactant protein A modulates the cellular response to smooth and rough lipopolysaccharides by interaction with CD14. J Immunol 1999; 163:387–395.
43. Murakami S, Iwaki D, Mitsuzawa H, et al. Surfactant protein A inhibits peptidoglycan-induced tumor necrosis factor-alpha secretion in U937 cells and alveolar macrophages by direct interaction with toll-like receptor 2. J Biol Chem 2002; 277:6830–6837.

44. Yamada C, Sano H, Shimizu T, et al. Surfactant protein A directly interacts with TLR4 and MD-2 and regulates inflammatory cellular response. Importance of supratrimeric oligomerization. J Biol Chem 2006; 281:21771–21780.

45. Ohya M, Nishitani C, Sano H, et al. Human pulmonary surfactant protein D binds the extracellular domains of Toll-like receptors 2 and 4 through the carbohydrate recognition domain by a mechanism different from its binding to phosphatidylinositol and lipopolysaccharide. Biochemistry 2006; 45:8657–8664.

46. Gardai SJ, Xiao YQ, Dickinson M, et al. By binding SIRPalpha or calreticulin/CD91, lung collectins act as dual function surveillance molecules to suppress or enhance inflammation. Cell 2003; 115:13–23.

47. Brinker KG, Garner H, Wright JR. Surfactant protein A modulates the differentiation of murine bone marrow-derived dendritic cells. Am J Physiol Lung Cell Mol Physiol 2003; 284:L232–L241.

48. Brinker KG, Martin E, Borron P, et al. Surfactant protein D enhances bacterial antigen presentation by bone marrow-derived dendritic cells. Am J Physiol Lung Cell Mol Physiol 2001; 281:L1453–L1463.

49. Wang JY, Kishore U, Lim BL, et al. Interaction of human lung surfactant proteins A and D with mite (Dermatophagoides pteronyssinus) allergens. Clin Exp Immunol 1996; 106:367–373.

50. Augusto LA, Synguelakis M, Johansson J, et al. Interaction of pulmonary surfactant protein C with CD14 and lipopolysaccharide. Infect Immun 2003; 71:61–67.

51. Nogee LM, Dunbar AE 3rd, Wert SE, et al. A mutation in the surfactant protein C gene associated with familial interstitial lung disease. N Engl J Med 2001; 344:573–579.

52. Schmidt R, Meier U, Yabut-Perez M, et al. Alteration of fatty acid profiles in different pulmonary surfactant phospholipids in acute respiratory distress syndrome and severe pneumonia. Am J Respir Crit Care Med 2001; 163:95–100.

53. McCormack FX, King TE Jr., Voelker DR, et al. Idiopathic pulmonary fibrosis. Abnormalities in the bronchoalveolar lavage content of surfactant protein A. Am Rev Respir Dis 1991; 144:160–166.

54. Hite RD, Seeds MC, Bowton DL, et al. Surfactant phospholipid changes after antigen challenge: a role for phosphatidylglycerol in dysfunction. Am J Physiol Lung Cell Mol Physiol 2005; 288:L610–L617.

55. Robinson PC, Watters LC, King TE, et al. Idiopathic pulmonary fibrosis. Abnormalities in bronchoalveolar lavage fluid phospholipids. Am Rev Respir Dis 1988; 137:585–591.

56. Wright JR. Immunomodulatory functions of surfactant. Physiol Rev 1997; 77:931–962.

57. Hashimoto M, Asai Y, Ogawa T. Treponemal phospholipids inhibit innate immune responses induced by pathogen-associated molecular patterns. J Biol Chem 2003; 278:44205–44213.

58. Kuronuma K, Mitsuzawa H, Takeda K, et al. Anionic pulmonary surfactant phospholipids inhibit inflammatory responses from alveolar macrophages and U937 cells by binding the lipopolysaccharide interacting proteins CD14 and MD2. J Biol Chem 2009; [Epub ahead of print] PMID: 19584052.

59. Mutti A, Corradi M, Goldoni M, et al. Exhaled metallic elements and serum pneumoproteins in asymptomatic smokers and patients with COPD or asthma. Chest 2006; 129: 1288–1297.

60. Devendra G, Spragg RG. Lung surfactant in subacute pulmonary disease. Respir Res 2002; 3:19.

61. Greene KE, Wright JR, Steinberg KP, et al. Serial changes in surfactant-associated proteins in lung and serum before and after onset of ARDS. Am J Respir Crit Care Med 1999; 160:1843–1850.

62. Takahashi H, Kuroki Y, Tanaka H, et al. Serum levels of surfactant proteins A and D are useful biomarkers for interstitial lung disease in patients with progressive systemic sclerosis. Am J Respir Crit Care Med 2000; 162:258–263.

63. Noah TL, Murphy PC, Alink JJ, et al. Bronchoalveolar lavage fluid surfactant protein-A and surfactant protein-D are inversely related to inflammation in early cystic fibrosis. Am J Respir Crit Care Med 2003; 168:685–691.

64. von Bredow C, Birrer P, Griese M. Surfactant protein A and other bronchoalveolar lavage fluid proteins are altered in cystic fibrosis. Eur Respir J 2001; 17:716–722.

65. Bufler P, Schmidt B, Schikor D, et al. Surfactant protein A and D differently regulate the immune response to nonmucoid Pseudomonas aeruginosa and its lipopolysaccharide. Am J Respir Cell Mol Biol 2003; 28:249–256.

66. Wang G, Myers C, Mikerov A, et al. Effect of cysteine 85 on biochemical properties and biological function of human surfactant protein A variants. Biochemistry 2007; 46:8425–8435.

67. Mariencheck WI, Alcorn JF, Palmer SM, et al. Pseudomonas aeruginosa elastase degrades surfactant proteins A and D. Am J Respir Cell Mol Biol 2003; 28:528–537.

68. Glasser SW, Senft AP, Whitsett JA, et al. Macrophage dysfunction and susceptibility to pulmonary Pseudomonas aeruginosa infection in surfactant protein C-deficient mice. J Immunol 2008; 181:621–628.

69. Baudouin SV. Exogenous surfactant replacement in ARDS—one day, someday, or never? N Engl J Med 2004; 351:853–855.

70. Markart P, Ruppert C, Wygrecka M, et al. Patients with ARDS show improvement but not normalisation of alveolar surface activity with surfactant treatment: putative role of neutral lipids. Thorax 2007; 62:588–594.

71. Selman M, Lin HM, Montano M, et al. Surfactant protein A and B genetic variants predispose to idiopathic pulmonary fibrosis. Hum Genet 2003; 113:542–550.

72. Saxena S, Kumar R, Madan T, et al. Association of polymorphisms in pulmonary surfactant protein A1 and A2 genes with high-altitude pulmonary edema. Chest 2005; 128:1611–1619.

73. Lofgren J, Ramet M, Renko M, et al. Association between surfactant protein A gene locus and severe respiratory syncytial virus infection in infants. J Infect Dis 2002; 185:283–289.

74. Lahti M, Lofgren J, Marttila R, et al. Surfactant protein D gene polymorphism associated with severe respiratory syncytial virus infection. Pediatr Res 2002; 51:696–699.

75. Floros J, Lin HM, Garcia A, et al. Surfactant protein genetic marker alleles identify a subgroup of tuberculosis in a Mexican population. J Infect Dis 2000; 182:1473–1478.

76. Whitsett JA, Wert SE, Trapnell BC. Genetic disorders influencing lung formation and function at birth. Hum Mol Genet 2004; 13(Spec No 2):R207–R215.

77. Whitsett JA, Weaver TE. Hydrophobic surfactant proteins in lung function and disease. N Engl J Med 2002; 347:2141–2148.

78. Amin RS, Wert SE, Baughman RP, et al. Surfactant protein deficiency in familial interstitial lung disease. J Pediatr 2001; 139:85–92.

79. Haczku A, Vass G, Kierstein S. Surfactant protein D and asthma. Clin Exp Allergy 2004; 34:1815–1818.

80. Cheng G, Ueda T, Numao T, et al. Increased levels of surfactant protein A and D in bronchoalveolar lavage fluids in patients with bronchial asthma. Eur Respir J 2000; 16:831–835.

81. Erpenbeck VJ, Schmidt R, Gunther A, et al. Surfactant protein levels in bronchoalveolar lavage after segmental allergen challenge in patients with asthma. Allergy 2006; 61:598–604.

82. Deb R, Shakib F, Reid K, et al. Major house dust mite allergens Dermatophagoides pteronyssinus 1 and Dermatophagoides farinae 1 degrade and inactivate lung surfactant proteins A and D. J Biol Chem 2007; 282:36808–36819.

83. Malhotra R, Haurum J, Thiel S, et al. Pollen grains bind to lung alveolar type II cells (A549) via lung surfactant protein A (SP-A). Biosci Rep 1993; 13:79–90.

84. Erpenbeck VJ, Malherbe DC, Sommer S, et al. Surfactant protein D increases phagocytosis and aggregation of pollen-allergen starch granules. Am J Physiol Lung Cell Mol Physiol 2005; 288:L692–L698.

85. Wang JY, Shieh CC, You PF, et al. Inhibitory effect of pulmonary surfactant proteins A and D on allergen-induced lymphocyte proliferation and histamine release in children with asthma. Am J Respir Crit Care Med 1998; 158:510–518.
86. Allen MJ, Harbeck R, Smith B, et al. Binding of rat and human surfactant proteins A and D to Aspergillus fumigatus conidia. Infect Immun 1999; 67:4563–4569.
87. Madan T, Kishore U, Singh M, et al. Surfactant proteins A and D protect mice against pulmonary hypersensitivity induced by Aspergillus fumigatus antigens and allergens. J Clin Invest 2001; 107:467–475.
88. Madan T, Kishore U, Shah A, et al. Lung surfactant proteins A and D can inhibit specific IgE binding to the allergens of Aspergillus fumigatus and block allergen-induced histamine release from human basophils. Clin Exp Immunol 1997; 110:241–249.
89. Malherbe DC, Erpenbeck VJ, Abraham SN, et al. Surfactant protein D decreases pollen-induced IgE-dependent mast cell degranulation. Am J Physiol Lung Cell Mol Physiol 2005; 289:L856–L866.
90. Borron PJ, Crouch EC, Lewis JF, et al. Recombinant rat surfactant-associated protein D inhibits human T lymphocyte proliferation and IL-2 production. J Immunol 1998; 161:4599–4603.
91. Kremlev SG, Umstead TM, Phelps DS. Effects of surfactant protein A and surfactant lipids on lymphocyte proliferation in vitro. Am J Physiol 1994; 267:L357–L364.
92. Woerndle S, Bartmann P. The effect of three surfactant preparations on in vitro lymphocyte functions. J Perinat Med 1994; 22:119–128.
93. Haczku A, Cao Y, Vass G, et al. IL-4 and IL-13 form a negative feedback circuit with surfactant protein-D in the allergic airway response. J Immunol 2006; 176:3557–3565.
94. Cheng G, Ueda T, Nakajima H, et al. Suppressive effects of SP-A on ionomycin-induced IL-8 production and release by eosinophils. Int Arch Allergy Immunol 1998; 117(suppl 1): 59–62.
95. Mahajan L, Madan T, Kamal N, et al. Recombinant surfactant protein-D selectively increases apoptosis in eosinophils of allergic asthmatics and enhances uptake of apoptotic eosinophils by macrophages. Int Immunol 2008; 20:993–1007.
96. Takeda K, Miyahara N, Rha YH, et al. Surfactant protein D regulates airway function and allergic inflammation through modulation of macrophage function. Am J Respir Crit Care Med 2003; 168:783–789.
97. Strong P, Townsend P, Mackay R, et al. A recombinant fragment of human SP-D reduces allergic responses in mice sensitized to house dust mite allergens. Clin Exp Immunol 2003; 134:181–187.
98. Hammad H, Lambrecht BN. Dendritic cells and epithelial cells: linking innate and adaptive immunity in asthma. Nat Rev Immunol 2008; 8:193–204.
99. Steinman RM, Hawiger D, Nussenzweig MC. Tolerogenic dendritic cells. Annu Rev Immunol 2003; 21:685–711.
100. Hansen S, Lo B, Evans K, et al. Surfactant protein D augments bacterial association but attenuates major histocompatibility complex class II presentation of bacterial antigens. Am J Respir Cell Mol Biol 2007; 36:94–102.
101. Heeley EL, Hohlfeld JM, Krug N, et al. Phospholipid molecular species of bronchoalveolar lavage fluid after local allergen challenge in asthma. Am J Physiol Lung Cell Mol Physiol 2000; 278:L305–L311.
102. Cochrane CG. Pulmonary surfactant in allergic inflammation: new insights into the molecular mechanisms of surfactant function. Am J Physiol Lung Cell Mol Physiol 2005; 288:L608–L609.
103. Cochrane CG, Revak SD. Pulmonary surfactant protein B (SP-B): structure-function relationships. Science 1991; 254:566–568.

104. Girod de Bentzmann S, Pierrot D, Fuchey C, et al. Distearoyl phosphatidylglycerol liposomes improve surface and transport properties of CF mucus. Eur Respir J 1993; 6:1156–1161.
105. Baker CS, Evans TW, Randle BJ, et al. Damage to surfactant-specific protein in acute respiratory distress syndrome. Lancet 1999; 353:1232–1237.
106. Notter RH. Lung surfactant dysfunction lung biology in health and disease. In: Lenfant C, ed. Lung Surfactants Basic Science and Clinical Applications. New York: Marcel Dekker, Inc., 2000:207–231.
107. Hohlfeld J, Fabel H, Hamm H. The role of pulmonary surfactant in obstructive airways disease. Eur Respir J 1997; 10:482–491.
108. Hohlfeld JM, Ahlf K, Enhorning G, et al. Dysfunction of pulmonary surfactant in asthmatics after segmental allergen challenge. Am J Respir Crit Care Med 1999; 159:1803–1809.
109. Hite RD, Seeds MC, Safta AM, et al. Lysophospholipid generation and phosphatidylglycerol depletion in phospholipase A(2)-mediated surfactant dysfunction. Am J Physiol Lung Cell Mol Physiol 2005; 288:L618–L624.
110. Seeds MC, Jones KA, Duncan Hite R, et al. Cell-specific expression of group X and group V secretory phospholipases A(2) in human lung airway epithelial cells. Am J Respir Cell Mol Biol 2000; 23:37–44.
111. Kim DK, Fukuda T, Thompson BT, et al. Bronchoalveolar lavage fluid phospholipase A2 activities are increased in human adult respiratory distress syndrome. Am J Physiol 1995; 269:L109–L118.
112. Anderson BO, Moore EE, Banerjee A. Phospholipase A2 regulates critical inflammatory mediators of multiple organ failure. J Surg Res 1994; 56:199–205.
113. Chilton FH, Averill FJ, Hubbard WC, et al. Antigen-induced generation of lyso-phospholipids in human airways. J Exp Med 1996; 183:2235–2245.
114. Kwatia MA, Doyle CB, Cho W, et al. Combined activities of secretory phospholipases and eosinophil lysophospholipases induce pulmonary surfactant dysfunction by phospholipid hydrolysis. J Allergy Clin Immunol 2007; 119:838–847.
115. Ackerman SJ, Kwatia MA, Doyle CB, et al. Hydrolysis of surfactant phospholipids catalyzed by phospholipase A2 and eosinophil lysophospholipases causes surfactant dysfunction: a mechanism for small airway closure in asthma. Chest 2003; 123:355S.
116. Blom M, Tool AT, Wever PC, et al. Human eosinophils express, relative to other circulating leukocytes, large amounts of secretory 14-kD phospholipase A2. Blood 1998; 91:3037–3043.
117. Henderson WR Jr., Chi EY, Bollinger JG, et al. Importance of group X-secreted phospholipase A2 in allergen-induced airway inflammation and remodeling in a mouse asthma model. J Exp Med 2007; 204:865–877.
118. Johnston SL. Overview of virus-induced airway disease. Proc Am Thorac Soc 2005; 2: 150–156.
119. Tauro S, Su YC, Thomas S, et al. Molecular and cellular mechanisms in the viral exacerbation of asthma. Microbes Infect 2008; 10:1014–1023.
120. MacDowell AL, Bacharier LB. Infectious triggers of asthma. Immunol Allergy Clin North Am 2005; 25:45–66.
121. Martin RJ. Infections and asthma. Clin Chest Med 2006; 27:87–98, vi.
122. Message SD, Johnston SL. The immunology of virus infection in asthma. Eur Respir J 2001; 18:1013–1025.
123. Gern JE. Mechanisms of virus-induced asthma. J Pediatr 2003; 142:S9–S13; discussion S13–S14.
124. Griese M. Respiratory syncytial virus and pulmonary surfactant. Viral Immunol 2002; 15:357–363.
125. Kerr MH, Paton JY. Surfactant protein levels in severe respiratory syncytial virus infection. Am J Respir Crit Care Med 1999; 159:1115–1118.

126. LeVine AM, Lotze A, Stanley S, et al. Surfactant content in children with inflammatory lung disease. Crit Care Med 1996; 24:1062–1067.
127. Alcorn JL, Stark JM, Chiappetta CL, et al. Effects of RSV infection on pulmonary surfactant protein SP-A in cultured human type II cells: contrasting consequences on SP-A mRNA and protein. Am J Physiol Lung Cell Mol Physiol 2005; 289:L1113–L1122.
128. Hall CB. Respiratory syncytial virus and parainfluenza virus. N Engl J Med 2001; 344:1917–1928.
129. LeVine AM, Gwozdz J, Stark J, et al. Surfactant protein-A enhances respiratory syncytial virus clearance in vivo. J Clin Invest 1999; 103:1015–1021.
130. LeVine AM, Elliott J, Whitsett JA, et al. Surfactant protein-d enhances phagocytosis and pulmonary clearance of respiratory syncytial virus. Am J Respir Cell Mol Biol 2004; 31:193–199.
131. LeVine AM, Hartshorn K, Elliott J, et al. Absence of SP-A modulates innate and adaptive defense responses to pulmonary influenza infection. Am J Physiol Lung Cell Mol Physiol 2002; 282:L563–L572.
132. Hartshorn K, Chang D, Rust K, et al. Interactions of recombinant human pulmonary surfactant protein D and SP-D multimers with influenza A. Am J Physiol 1996; 271:L753–L762.
133. Hartshorn KL, Reid KB, White MR, et al. Neutrophil deactivation by influenza A viruses: mechanisms of protection after viral opsonization with collectins and hemagglutination-inhibiting antibodies. Blood 1996; 87:3450–3461.
134. Hawgood S, Brown C, Edmondson J, et al. Pulmonary collectins modulate strain-specific influenza a virus infection and host responses. J Virol 2004; 78:8565–8572.
135. Hartshorn KL, Webby R, White MR, et al. Role of viral hemagglutinin glycosylation in anti-influenza activities of recombinant surfactant protein D. Respir Res 2008; 9:65.
136. White MR, Crouch E, van Eijk M, et al. Cooperative anti-influenza activities of respiratory innate immune proteins and neuraminidase inhibitor. Am J Physiol Lung Cell Mol Physiol 2005; 288:L831–L840.
137. LeVine AM, Whitsett JA, Hartshorn KL, et al. Surfactant protein D enhances clearance of influenza A virus from the lung in vivo. J Immunol 2001; 167:5868–5873.
138. Gern JE, Busse WW. Relationship of viral infections to wheezing illnesses and asthma. Nat Rev Immunol 2002; 2:132–138.
139. Cosentini R, Tarsia P, Canetta C, et al. Severe asthma exacerbation: role of acute Chlamydophila pneumoniae and Mycoplasma pneumoniae infection. Respir Res 2008; 9:48.
140. Johnston SL, Martin RJ. Chlamydophila pneumoniae and Mycoplasma pneumoniae: a role in asthma pathogenesis? Am J Respir Crit Care Med 2005; 172:1078–1089.
141. Sutherland ER, Martin RJ. Asthma and atypical bacterial infection. Chest 2007; 132: 1962–1966.
142. Chiba H, Pattanajitvilai S, Evans AJ, et al. Human surfactant protein D (SP-D) binds Mycoplasma pneumoniae by high affinity interactions with lipids. J Biol Chem 2002; 277:20379–20385.
143. Hickman-Davis JM, Gibbs-Erwin J, Lindsey JR, et al. Role of surfactant protein-A in nitric oxide production and mycoplasma killing in congenic C57BL/6 mice. Am J Respir Cell Mol Biol 2004; 30:319–325.
144. Sinha SK, Lacaze-Masmonteil T, Valls i Soler A, et al. A multicenter, randomized, controlled trial of lucinactant versus poractant alfa among very premature infants at high risk for respiratory distress syndrome. Pediatrics 2005; 115:1030–1038.
145. Jobe AH. Pulmonary surfactant therapy. N Engl J Med 1993; 328:861–868.
146. Erpenbeck VJ, Krug N, Hohlfeld JM. Therapeutic use of surfactant components in allergic asthma. Naunyn Schmiedebergs Arch Pharmacol 2009; 379:217–224.

147. Madan T, Reid KB, Singh M, et al. Susceptibility of mice genetically deficient in the surfactant protein (SP)-A or SP-D gene to pulmonary hypersensitivity induced by antigens and allergens of Aspergillus fumigatus. J Immunol 2005; 174:6943–6954.
148. Hills BA, Chen Y. Suppression of neural activity of bronchial irritant receptors by surface-active phospholipid in comparison with topical drugs commonly prescribed for asthma. Clin Exp Allergy 2000; 30:1266–1274.
149. Kurashima K, Ogawa H, Ohka T, et al. A pilot study of surfactant inhalation in the treatment of asthmatic attack. Arerugi 1991; 40:160–163.
150. Babu KS, Woodcock DA, Smith SE, et al. Inhaled synthetic surfactant abolishes the early allergen-induced response in asthma. Eur Respir J 2003; 21:1046–1049.
151. Oetomo SB, Dorrepaal C, Bos H, et al. Surfactant nebulization does not alter airflow obstruction and bronchial responsiveness to histamine in asthmatic children. Am J Respir Crit Care Med 1996; 153:1148–1152.
152. Erpenbeck VJ, Hagenberg A, Dulkys Y, et al. Natural porcine surfactant augments airway inflammation after allergen challenge in patients with asthma. Am J Respir Crit Care Med 2004; 169:578–586.

11
Host Defense Responses

HONG W. CHU and FABIENNE GALLY
National Jewish Health, Denver, Colorado, U.S.A.

I. Introduction

Airway infection is an important contributor to asthma pathobiology. Various pathogens including viruses and bacteria have been found in the airways of asthmatics (1). Host response to the invading pathogens is critical to terminate the infectious process. Any aberrant responses to the respiratory pathogens could lead to asthma exacerbations and/ or persistent infections.

Innate and adaptive immune responses represent the two pivotal components of host responses to any given pathogen. Innate immunity effects immediately or in hours after the infection and serves as the first line of host defense against the pathogens. Unlike innate immunity, adaptive immunity is induced after several days (usually three days) of the infection and provides a specific defense mechanism. Cooperation between the innate and adaptive immunities results in more efficient clearance of the invading pathogens. However, the persistent and repeated nature of infections in chronic asthma indicates an abnormal interaction of innate and adaptive immunities in the context of an allergic airway milieu. This chapter will focus on the nature of innate and adaptive immune responses to bacterial and viral infections, and the impact of an established adaptive (i.e., allergic) airway milieu on innate immunity of lung-resident cells such as airway epithelial cells and dendritic cells (DCs).

II. Innate Immunity and Its Function in Respiratory Infection

Several types of lung-resident and inflammatory cells actively participate in innate immune responses to infections of microorganisms such as bacteria and viruses. These include airway and alveolar epithelial cells, alveolar macrophages, DCs, natural killer (NK) cells, mast cells, and neutrophils. While each of these cells is essential to the intact innate immune system, we will focus on airway epithelial cells and DCs in this chapter.

A. Airway Epithelial Cells

Airway epithelial cells represent the very first line of host defense against the invading pathogens including bacteria and viruses in the lung. They respond to typical bacteria (e.g., *Pseudomonas aeruginosa*) by producing various mediators such as proinflammatory cytokines, mucins, and antimicrobial substances including peptides (β-defensins and LL-37) and proteins (lysozyme and lactoferrin) (2). An array of epithelial cell–derived cytokines recruit inflammatory cells (e.g., neutrophils) to the sites of infection to combat the pathogen. Mucins can trap the pathogens and facilitate airway epithelial mucociliary

Table 1 TLRs and Their Ligands

TLRs	Ligands
TLR1	Triacyl lipoproteins, soluble bacterial factors
TLR2	Peptidoglycans, lipoproteins, zymosan (fungal), glycosylphosphoinositols, glycolipids, lipoteichoic acid, porins, heat shock protein (HSP70) (host)
TLR3	dsRNA (viral)
TLR4	Lipopolysaccharide, taxol (plant), HSP60 (bacterial), fibronectin, hyaluronic acid, heparan sulfate, fibrinogen
TLR5	Flagellin
TLR6	Diacyl lipopeptide (*Mycoplasma*), zymosan (fungal)
TLR7	ssRNA (influenza)
TLR8	ssRNA (mostly viral), imidazoquinoline
TLR9	Unmethylated CpG DNA (mostly bacterial)
TLR10	Unknown; alleles linked to asthma susceptibility
TLR11	Uropathogenic bacteria

Abbreviation: TLR, toll-like receptor.

clearance. Antimicrobial substances exert bactericidal effects or inhibit bacterial growth. Coordination of phagocytosis, mucociliary clearance, and antimicrobial activity will ultimately eliminate the pathogen and restore the lung homeostasis.

How airway epithelial cells recognize the pathogen has been an area of active investigation. One of the mechanisms by which epithelial cells recognize pathogens and subsequently produce host defense molecules is through the toll-like receptor (TLR) pathway. TLRs are pattern recognition receptors for different microorganisms. Airway epithelial cells are known to express all the 11 TLRs described so far (3,4) (Table 1). For example, TLR2 and TLR4 are involved in the signal transduction of Gram-positive and Gram-negative bacteria and their components, respectively. On the other hand, TLR3 and TLR7 are necessary for viral recognition.

Our clinical studies have demonstrated that nearly 42% of chronic stable asthmatics are positive for atypical bacterium *Mycoplasma pneumoniae* (Mp). Since a previous study suggests that MALP-2, a lipoprotein from *M. fermentans*, activates macrophages through TLR2 signaling, we investigated the role of TLR2 in airway epithelial response to Mp infection. TLR2 is a transmembrane protein that signals as a heterodimer with either TLR1 or TLR6. Ligand binding to the TLR2 complex induces the TLR cytoplasmic domain to recruit and activate the adapter protein MyD88 and MyD88 adapter-like (Mal) protein or toll/IL-1 receptor (TIR) domain–containing adapter protein (TIRAP) (5). MyD88/Mal will bind to the death domain of a serine/threonine kinase, usually IL-1 receptor–associated kinase (IRAK). IRAK further activates TNF receptor–associated factor (TRAF) family, TRAF6, which eventually leads to the activation of nuclear factor kappa B (NF-κB) and mitogen-activated protein (MAP) kinases and transcription of target genes including proinflammatory cytokines (e.g., IL-6 and antimicrobial substances such as β-defensins) (6). The above process is referred to as TLR2 pathway activation— the binding of TLR2 to its ligands and eventual activation of transcription factors (e.g., NF-κB) and production of mediators including proinflammatory cytokines and antimicrobial substances. It is noteworthy that MyD88-dependant signaling is the predominant pathway for all the TLRs except TLR3 that utilizes the MyD88-independent signaling pathway involving the activation of TRAM, a TIR domain–containing adapter molecule. TRAM binds and activates TRIF, another TIR domain–containing adapter protein (7). TRIF then interacts with and activates two IκK homologs, TANK-binding kinase 1 (TBK1) and IKKε. This leads to the phosphorylation of interferon regulatory factor 3 (IRF3), its translocation to the nucleus, and subsequent regulation of the expression of type I interferon (IFN) genes (8). MyD88-independent signaling pathway can also culminate in the activation of NF-κB when TRIF binds to TRAF6 or receptor interacting protein 1 (RIP1) (9,10).

We have demonstrated that Mp activates TLR2 pathway including IL-6 production and NF-κB activation, which is critical for Mp-induced airway epithelial mucin production in allergen-naive mice (11). TLR2-deficient mice demonstrated impaired lung Mp clearance accompanied by reduced IL-6 production and NF-κB activation in the lung compared with the wild-type mice. We further cultured mouse tracheal epithelial cells under the air-liquid interface culture conditions and found that TLR2-deficient mouse epithelial cells demonstrated low level of IL-6 response to Mp or TLR2 agonist Pam3CSK4. Collectively, our studies suggest that activation of epithelial TLR2 signaling promotes bacterial clearance.

Other groups of investigators also reveal a pivotal role of airway epithelial cells in host defense against bacteria and viruses that are relevant to asthma pathogenesis. For example, human airway epithelial cells produce granulocyte-macrophage colony-stimulating factor (GM-CSF) upon *Chlamydia pneumoniae* infection (12). Respiratory syncytial virus (RSV) and rhinovirus (RV) are known to be involved in asthma inception and/or exacerbations. Monick and colleagues have shown that RSV synergizes with T helper 2 (T_h2) cytokines IL-4 and IL-13 to induce epithelial expression of thymus- and activation-regulated chemokine (TARC) that is able to recruit T_h2 cells to sites of infection (13). A variety of host defense molecules such as IL-8 and type I IFNs are released from primary human bronchial epithelial cells following RV infection (14,15). Interestingly, RV-infected bronchial epithelial cells from asthmatics produced less IFN-β than those from normal subjects, suggesting that a deficient epithelial function may account for the increased susceptibility of asthmatics to viral infections (16).

B. Dendritic Cells

In case airway epithelial cells fail to completely eliminate the invading pathogen, DCs represent another critical line of host defense mechanism. DCs reside within airway epithelium and other compartments of the lung such as alveolar and connective tissue. Interestingly, DCs within the airway epithelial layer have an immature phenotype, while DCs in other compartments express a mature phenotype (17). As compared with mature DCs, immature DCs have more potent antigen uptake and processing capacity and express high levels of TLRs (e.g., TLR2, TLR4) but low levels of costimulatory molecules [e.g., CD80, CD86, and major histocompatibility complex (MHC) class II]. The phenotypic differences of DCs in different lung compartments suggest that DCs within the airway epithelium serve as sentinels to process the antigens of infectious agents.

DCs express various receptors and costimulatory molecules to cope with danger signals including pathogens (Table 2). In response to bacterial and viral infections, DCs produce host defense cytokines including IL-1β, IL-6, IFN-γ, and IL-12 (18). Another major function of DCs is to bridge the innate and adaptive immunities. In the lung, pathogen-activated DCs migrate to local lymph nodes, become matured, and activate T cells. In bacterial and viral infections, DCs usually induce T cell differentiation into

Table 2 DC Subsets and the Expression Level of Their Surface Markers

	CD11c	CD8	CD11b	CD4	CD205	Class II	B220
Myeloid DCs	+++	−	+++	+/−	−	+++	−
Lymphoid DCs	+++	+++	−	−	++	+++	−
Plasmacytoid DCs	+++	+/−	−	−	−	+++	++
Tissue-resident DCs	+++	+	++	−	++	+++	−

+++, high; ++, intermediate; +, low; and −, negative.
Abbreviation: DC, dendritic cell.

T_h1 cells via IL-12 production. However, in parasitic and fungal infections, DCs direct naive T cells into T_h2 differentiation (IL-4, IL-13, and IL-5). It has been proposed that DCs may produce IL-10 and induce regulatory T cells (Tregs) to suppress the T-cell activation process. What we have learned about the role of DCs in host defense is largely obtained from mouse models. How DCs directly interact with bacteria or viruses in human lung diseases such as asthma remains poorly understood.

Previous studies in animals suggest that activation of lung DCs following bacterial or viral infection is a critical step in host defense. An increased number of DCs have been reported in rat tracheal mucosa after *M. pulmonis* (a nonhuman pathogen) infection (19). We have demonstrated upregulation of TLR2 expression in pulmonary DCs, which produce high levels of IL-6 upon Mp infection or TLR2 agonist Pam3CSK4 stimulation. RV infection in mouse models induces the production of DC chemokine MIP-3α (20). DCs can be categorized into plasmacytoid DCs (pDCs) and conventional or myeloid DCs. Depletion of DCs, especially pDCs, abrogates the protective role of DCs in RSV infection in mice (21). These studies suggest that activation of DCs following bacterial or viral infection in mice is essential to timely eliminate the invading pathogen from host lungs.

There are fewer studies in human subjects to dissect the role of lung DCs in host (e.g., asthmatic) defense against infections. DCs isolated from normal regions of resected lungs of cancer and chronic obstructive pulmonary disease (COPD) patients respond to influenza A or lipopolysaccharide (LPS) by producing IFN-α or MIP-1α (macrophage inflammatory protein-1α) and IL-6, respectively. Increased number of DCs has been described in the bronchial mucosal tissue of atopic asthmatic patients, which is effectively reduced by inhaled corticosteroids (22). So far, there is no study examining the number and activity of airway DCs in asthma exacerbations or in chronic asthma associated with bacterial or viral infections. Future studies are imperative to understand the role of DCs in human airways or lungs under pathological conditions. If deficient functions of DCs in asthmatic lungs can be verified, DC-based immunotherapy (or vaccines) would be a powerful and novel approach to treat persistent infections in asthma. For example, autologous peripheral blood monocyte–derived DCs could be activated in vitro by stimulation with relevant TLR agonists and then delivered (e.g., inhalation) to the patient lung.

III. Adaptive Immunity and Its Function in Respiratory Infection

After DCs uptake and process the pathogen in the lung, they migrate to local lymph nodes where they present antigens to T cells to initiate the adaptive immune response.

Activated T cells produce a variety of mediators or cytokines to promote pathogen clearance from the host and also induce immunoglobulin (Ig) production to further enhance host defense functions. However, a dysregulated adaptive immune response could cause asthma exacerbations. In this chapter, we focus on the role of T-cell activation as well as humoral response in host defense against respiratory bacterial and viral infections, and their impact on asthma pathogenesis.

A. Role of T Cells in Respiratory Infections and Asthma

T cells are critical to the pathogenesis of asthma, especially allergic asthma. A predominant T_h2 response is considered as a hallmark of airway allergic inflammation in asthma. The impact of infection-induced adaptive immunity on established asthma is complex and varies depending on several factors such as the dose of the pathogen, the timing of the infection, and host genetic susceptibility to the infection. To simplify our understanding of the role of T cells in asthma in the context of an infection, we will discuss the role of various subsets of T cells and the mechanisms underlying their induction.

T_h1 Cells

T_h1 cells are typically defined as $CD4^+$ T cells producing cytokines IFN-γ and TNF-β (23). T_h1 cell differentiation and subsequent T_h1 cytokine production are under the control of IL-12 from antigen-presenting cells such as DCs. The function of T_h1 cytokines is to enhance host antimicrobial activities against intracellular bacterial and viral infections through various mechanisms including recruitment of phagocytes (e.g., neutrophils), activation of lung macrophages, and production of antimicrobial substances.

In normal lungs, viral and bacterial infections induce a T_h1 response, which is critical for quick removal of the invading pathogen and subsequent resolution of inflammation. In the absence of allergic inflammation, virtually all the viral and bacterial infections involved in asthma inception, maintenance, or exacerbations induce a T_h1 response characterized by higher levels of IFN-γ and IL-12. Mild but not severe RSV infection in children increases IFN-γ in peripheral blood monocytes (24). Bacterial (e.g., Mp) infection in human subjects also increases serum IFN-γ levels (25).

Viral infections in asthmatics fail to induce sufficient T_h1 cytokines (26), which is associated with asthma exacerbations. Therefore, therapeutic approaches to enhance IFN-γ production have been investigated. Recombinant IFN-γ protein appears to inhibit allergic response in mice (27,28). However, treatment of steroid-dependent asthma with recombinant IFN-γ has not been shown to be effective in improving lung function (29). It is worthy of noting that upregulation of a T_h1 response has been reported in asthma, especially severe asthma (30). These results suggest that an enhanced T_h1 response associated with an infection is not necessarily good for asthma. In line with this observation, IFN-γ has been shown to directly induce airway epithelial cell apoptosis and injury, which may cause airway hyperresponsiveness (31,32).

T_h2 Cells

T_h2 cells produce T_h2 cytokines IL-4, IL-5, IL-9, and IL-13, thus significantly contributing to allergic responses in asthma. The classical function of T_h2 cells is to activate B cells and promote antibody production. The effect of a respiratory infection on T_h2 responses in asthma remains controversial. Infection alone in healthy or nonallergic lungs generally does not or minimally induces a T_h2 response. However, in allergic lungs, an ensuing viral or bacterial infection could further enhance or exacerbate the allergic responses in both humans and mice. Infections with RSV, influenza virus, and parainfluenza virus during early infancy (e.g., within three months) preferentially promote a T_h2-like response in the nose with local production of IL-4, IL-5, and infiltration and activation of eosinophils (33). We have shown that asthmatics with evidence of airway Mp have more mast cells in airways (34). In a mouse model of allergic inflammation, lung infection with Mp after allergen challenges increases IL-4 levels in bronchoalveolar lavage fluid (35).

The role of T_h2 cells in host defense against pathogens in asthma is poorly understood. Since eosinophils are recruited into the allergic sites following IL-5 production, they may promote pathogen clearance. It is well known that eosinophils are critical for host defense against parasite infection. In IL-5 transgenic mouse model, eosinophils are shown to promote lung RSV clearance, which is mediated through TLR-7-MyD88 pathway activation and subsequent production of antiviral mediators including IFN-β and nitric oxide production (36). However, because of the release of cytotoxic substances from the granules, eosinophils may damage airway mucosal tissue and subsequently dampen the host defense functions.

T_h17 Cells

T_h17 cells (i.e., IL-17-producing T_h cells) mainly produce IL-17A and IL-17F. These cells are involved in the pathogenesis of autoimmune diseases, including rheumatoid arthritis (37). IL-17A exerts its lung defense function against extracellular pathogens through the recruitment of neutrophils and induction of airway epithelial cell antimicrobial substance production such as β-defensin 2 (38).

Increased expression of IL-17A is found in asthmatic sputum samples and nasal polyps and does not appear to be suppressed by corticosteroid treatment (39,40). The cause of increased T_h17 cells in human asthmatic lungs remains unclear. Animal models have suggested that bacterial infection increases IL-17A production (41). We have found that Mp infection in mice increases IL-17A and IL-17F production, which is critical to neutrophil function and eventual bacterial clearance (42). RSV infection has not been reported to induce IL-17 production (43). In contrast, bacteria-induced IL-17 is inhibited by viral infection (44). The role of T_h17 cells in asthma in the context of viral and bacterial infections deserves further studies.

Regulatory T Cells

Tregs, consisting mainly of naturally occurring $CD25^+$ Tregs and adaptive Tregs, suppress T_h1 and T_h2 responses in large part through production of TGF-β and IL-10 (45,46). Transcription factor Foxp3 is essential for the development of Tregs. Functional deficiency of Tregs has been reported in allergic asthma (47). Because of their ability to inhibit the T_h2 response, Tregs have been considered as a promising approach to treat allergic asthma.

Chronic persistent infections by human pathogens such as parasites, viruses, and (myco)bacteria increase Tregs (48). Unlike the chronic infection, an acute infection or stimulation with bacterial components (e.g., TLR2 agonists) may attenuate the suppressive activity of Tregs (49). Since induction of Tregs could compromise host defense against infections, functional suppression of Tregs in the acute phase of infection may promote pathogen clearance. However, increased Tregs in chronically infected hosts may attempt to dampen the T_h2 response at the cost of a low level of persistent infection.

Future studies are needed to elucidate whether an infection in human asthmatics affects the number or activity of Tregs. In mice, parasite infection induces lung Tregs, which are responsible for inhibition of allergic responses (50). In contrast, TLR2 agonist ameliorates established allergic airway inflammation in mice by promoting T_h1 response but not Tregs (51).

Mechanisms of Induction of Various T-Cell Subsets Following an Infection

It appears that different subsets of T cells (T_h1, T_h2, T_h17, and Treg) are induced following the infection of various pathogens. These T cell subsets function synergistically or antagonistically in host defense against the invading pathogens. It is critical to understand why infections lead to a diverse T-cell response. With a better understanding of T_h cell polarization, we will be able to develop therapeutic strategies to tune the adaptive immunity so that a beneficial T_h subset can be induced to eliminate pathogens from allergic airways.

The mechanisms by which a polarized T_h cell is developed from the naive precursor following an infection in the absence and, particularly, the presence of an allergic airway milieu or asthma remain to be determined. Current literature suggests that multiple factors determine if a subset of T_h cells are developed. These include the dominant cytokine microenvironment, costimulatory molecules, type and load of antigen (pathogen) presented to T cells, and the involved signaling pathways (23). The following figure (Fig. 1) proposes how a pathogen could influence the function of airway epithelial cells and DCs and subsequently polarize T_h differentiation.

Although it is believed that different types of pathogens elicit a predominant subset of T_h cells, the same type of pathogen may generate different T_h subsets during the course of an infection. One could postulate that in a normal host an early robust induction of T_h17 cells, followed by T_h1 cell recruitment and activation, is necessary to initiate effective host-adaptive immunity against the infection of extracellular bacteria. Later in infection, predominance of Tregs would be critical to suppress the T_h1 and/or T_h17 responses, thus maintaining homeostasis.

One of the important determinants in T_h differentiation is the dose of a pathogen or its components. For example, LPS inhaled at a low dose in ovalbumin-challenged mice triggers T_h2 polarization and acts as an adjuvant for T_h2 sensitization to induce an allergic airway response. In contrast, LPS at doses 1000-fold higher than those promoting T_h2 responses induces a T_h1-predominent response and prevents airway eosinophilic inflammation (52). Moreover, a repeated low-grade, but not a high-grade, RSV infection has been shown to promote a T_h2 response in allergic mice (53).

B. Role of Humoral Response in Respiratory Infections and Asthma

Respiratory infections generate varying degree of B cell activation and antibody production. In asthma, viral and bacterial infections do not seem to produce effective antibodies in the serum or at mucosal surface that prevent the ensuing infections. A typical example is that RSV infection in all age groups does not result in a protection against future infections (54). Our studies also suggest a deficient production of serum IgG and IgM in asthmatics with Mp in the lung (34). Therefore, vaccination against respiratory infections in asthma remains to be a challenge.

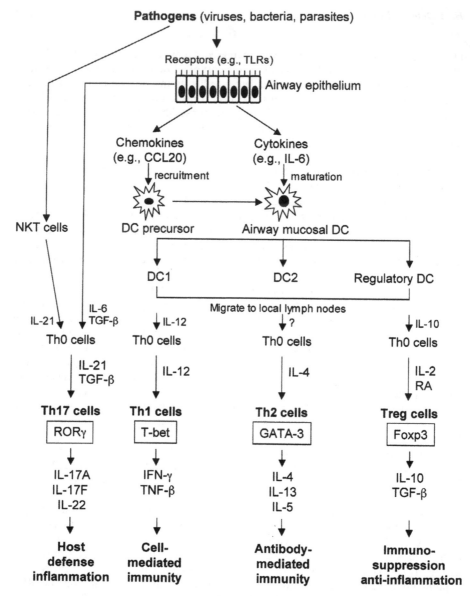

Figure 1 Respiratory viral, bacterial, or parasitic infection induces the development of different T_h cells. Airway epithelial cells respond to the invading pathogens to produce chemokines and cytokines through various receptors such as TLRs, which leads to the recruitment of DC precursors to the airways and activation of airway mucosal resident DCs. Because of their selective expression of cytokines, coreceptors, and T_h polarizing signals, DCs are classified as DC1, DC2, and regulatory DC, which promote the development of T_h1, T_h2, and Treg cells, respectively. Differentiation of T_h0 cells into T_h17 does not depend on DCs. Instead, IL-6, TGF-β, and IL-21 from airway epithelial cells and NKT cells act on T_h0 cells in a synergistic manner to induce T_h17 cell differentiation. *Abbreviations*: T_h, T helper; DC, dendritic cell; TLR, toll-like receptor; Treg, regulatory T; NKT, natural killer T; CCL20, chemokine ligand 20; RA, retinoic acid; RORγ, retinoic acid receptor–related orphan receptor γ.

An alternative approach to vaccination is to enhance airway mucosal immunity such as secretory IgA (S-IgA) production. S-IgA in the mucociliary blanket affords protection to mucosal surfaces by neutralizing or preventing the attachment of viruses, bacteria, and toxins to the mucosal epithelium (55). S-IgA can be produced in a T cell–independent manner. For example, airway epithelial cell mediators such as IL-2, TGF-β, IL-6, and IL-10 are sufficient for B cell clonal proliferation, IgA isotype switch, and differentiation into IgA-producing plasma cells (56). An increase in allergic disorders and asthma has been reported in patients with known IgA deficiency (57,58). While some IgA-deficient subjects may present with allergy/asthma, others may suffer from recurrent respiratory infections, bronchiectasis, or autoimmune disorders. Further, S-IgA levels are positively correlated with lung function in asthmatics (59). Thus, mucosal immunization with inactivated pathogen in combination with an adjuvant [e.g., CpG oligodeoxynucleotide (ODN)] could serve as an efficient therapy to increase pathogen removal from the airways (60).

IV. Impact of Allergic Inflammation on Host Innate Immunity

Previous work has centered on the impact of respiratory infections on allergic responses or asthma exacerbations. An important, but unanswered research question is: once the airway allergic inflammation has been established following allergen exposure with or without an infection, does the established allergic inflammation suppress host innate immunity and subsequently hinder the elimination of an infectious organism from the airways?

Until recently, studies have started to reveal the impact of allergic inflammation or T_h2 cytokines on host susceptibility to infections. Pitzurra and colleagues examined the relationship between TLR expression and detection of typical bacterial and fungal infection in patients with nasal polyps (61). As compared with nasal mucosa from patients without infection, nasal polyp tissues from patients with either bacterial or fungal infection have higher levels of IL-4 and IL-13 mRNA. Moreover, TLR2, TLR4, TLR5, and TLR9 mRNA expression in nasal polyp tissues is markedly reduced in infected patients as compared with noninfected patients. These results clearly suggest that mucosal infection in allergic subjects is associated with impaired TLR expression (e.g., TLR2) and high levels of T_h2 cytokines (i.e., IL-4 and IL-13). Several other human studies suggest that deficient expression of antimicrobial peptides (e.g., LL-37, β-defensins 2 and 3) may contribute to the increased susceptibility of patients with atopic dermatitis to *Staphylococcus aureus* infection (62,63). We have found that IL-13 directly decreases the expression and secretion of short palate, lung, and nasal epithelium clone 1 (SPLUNC1) protein in human primary airway epithelial cells (64). SPLUNC1 has been shown to exert antimicrobial effects such as inhibition of Mp and *P. aeruginosa* (64,65). Further, SPLUNC1 levels are significantly lower in allergic mice than in nonallergic mice (64).

To reveal the molecular mechanisms, we have determined whether allergic inflammation or T_h2 cytokines inhibit TLR2 signaling, thus impairing bacterial clearance from the lung. We have found that the established ovalbumin-induced allergic airway inflammation and the prominent T_h2 cytokines IL-4 and IL-13 reduce Mp-induced TLR2 expression and subsequent production of IL-6 and eventually impair *mycoplasma pneumoniae* (Mp) clearance from the allergic lungs (66). This cascade is partly mediated by inhibition of NF-κB activation through the signal transducer and activator of transcription 6 (STAT6) signaling pathway. Collectively, our animal model data indicate that attenuation of TLR2-mediated innate immune responses by T_h2 cytokines renders the allergic lungs more susceptible to respiratory bacterial infections (66). A T_h2 cytokine milieu may also predispose the host to viral infections. For example, asthmatics are known to be more susceptible to RV infection, which may be caused by deficient production of type III IFN-λ production in airway epithelial cells and alveolar macrophages (67). Moreover, IL-4 overexpression in mice delays RSV clearance from the lungs (68). Future clinical studies are warranted to explore if asthmatics have a broad range of impaired innate immunity. These studies should provide guidance to basic scientists to define which innate pathways are responsible for various (e.g., bacterial, viral, and fungal) infections. Such translational research will lead to novel targets for prevention and treatment of infections in asthma.

V. Conclusions

Host defense responses to respiratory infections involve both innate and adaptive immunities. With its constitutive expression, broad antimicrobial activity, and instant availability, innate immunity provides a great potential for fortifying host defense functions. A growing literature is beginning to reveal deficiency of innate immunity in asthmatics who are more susceptible to infections of bacteria, viruses, and other pathogens. Impaired innate immunity can be partly caused by the existing allergic inflammation or T_h2 cytokines. Genetic alterations such as single-nucleotide polymorphisms (SNPs) of genes (e.g., TLR2 and TLR4) involved in innate immunity continue to be described in asthma patients and are associated with asthma prevalence (69,70). It is imperative to dissect the role of innate gene SNPs in shaping host defense functions in the context of an allergic airway milieu. Adaptive immune responses to pathogens are very complicated, involving various subsets of T cells as well as antibodies from B cells. It appears that asthmatics also present evidence of insufficient adaptive immune responses to the invading pathogens. Understanding of switch to different subsets of T_h cells will be instrumental in developing effective therapies in asthma. Since asthmatics do not generate robust systemic Ig production against viral or bacterial infections, great efforts should be made to enhance airway mucosal S-IgA production or function to quickly and efficiently eliminate the respiratory pathogens.

References

1. Busse WW. The role of respiratory infections in airway hyperresponsiveness and asthma. Am J Respir Crit Care Med 1994; 150(5 pt 2):S77–S79.
2. Bals R, Hiemstra PS. Innate immunity in the lung: how epithelial cells fight against respiratory pathogens. Eur Respir J 2004; 23(2):327–333.
3. Schaefer L, Babelova A, Kiss E, et al. The matrix component biglycan is proinflammatory and signals through Toll-like receptors 4 and 2 in macrophages. J Clin Invest 2005; 115(8): 2223–2233.
4. Moynagh PN. TLR signalling and activation of IRFs: revisiting old friends from the NF-kappaB pathway. Trends Immunol 2005; 26(9):469–476.
5. Horng T, Barton GM, Medzhitov R. TIRAP: an adapter molecule in the Toll signaling pathway. Nat Immunol 2001; 2(9):835–841.
6. Kumar A, Zhang J, Yu FS. Toll-like receptor 2-mediated expression of beta-defensin-2 in human corneal epithelial cells. Microbes Infect 2006; 8(2):380–389.
7. Yamamoto M, Sato S, Hemmi H, et al. Role of adaptor TRIF in the MyD88-independent toll-like receptor signaling pathway. Science 2003; 301(5633):640–643.

8. Nakaya T, Sato M, Hata N, et al. Gene induction pathways mediated by distinct IRFs during viral infection. Biochem Biophys Res Commun 2001; 283(5):1150–1156.
9. Sato S, Sugiyama M, Yamamoto M, et al. Toll/IL-1 receptor domain-containing adaptor inducing IFN-beta (TRIF) associates with TNF receptor-associated factor 6 and TANK-binding kinase 1, and activates two distinct transcription factors, NF-kappa B and IFN-regulatory factor-3, in the Toll-like receptor signaling. J Immunol 2003; 171(8):4304–4310.
10. Meylan E, Burns K, Hofmann K, et al. RIP1 is an essential mediator of Toll-like receptor 3-induced NF-kappa B activation. Nat Immunol 2004; 5(5):503–507.
11. Chu HW, Jeyaseelan S, Rino JG, et al. TLR2 signaling is critical for *Mycoplasma pneumoniae*-induced airway mucin expression. J Immunol 2005; 174(9):5713–5719.
12. Krüll M, Bockstaller P, Wuppermann FN, et al. Mechanisms of *Chlamydophila pneumoniae*-mediated GM-CSF release in human bronchial epithelial cells. Am J Respir Cell Mol Biol 2006; 34(3):375–382.
13. Monick MM, Powers LS, Hassan I, et al. Respiratory syncytial virus synergizes with Th2 cytokines to induce optimal levels of TARC/CCL17. J Immunol 2007; 179(3):1648–1658.
14. Edwards MR, Slater L, Johnston SL. Signalling pathways mediating type I interferon gene expression. Microbes Infect 2007; 9(11):1245–1251.
15. Newcomb DC, Sajjan US, Nagarkar DR, et al. Cooperative effects of rhinovirus and TNF-α on airway epithelial cell chemokine expression. Am J Physiol Lung Cell Mol Physiol 2007; 293(4):L1021–L1028.
16. Wark PA, Johnston SL, Bucchieri F, et al. Asthmatic bronchial epithelial cells have a deficient innate immune response to infection with rhinovirus. J Exp Med 2005; 201(6):937–947.
17. Lipscomb MF, Masten BJ. Dendritic cells: immune regulators in health and disease. Physiol Rev 2002; 82(1):97–130.
18. Lambrecht BN. Lung dendritic cells: targets for therapy in allergic disease. Curr Mol Med 2008; 8(5):393–400.
19. Umemoto EY, Brokaw JJ, Dupuis M, et al. Rapid changes in shape and number of MHC class II expressing cells in rat airways after *Mycoplasma pulmonis* infection. Cell Immunol 2002; 220(2):107–115.
20. Bartlett NW, Walton RP, Edwards MR, et al. Mouse models of rhinovirus-induced disease and exacerbation of allergic airway inflammation. Nat Med 2008; 14(2):199–204.
21. Smit JJ, Lindell DM, Boon L, et al. The balance between plasmacytoid DC versus conventional DC determines pulmonary immunity to virus infections. PLoS ONE 2008; 3(3):e1720.
22. Möller GM, Overbeek SE, Van Helden-Meeuwsen CG, et al. Increased numbers of dendritic cells in the bronchial mucosa of atopic asthmatic patients: downregulation by inhaled corticosteroids. Clin Exp Allergy 1996; 26(5):517–524.
23. Kaiko GE, Horvat JC, Beagley KW, et al. Immunological decision-making: how does the immune system decide to mount a helper T-cell response? Immunology 2008; 123(3):326–338.
24. Pinto RA, Arredondo SM, Bono MR, et al. T helper 1/T helper 2 cytokine imbalance in respiratory syncytial virus infection is associated with increased endogenous plasma cortisol. Pediatrics 2006; 117(5):e878–e886.
25. Tanaka H, Narita M, Teramoto S, et al. Role of interleukin-18 and T-helper type 1 cytokines in the development of *Mycoplasma pneumoniae* pneumonia in adults. Chest 2002; 121(5): 1493–1497.
26. Message SD, Laza-Stanca V, Mallia P, et al. Rhinovirus-induced lower respiratory illness is increased in asthma and related to virus load and Th1/2 cytokine and IL-10 production. Proc Natl Acad Sci U S A 2008; 105(36):13562–13567.
27. Yoshida M, Leigh R, Matsumoto K, et al. Effect of interferon-gamma on allergic airway responses in interferon-gamma-deficient mice. Am J Respir Crit Care Med 2002; 166(4):451–456.
28. Hofstra CL, Van Ark I, Hofman G, et al. Differential effects of endogenous and exogenous interferon-gamma on immunoglobulin E, cellular infiltration, and airway responsiveness in a murine model of allergic asthma. Am J Respir Cell Mol Biol 1998; 19(5):826–835.

29. Boguniewicz M, Schneider LC, Milgrom H, et al. Treatment of steroid-dependent asthma with recombinant interferon-gamma. Clin Exp Allergy 1993; 23(9):785–790.

30. Shannon J, Ernst P, Yamauchi Y, et al. Differences in airway cytokine profile in severe asthma compared to moderate asthma. Chest 2008; 133(2):420–426.

31. Tesfaigzi Y. Roles of apoptosis in airway epithelia. Am J Respir Cell Mol Biol 2006; 34(5): 537–547.

32. Kim YK, Oh SY, Jeon SG, et al. Airway exposure levels of lipopolysaccharide determine type 1 versus type 2 experimental asthma. J Immunol 2007; 178(8):5375–5382.

33. Kristjansson S, Bjarnarson SP, Wennergren G, et al. Respiratory syncytial virus and other respiratory viruses during the first 3 months of life promote a local TH2-like response. J Allergy Clin Immunol 2005; 116(4):805–811.

34. Martin RJ, Kraft M, Chu HW, et al. A link between chronic asthma and chronic infection. J Allergy Clin Immunol 2001; 107(4):595–601.

35. Chu HW, Honour JM, Rawlinson CA, et al. Effects of respiratory *Mycoplasma pneumoniae* infection on allergen-induced bronchial hyperresponsiveness and lung inflammation in mice. Infect Immun 2003; 71(3):1520–1526.

36. Phipps S, Lam CE, Mahalingam S, et al. Eosinophils contribute to innate antiviral immunity and promote clearance of respiratory syncytial virus. Blood 2007; 110(5):1578–1586.

37. Lubberts E. IL-17/Th17 targeting: on the road to prevent chronic destructive arthritis? Cytokine 2008; 41(2):84–91.

38. Kao CY, Chen Y, Thai P, et al. IL-17 markedly up-regulates beta-defensin-2 expression in human airway epithelium via JAK and NF-kappaB signaling pathways. J Immunol 2004; 173(5):3482–3491.

39. Bullens DM, Truyen E, Coteur L, et al. IL-17 mRNA in sputum of asthmatic patients: linking T cell driven inflammation and granulocytic influx? Respir Res 2006; 7(1):135–143.

40. Molet SM, Hamid QA, Hamilos DL. IL-11 and IL-17 expression in nasal polyps: relationship to collagen deposition and suppression by intranasal fluticasone propionate. Laryngoscope 2003; 113(10):1803–1812.

41. Ye P, Garvey PB, Zhang P, et al. Interleukin-17 and lung host defense against Klebsiella pneumoniae infection. Am J Respir Cell Mol Biol 2001; 25(3):335–340.

42. Wu Q, Martin RJ, Rino JG, et al. IL-23-dependent IL-17 production is essential in neutrophil recruitment and activity in mouse lung defense against respiratory *Mycoplasma pneumoniae* infection. Microbes Infect 2007; 9(1):78–86.

43. Hashimoto K, Durbin JE, Zhou W, et al. Respiratory syncytial virus infection in the absence of STAT 1 results in airway dysfunction, airway mucus, and augmented IL-17 levels. J Allergy Clin Immunol 2005; 116(3):550–557.

44. Yang J, Yang M, Htut TM, et al. Epstein-Barr virus-induced gene 3 negatively regulates IL-17, IL-22 and RORgamma. Eur J Immunol 2008; 38(5):1204–1214.

45. Robinson DS, Larché M, Durham SR. Tregs and allergic disease. J Clin Invest 2004; 114 (10):1389–1397.

46. van Oosterhout AJ, Bloksma N. Regulatory T-lymphocytes in asthma. Eur Respir J 2005; 26 (5):918–932.

47. Lin YL, Shieh CC, Wang JY. The functional insufficiency of human CD4+CD25 high T-regulatory cells in allergic asthma is subjected to TNF-alpha modulation. Allergy 2008; 63(1):67–74.

48. Joosten SA, Ottenhoff TH. Human CD4 and CD8 regulatory T cells in infectious diseases and vaccination. Hum Immunol 2008; 69(11):760–770.

49. Liu H, Komai-Koma M, Xu D, et al. Toll-like receptor 2 signaling modulates the functions of CD4+ CD25+ regulatory T cells. Proc Natl Acad Sci U S A 2006; 103(18):7048–7053.

50. Dittrich AM, Erbacher A, Specht S, et al. Helminth infection with Litomosoides sigmodontis induces regulatory T cells and inhibits allergic sensitization, airway inflammation, and hyperreactivity in a murine asthma model. J Immunol 2008; 180(3):1792–1799.

51. Patel M, Xu D, Kewin P, et al. TLR2 agonist ameliorates established allergic airway inflammation by promoting Th1 response and not via regulatory T cells. J Immunol 2005; 174(12):7558–7563.
52. Eisenbarth SC, Piggott DA, Huleatt JW, et al. Lipopolysaccharide-enhanced, toll-like receptor 4-dependent T helper cell type 2 responses to inhaled antigen. J Exp Med 2002; 196(12): 1645–1651.
53. Kondo Y, Matsuse H, Machida I, et al. Effects of primary and secondary low-grade respiratory syncytial virus infections in a murine model of asthma. Clin Exp Allergy 2004; 34(8): 1307–1313.
54. van Drunen Littel-van den Hurk S, Mapletoft JW, Arsic N, et al. Immunopathology of RSV infection: prospects for developing vaccines without this complication. Rev Med Virol 2007; 17(1):5–34.
55. Renegar KB, Small PA Jr., Boykins LG, et al. Role of IgA versus IgG in the control of influenza viral infection in the murine respiratory tract. J Immunol 2004; 173(3):1978–1986.
56. Salvi S, Holgate ST. Could the airway epithelium play an important role in mucosal immunoglobulin A production? Clin Exp Allergy 1999; 29(12):1597–1605.
57. Chapel H, Geha R, Rosen F, et al. Primary immunodeficiency diseases: an update. Clin Exp Immunol 2003; 132(1):9–15.
58. Edwards E, Razvi S, Cunningham-Rundles C. IgA deficiency: clinical correlates and responses to pneumococcal vaccine. Clin Immunol 2004; 111(1):93–97.
59. Balzar S, Strand M, Nakano T, et al. Subtle immunodeficiency in severe asthma: IgA and IgG2 correlate with lung function and symptoms. Int Arch Allergy Immunol 2006; 140(2): 96–102.
60. Lee CJ, Lee LH, Gu XX. Mucosal immunity induced by pneumococcal glycoconjugate. Crit Rev Microbiol 2005; 31(3):137–144.
61. Pitzurra L, Bellocchio S, Nocentini A, et al. Antifungal immune reactivity in nasal polyposis. Infect Immun 2004; 72(12):7275–7281.
62. Ong PY, Ohtake T, Brandt C, et al. Endogenous antimicrobial peptides and skin infections in atopic dermatitis. N Engl J Med 2002; 347(15):1151–1160.
63. Nomura I, Goleva E, Howell MD, et al. Cytokine milieu of atopic dermatitis, as compared to psoriasis, skin prevents induction of innate immune response genes. J Immunol 2003; 171 (6):3262–3269.
64. Chu HW, Thaikoottathil J, Rino JG, et al. Function and regulation of SPLUNC1 protein in *Mycoplasma* infection and allergic inflammation. J Immunol 2007; 179(6):3995–4002.
65. Zhou HD, Li XL, Li GY, et al. Effect of SPLUNC1 protein on the Pseudomonas aeruginosa and Epstein-Barr virus. Mol Cell Biochem 2008; 309(1–2):191–197.
66. Wu Q, Martin RJ, Lafasto S, et al. Toll-like receptor 2 down-regulation in established mouse allergic lungs contributes to decreased Mycoplasma clearance. Am J Respir Crit Care Med 2008; 177(7):720–729.
67. Contoli M, Message SD, Laza-Stanca V, et al. Role of deficient type III interferon-lambda production in asthma exacerbations. Nat Med 2006; 12(9):1023–1026.
68. Fischer JE, Johnson JE, Kuli-Zade RK, et al. Overexpression of interleukin-4 delays virus clearance in mice infected with respiratory syncytial virus. J Virol 1997; 71(11):8672–8677.
69. Eder W, Klimecki W, Yu L, et al. Toll-like receptor 2 as a major gene for asthma in children of European farmers. J Allergy Clin Immunol 2004; 113(3):482–488.
70. Kormann MS, Depner M, Hartl D, et al. Toll-like receptor heterodimer variants protect from childhood asthma. J Allergy Clin Immunol 2008; 122(1):86–92.

12

Antimicrobial and Anti-inflammatory Effects of Antibiotics: A Role in Asthma Therapy

DRUHAN HOWELL and MONICA KRAFT
Duke University Medical Center, Durham, North Carolina, U.S.A.

I. Introduction

Asthma affects over 22 million Americans. The prevalence of asthma has increased dramatically over the last several decades, although the reason for this continuing increase remains unclear (1). It is likely that the etiology is multifactorial, which has led to research regarding novel mechanisms and therapeutic modalities. One of these avenues has been the impact of infection on both the development and exacerbation of asthma symptoms. While the in-depth role of bacterial and viral infections in asthma is discussed in other chapters in this text, active viral illnesses have been identified as precipitants to acute exacerbations in adult and pediatric populations in numerous studies (2–4). However, the role of bacterial infections in asthma has remained far more controversial. In a comprehensive review, Johnston and Martin highlighted the role of atypical infections in both acute and chronic asthma settings as well as the effect of treatment with macrolide antibiotics may have in ameliorating the impact of these infections on asthmatic patients. They concluded that a general increased susceptibility to infections is associated with asthma and that atypical infection in this population plays a direct role in the proinflammatory state (5). Blasi and Johnston cited increasing evidence for the role of atypical pathogens in ongoing inflammation and possibly contributing to airway remodeling in both acute exacerbations as well as chronic stable asthma (6).

Given the implications of atypical infection development, exacerbation, and chronicity of asthma, research has focused on the treatment of these infections, specifically with macrolide antibiotics, the most studied class of antibiotics in the treatment of acute and chronic asthma. Macrolides are a well-established class of antibiotics isolated from *Streptomycetes*. In 1952, erythromycin A was isolated from *Streptomyces erythraea* in a Philippine soil sample and subsequently introduced into clinical practice (7). Functionally, macrolides reversibly bind to the 50S ribosomal subunit of susceptible pathogens, thereby inhibiting RNA-dependent protein synthesis (8). Since the 1950s, the macrolide antibiotic class has expanded to consist of 14-, 15-, and 16-member macrolactam ring antimicrobials.

While the antimicrobial effects of macrolides have been well described, the immunomodulatory effects of macrolides are still being elucidated. Interest in their immunomodulatory effects began in the 1960s with the observation that the 14-member macrolactam ring antibiotic, troleandomycin, was an effective "steroid-sparing" agent when used to treat patients with severe asthma (9). Use of macrolides as immunomodulators became mainstream when azithromycin became standard treatment for cystic fibrosis patients (10). Additionally, in the late 1980s, the use of macrolides became the standard of care in diffuse panbronchiolitis (DPB) when it was discovered that its use dramatically changed life expectancy (11,12). With this revelation, the investigation of macrolides as a therapeutic option in the care of patients with airway disease has progressed extensively and will be discussed herein.

II. Acute Asthma

A. Role of Atypical Bacterial Infection in Asthma

Viral and bacterial infections have been implicated in the pathogenesis of asthma and the exacerbation of acute illness. Of particular interest is the specific role of atypical bacteria, specifically *Chlamydophila pneumoniae* and *Mycoplasma pneumoniae*. Despite some evidence that bacterial pathogens may be important in asthma, antibiotic use in acute asthma exacerbations has fallen out of favor because of the high prevalence of viral infections and lack of documented improved outcome (13–15). Furthermore, antibiotics are not recommended in the new National Asthma Education and Prevention Program guidelines because of implications of viral illnesses and allergens in acute exacerbations (16). However, atypical pathogens and treatment with macrolide antibiotics may, in fact, play a significant role in the treatment of acute asthma exacerbations. Johnston and Martin's review commented on twelve studies regarding *C. pneumoniae* and *M. pneumoniae* infections and acute asthma exacerbations. Nine of the twelve studies demonstrated a significant relationship between infection and asthma exacerbation (5). A small selection of these studies is discussed here, with the addition of several other key research endeavors.

Biscoine et al. prospectively followed a spouse pair cohort of atopic asthmatics and nonatopic nonasthmatic subjects. Nasal secretions were obtained from October through December. Using reverse transcriptase polymerase chain reaction (RT-PCR), a significantly higher rate of *C. pneumoniae* was noted in the asthmatic population versus nonasthmatic controls, 22% versus 9% (17). In a longitudinal study of *M. pneumoniae* in the pediatric population, which included both asthmatics and nonasthmatics, patients aged 0 to 20 years had serum samples analyzed for *M. pneumoniae* antibody titers and cytokines (18). As expected, infection rates increased in the winter months (November–March), with seropositivity ranging from 6.3% to 23.8% and peak age ranging from three to seven years depending on the year. In seropositive patients, serum interleukin (IL)-1α, IL-1β, IL-4, IL-5, IL-6, IL-8, IL-10, interferon (IFN)-γ, and tumor necrosis factor (TNF)-α were elevated in relation to established normal values. When presenting with evidence of lower respiratory tract infection, children had higher levels of proinflammatory cytokines IL-1α, IL-4, IL-6, IL-8, and IL-10 compared with normal values or patients with upper respiratory tract infections, suggestive of a T_H2-like cytokine response to *M. pneumoniae* infection. Similarly, in BALB/c mice, Pietsch et al. found elevations in IL-1, IL-6, IFN-γ, and TNF-α during the acute phase of *M. pneumoniae* infection. Upon reinfection, a 10-fold increase in IL-6 and TNF-α and a 50-fold increase in IFN-γ were noted (18). In a single patient, cytokine levels were measured following treatment with clarithromycin, and proinflammatory cytokines IL-1α and IL-6 were found to be dramatically decreased (19).

To evaluate the relationship between atypical infection, first wheezing episode, and subsequent development of asthma, Zaitsu et al. compared 103 first-time wheezing infants and toddlers with 64 healthy controls. Seroconversion to *C. pneumoniae* was significantly higher in the wheezing subjects versus healthy controls (44.7% and 17.2%, respectively).

Among the wheezing patient population, those who progressed to developing asthma were statistically more likely to have a family history of allergic diseases, higher eosinophil counts, higher total IgE, and higher elevations in IgM *C. pneumoniae* titers. Furthermore, wheezing patients with *C. pneumoniae* infection were more likely to develop asthma than those without infection (relative risk 2.9) (20). However, in a 15-year prospective study, Pasternack et al. were unable to demonstrate a correlation between *C. pneumoniae* sero-positivity and the risk of developing asthma (21).

As evidence of the role atypical infections play in acute asthma, Biscardi et al. prospectively studied children admitted to the hospital with severe acute asthma exacerbations. Nasopharyngeal samples were obtained at admission and evaluated for the presence of a variety of respiratory viruses and for *C. pneumoniae* and *M. pneumoniae*. Acute infection was diagnosed by either elevation of specific IgM at initial serology or fourfold increase in IgG titers at follow-up. For data analysis, study subjects were divided into two groups and controls. Group 1 consisted of known asthmatics; group 2 subjects were presenting with their first episode of wheezing; and control subjects were known asthmatics followed in outpatient clinic, who had not had an exacerbation in the previous six months. In group 1, respiratory syncytial virus (RSV) or influenza A/B was detected in 18 of 119 subjects. *M. pneumoniae* was found in 24 subjects (20%), and *C. pneumoniae* was detected in four (3.4%) subjects in this cohort. Interestingly, in group 2, there was no influenza detected, and RSV was found in only 2 of 51 subjects, although *M. pneumoniae* was found in 26 subjects (50%), a statistically significant difference when compared with group 1. *C. pneumoniae* was detected in three (6%). At one-year follow-up, 62% of subjects in group 2 who had been diagnosed with an atypical infection had recurrence of asthma, compared with only 27% of noninfected subjects (22).

In a study of mild to moderate adult asthmatics with acute exacerbations in the outpatient setting, Allegra et al. noted that 20% of subjects had seroconverted to one or more pathogens during the study as evidenced by a fourfold increase in titers during the six-month study period. Almost half (7%) of subjects who had seroconversion were found to be infected by a virus. However, 8% seroconverted to *C. pneumoniae* and 2% to *M. pneumoniae,* suggesting that these pathogens may play a more prominent role in acute exacerbations (23). Cunningham et al. evaluated 108 children with asthma and obtained sera and nasal aspirates if there was a significant fall in peak flow or an increase in respiratory symptoms. Compared with 39% of control subjects, 45% of asthmatic children had specimens positive for *C. pneumoniae* by RT-PCR and were more likely to remain positive at subsequent testing, suggestive of chronic infection (13). In a similar study of adult patients admitted with acute exacerbations over a 12-month period, subjects had a significantly higher rate of *M. pneumoniae* infection diagnosed by a rise in titers compared with hospitalized controls (24). Miyashita et al. found a statistically significant increase in *C. pneumoniae*–specific IgG and IgA in adult asthmatics when compared with age-, gender-, and tobacco-matched controls (25).

Taken together, these studies suggest that *C. pneumoniae* and *M. pneumoniae* infections are frequently present in acute exacerbations. These infections correlate with an increasing risk of developing asthma. Compared with healthy matched controls, asthmatic patients' airways are more likely to be colonized with *C. pneumoniae* and *M. pneumoniae*. Infections with these atypical pathogens are also more likely to become chronic. These findings reflect a higher burden of disease related to atypical infections than what has been previously suspected.

B. Role of Antibiotics in Acute Asthma

Despite the strong implications that *C. pneumoniae* and *M. pneumoniae* infections are present in acute exacerbations and that treatment with an antibiotic, most likely a macrolide, would be a part of the standard of care, there are very few studies that evaluate the direct role of macrolides in acute exacerbations. Instead, investigators have tended to focus on chronic asthma and airway hyperresponsiveness as surrogate models for acute exacerbation. Three studies that specifically evaluated the effects of treatment in acute exacerbations are discussed here in detail. The most prominent of these is the Telithromycin, *Chlamydophila*, and Asthma Trial (TELICAST), a double-blind placebo-controlled study, which evaluated the use of telithromycin, a ketolide, for acute asthma exacerbation in adults presenting to outpatient clinic. In the telithromycin treatment arm, symptom scores decreased by 40.4%, compared with a 26.5% reduction in controls with a higher proportion of symptom-free days in the treatment arm, 16% versus 8%, respectively. However, morning peak expiratory flow was unchanged between groups. On completion of telithromycin therapy, forced expiratory volume in one second (FEV$_1$), forced vital capacity (FVC), and forced expiratory flow at 25% to 75% of FVC (FEF$_{25-75\%}$) had improved significantly in the treatment group. This effect disappeared at the six-week follow-up visit. Finally, in evaluation of the telithromycin group, investigators noted that patients with evidence of infection had significant improvement in FEV$_1$ compared with those in the placebo group. If there was no evidence of infection, then a change in FEV$_1$ was not demonstrated (26).

However, the presence of either *M. pneumoniae or C. pneumoniae* via PCR analysis of upper airway samples did not predict response to treatment. This observation supports work by Kraft et al. who observed that only PCR positivity of lower airway samples obtained by bronchoscopy predicted response to clarithromycin (27).

Fonseca-Aten et al. followed 43 children who were enrolled in a double-blind placebo-controlled trial. Children were enrolled when they presented to the emergency room within 72 hours of an acute exacerbation of wheeze. Nasopharyngeal samples from subjects revealed *C. pneumoniae* in 12 (28%), *M. pneumoniae* in 20 (48%), and coinfection in 9 by PCR and/or serology. Interestingly, clarithromycin offered no clinical benefit when compared with placebo therapy; however, both groups were treated with systemic steroids and β-agonists (28). In a prospective observational study, Emre et al. followed 118 subjects with an acute wheezing episode and 41 age- and gender-matched controls. *C. pneumoniae* was isolated in culture in 13 (11%) of wheezing subjects and in 2 (4.9%) of controls. When *C. pneumoniae* infection was identified via culture, subjects were treated with erythromycin or clarithromycin, and they demonstrated clinical improvement with resolution of symptoms (29).

Treatment of acute asthma exacerbations with non-macrolide antibiotics has not been extensively studied. In the last five years, only one article has been published specifically focusing on asthma, excluding the TELICAST study described above (30). However, the literature regarding chronic obstructive pulmonary disease and chronic bronchitis is slightly broader. Horiguchi et al. evaluated the efficacy of sparfloxacin in asthmatics with a recent flare in symptoms and positive titers for *C. pneumoniae*. Titers remained unchanged over the 21 days of treatment. However, asthma symptoms, morning peak expiratory flow, and frequency of β-agonist use all improved significantly (30). This study suggests that other antibiotics with atypical pathogen coverage may also be beneficial in treatment of exacerbations.

III. Chronic Asthma

A. Role of Bacteria in Chronic Asthma

In addition to the role atypical infections play in acute exacerbations, there is mounting evidence that chronic infection can significantly impact asthma severity. Over 30 studies have been published in this area, and 19 are highlighted in review by Johnston and Martin (5). Literature suggests a relationship between infection and chronic asthma pathobiology. Brief reviews of pertinent studies are detailed here. In a retrospective study of adults with mild asthma, subjects were noted to have significant elevations in IgA titers to *C. pneumoniae* compared with controls (72% vs. 44%, respectively) (31). As further evidence of the burden of atypical infections in asthmatics, 55 chronic asthmatic subjects and 11 normal controls were evaluated for evidence of ongoing infection via sampling from upper and lower airways as well as serology. PCR analysis of upper and lower airway samples revealed that 23 of 55 asthmatic subjects were positive for *M. pneumoniae* and 7 of 55 were positive for *C. pneumoniae* compared with 1 of 11 and 0 of 11 controls, respectively. In addition, *M. pneumoniae* serology was negative in all subjects and controls, while *C. pneumoniae* serology was positive in 18 asthmatics and 1 control. Of the seven asthma subjects positive for *C. pneumoniae* by PCR, only three were noted to be seropositive (32). In the follow-up treatment trial, antibiotic therapy was initiated in this cohort of asthmatics where 23 of 55 demonstrated PCR positivity for *M. pneumoniae* and 7 of 55 demonstrated PCR positivity for *C. pneumoniae*.

In a prospective study of a Finnish cohort, subjects with asthma and serologic evidence of *C. pneumoniae* had a more rapid decline in FEV1 compared with matched asthma subjects. In subanalysis, this correlation only held true for nonatopic asthmatics (22). In a comparison of asthmatics with high titers to *C. pneumoniae* (defined as IgG $\geq$ 1:64 or IgA $\geq$ 1:16) to asthmatics with low titers, moderate- to high-dose inhaled corticosteroids use was associated with high titers. FEV_1 percent predicted was inversely proportional to IgG and IgA titers (33).

B. Antibiotic Trials in Chronic Asthma

Of the trials evaluating the role of bacterial infection in chronic asthma, there are six studies in which treatment with antibiotics was initiated (6,32,34–37). Given the limited data on the effect of macrolides in acute exacerbations, a beneficial surrogate for acute exacerbation of the chronic asthma state may be airway hyperresponsiveness. Additionally, this study design is more readily replicated than acute exacerbations, which are variably triggered. Miyatake et al. evaluated the change in histamine provocation concentration producing a fall in the FEV_1 of 20% (PC_{20}) in asymptomatic asthmatics before and after 10 weeks of erythromycin therapy. A significant increase in PC_{20} in the treatment arm was observed. Furthermore, FEV_1, FEV_1 percent predicted, and theophylline levels were not significantly changed during the study (38). Similar increase in histamine PC_{20} was demonstrated in chronically hospitalized children with asthma when treated with roxithromycin for eight weeks (39). A follow-up study revealed an increase in the cough threshold at weeks 4 and 8 of roxithromycin treatment, which was unrelated to bronchodilation, theophylline levels, or steroid-sparing effects (40). Koh et al. found similar results regarding FEV_1 and provocative cumulative dose producing a 20% fall in FEV_1 (PD_{20}) and in a double-blind placebo-controlled study of roxithromycin therapy in bronchiectasis (Figs. 1 and 2). Additionally, they noted a significant decrease in sputum purulence and leukocyte scores (41).

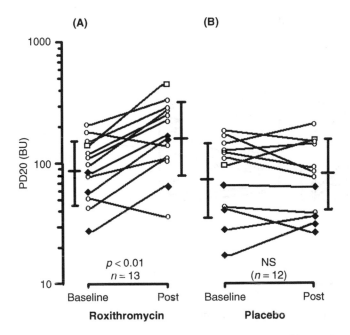

Figure 1 (**A**) Subject PD_{20} values at baseline and post roxithromycin treatment for 12 weeks. (**B**) Subject PD_{20} values at baseline and post placebo treatment for 12 weeks. Means and 1 SD are indicated with horizontal bars. ◆, asthmatic subject; □, atopic nonasthmatic subject; ○, nonatopic nonasthmatic subject. *Abbreviations*: PD_{20}, provocative cumulative dose producing a 20% fall in FEV_1; NS, nonsignificant; BU, breath unit (1 BU denotes one inhalation of 1 mg/mL methacholine). *Source*: Adapted from Ref. 41.

In a placebo-controlled study by Amayasu et al., clarithromycin treatment for eight weeks significantly increased PC_{20} when compared with baseline values and placebo subjects, although no significant change was noted in either FVC or FEV_1. Additionally, symptom scores were significantly increased in the treatment phase of the study (42). Clarithromycin treatment in a double-blind placebo-controlled study demonstrated similar increased PD_{20} values without significant alteration in the remainder of pulmonary function tests (43). In a study of mild asthmatics, azithromycin was given twice a week for eight weeks, with histamine challenges at baseline, week 4, and post treatment. The increase in PC_{20} trended toward significance by week 4 and was statistically significant post treatment. Again, no change in FEV_1 was noted throughout the study (44).

Furthermore, several studies of macrolides in the treatment of chronic asthma, both with and without documentation of atypical pathogens, have been reported (32,34–37,45). Hahn et al. treated 46 patients with moderate to severe, stable chronic asthma with four weeks of doxycycline, azithromycin, or erythromycin and evaluated the change in pulmonary function and symptoms scores. All patients were seroreactive (defined by an IgA titer greater than 1:16), and eight had evidence of acute infection. Slightly more than half (54%) of patients responded to treatment demonstrated by an improvement in pulmonary function. Interestingly, 7 of the 46 patients had complete remission of asthma

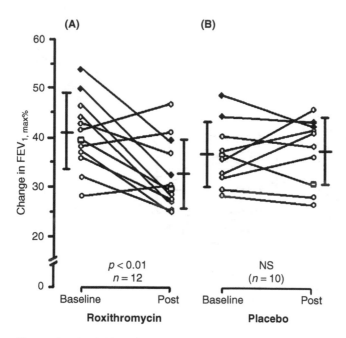

Figure 2 (A) Subject $\Delta FEV_{1,max}$ values at baseline and post roxithromycin treatment for 12 weeks. (B) Subject $\Delta FEV_{1,max}$ values at baseline and post placebo treatment for 12 weeks. Means and 1 SD are indicated with horizontal bars. ♦, asthmatic subject; □, atopic nonasthmatic subject; ○, nonatopic nonasthmatic subject. *Abbreviations*: NS, nonsignificant; $FEV_{1,max}$, maximal response to methacholine expressed as the percentage fall in forced expiratory volume in one second. *Source*: Adapted from Ref. 41.

as defined by resolution of symptoms and a normalization of pulmonary function. This remission was sustained in the long term in one patient (36).

In a randomized, double-blind, placebo-controlled trial by Kraft et al., subjects were randomized to treatment with clarithromycin versus placebo, and PCR was then performed on upper and lower airway samples. In the treatment arm, fourteen subjects were positive for *M. pneumoniae or C. pneumoniae,* and nine were PCR negative at the end of treatment, documenting clearance of infection. In the placebo arm, 13 patients were positive for *M. pneumoniae or C. pneumoniae.* After treatment, subjects receiving clarithromycin who were positive by PCR had a significant increase in FEV_1. Similar increases were not observed in the placebo groups, whether PCR positive or negative, or in the PCR-negative treatment group (17).

As further evidence of this causal relationship, a double-blind, placebo-controlled trial performed by Black et al. demonstrated that asthmatics with elevated *C. pneumoniae* titers who were treated with roxithromycin for six weeks had a significantly increased mean morning peak expiratory flow of 14 L/min when compared with 8 L/min in subjects receiving placebo. After discontinuation of therapy, a six-month follow-up revealed that this effect had disappeared. However, symptom scores, FEV_1, and use of rescue inhalers remained unchanged (34). In a case series, three elderly prednisone-dependent patients were treated with clarithromycin. Each patient experienced improvement in asthma symptoms, noted by improvements in FEV_1, FVC, and frequency of exacerbations. Two were able to be successfully weaned from prednisone in the long term (35).

In a recent study of azithromycin and the inhaled corticosteroid, budesonide, Strunk et al. evaluated children with moderate to severe asthma aged 6 to 18 years who were treated at one of five Childhood Asthma Research and Education (CARE) Network centers (45). Patients were transitioned to equivalent doses of budesonide and salmeterol twice daily, and budesonide dosing was increased if control was inadequate during the run-in period. After run-in, patients were randomized to three treatment arms: (*i*) placebo; (*ii*) azithromycin 250 or 500 mg, as determined by weight-based dosing, with montelukast placebo; or (*iii*) montelukast 5 or 10 mg, on the basis of age and azithromycin placebo. After randomization, patients underwent four six-week periods of steroid dosing. During first six weeks, budesonide dosing was unchanged. Budesonide dosing was decreased by 25% at the beginning of each of the subsequent six-week periods to 75%, 50%, and 25% of the original dose, respectively. The study was discontinued early after futility analysis demonstrated that it was highly unlikely that either montelukast or azithromycin would provide a steroid-sparing effect for inhaled budesonide (45).

Noneosinophilic asthma (NEA) is often associated with difficult-to-treat steroid-resistant asthma. In a recent study of refractory asthmatics who were optimized on medical therapy with inhaled corticosteroids and long-acting β-agonists, the use of clarithromycin therapy was investigated in a randomized, double-blind, placebo-controlled trial (37). Forty-six patients were enrolled and categorized as having an eosinophilic, paucigranulocytic, or neutrophilic phenotype at screening. Subjects in the treatment arm experienced a significant reduction in airway IL-8 levels from a median of 6.6 ng/mL prior to treatment to 3.9 ng/mL following therapy. Additionally, subjects had a significant reduction in total neutrophil numbers and neutrophil activation. Quality-of-life scores and self-report of wheezing improved in the treatment arm. A subanalysis of NEA patients receiving clarithromycin revealed that the decrease in IL-8 levels was most pronounced in this subgroup of patients. Additionally, the NEA subtype had a more significant improvement in quality of life scores. IL-8 acts as potent chemoattractant and activator of neutrophils and has been demonstrated to be significantly elevated in NEA, which may explain the effects seen with clarithromycin therapy. (37). When results of NEA and chronic asthma studies are compiled, evidence strongly suggests that atypical pathogens are important in the severity of disease, the degree of airway hyper-responsiveness, and asthma chronicity. Furthermore, treatment with macrolide antibiotics appears to be of significant benefit in difficult-to-treat populations of asthmatics.

IV. Immunomodulatory Role of Antibiotics in Asthma

A. Clinical Steroid-Sparing Effects of Antibiotics in Asthma

The steroid-sparing effect of macrolides has been extensively studied since the 1960s. Itkin et al. reported on 12 hospitalized asthmatic patients who were given troleandomycin (TAO), oleandomycin, tetracycline, and placebo for two weeks in random order after a two-week run-in period. TAO significantly decreased blood eosinophil percentage as well as absolute numbers. TAO and oleandomycin also significantly increased the absolute neutrophil count. Three of the twelve patients were noted to have ≥35% increase in FEV_1 on TAO (46). Similar results were seen in a study by Spector et al. (47). In two studies by Zeiger et al. and Siarcua et al., subjects receiving methylprednisolone and TAO experienced increase in FEV_1 and peak expiratory flow as well as a decrease in acute exacerbations. However, steroid-related adverse events were increased in both studies (48,49).

The mechanism of this effect was unclear at the time, but has been further elucidated. On the basis of the above findings, Szefler et al. investigated the role of TAO on methylprednisolone elimination. Ten severe asthmatics, four children and six adults, were given TAO for one week. Methylprednisolone clearance was decreased and half-life was increased significantly after one week of therapy (50). Interestingly, prednisone and prednisolone did not have similar decrease in clearance and increased half-life when used in combination with TAO. On the basis of this and other similar studies, TAO's effect appeared to be related to decreased steroid clearance. However, in a pediatric case report, combination treatment with TAO and methylprednisolone allowed for discontinuation of steroid dosing and TAO use as monotherapy, which suggests an immunomodulatory effect (51). An effect was further evidenced in a double-blind, placebo-controlled trial using low-dose TAO in combination with either methylprednisolone or prednisone or methylprednisolone alone for 12 weeks in children with asthma. A significant reduction in steroid dosing was observed across all arms of the study. Pulmonary functions improved slightly across all groups (52).

In vitro studies of peripheral blood mononuclear cells (PBMCs) isolated from patients, who were defined as either steroid sensitive or steroid resistant, demonstrated that macrolides increase sensitivity to corticosteroids. Initially, Sher et al. reported a significant reduction in glucocorticoid binding affinity, which was not induced by glucocorticoid therapy, in steroid-resistant subjects. Furthermore, they found that this effect was limited to the T-cell population (53). Spahn et al. expanded these findings by demonstrating that clarithromycin improved the ability of dexamethasone to suppress in vitro phytohemaglutinin (PHA)-induced proliferation of PBMCs from seven mild to moderate asthmatics. Subjects were then treated with a 10-day course of clarithromycin, and studies were repeated. Interestingly, lymphocytes were noted to have significantly suppressed response to PHA with clarithromycin alone and required lower doses of dexamethasone before significant PHA proliferation suppression was achieved (54). Erythromycin and clarithromycin in concomitant use with methylprednisolone resulted in reduction of methylprednisolone clearance and a longer half-life (55,56). For clarithromycin, this effect is not observed when prednisone is used concomitantly (55). As mentioned previously, concomitant use of azithromycin with inhaled budesonide failed to provide any steroid-sparing effect (45). Of note, only in vitro changes in steroid sparing were appreciated in these studies, and no conclusion was made regarding the ability to decrease clinical administration of steroids.

B. Anti-inflammatory Role of Macrolide Antibiotics
Mechanism of Action for Immunomodulatory Effects

The synthesis and release of proinflammatory cytokines are affected by the administration of macrolide antibiotics, especially the 14-member ring family. Although studies have shown variable effects, the evidence is compelling that macrolides have anti-inflammatory effects apart from their steroid-sparing properties. Additionally, in terms of airway physiology, macrolides exert significant effects on a variety cell types that compose the airway (Fig. 3).

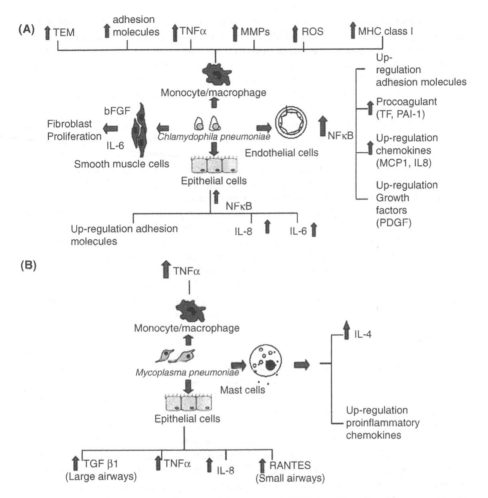

Figure 3 Interaction between *Chlamydophila pneumoniae* (**A**) and *Mycoplasma pneumoniae* (**B**) and different cell types present in the airways. *Abbreviations*: TEM, transendothelial migration; MMPs, matrix metalloproteinases; ROS, reactive oxygen species; MHC, major histocompatibility; NF, nuclear factor; MCP, monocyte chemotatic protein; PDGF, platelet-derived growth factor; bFGF, basic fibroblast growth factor; TF, tissue factor; PAI, plasminogen activator inhibitor; TNF, tumor necrosis factor; TGF, transforming growth factor; RANTES, regulated upon activation normal T cell expressed and secreted; IL, interleukin.

Interleukin-8

IL-8 is known to be a potent neutrophil chemoattractant and an activation factor. Therefore, there has been particular interest in the role of IL-8 in asthma as well as the modulation of its effects. In an in vitro study of eosinophils from atopic dermatitis or allergic asthmatic patients, erythromycin and clarithromycin suppressed the constitutive release of IL-8 as well as the inducible release of IL-8 by IL-1α, whereas josamycin, cefazolin, and tetracycline had no effect. Furthermore, erythromycin did not change IL-8 mRNA expression, suggesting an inhibition of IL-8 release (57,58). However, in a small study of five patients with chronic airway disease who received erythromycin or clarithromycin for more than three months, IL-8 mRNA in the airway was significantly reduced in the postbronchoscopy samples of four patients (58). IL-8 inhibition by roxithromycin has also be demonstrated to function in a dose-dependent fashion before and post stimulation with IL-1α (59).

In in vitro neutrophil studies, therapeutic doses of erythromycin and clarithromycin mildly suppressed production of IL-8 following treatment with lipopolysaccharide (LPS). This effect was also seen when dexamethasone was used but not with josamycin or ampicillin. Additionally, no increase or change in the rate of neutrophil apoptosis was demonstrated (60). These findings suggest that clarithromycin and erythromycin therapy results in neutrophil downregulation.

Nuclear factor kappa B (NF-κB) is the transcription factor for genes encoding many proinflammatory cytokines such as IL-1, IL-6, IL-8, and TNF-α. Given the reduction in IL-8 release seen in macrolide-treated subjects, investigation of the transcriptional regulation of proinflammatory cytokines gene expression has been evaluated. Erythromycin treatment of T cells inhibited transcription of IL-8 via NF-κB pathway but not nuclear factor of activated T cells (NFAT) (61). Further evidence of this effect was seen in PBMC and epithelial cells treated with clarithromycin. NF-κB expression and activation were significantly decreased following clarithromycin therapy (62).

Additional Proinflammatory Cytokines

In addition to IL-8, many other proinflammatory cytokines play a role in asthma. The effect of macrolides on these cytokines is multifaceted. Evaluation of the effects of LPS on monocytes isolated from healthy-donor PBMCs demonstrated production and release of IL-1α, IL-1β, IL-6, IL-10, and TNF-α. Following treatment with telithromycin, clarithromycin, or azithromycin and subsequent stimulation with LPS, IL-1α, and TNF-α, release was significantly inhibited (63–65). When compared with dexamethasone, fosfomycin and clarithromycin had similar suppression of IL-1α, IL-1β, and TNF-α production in LPS-stimulated monocytes in a concentration-dependent manner. However, fosfomycin enhanced production of IL-6 and IL-10 and clarithromycin enhanced production of only IL-10, while dexamethasone, in significant contrast, dramatically suppressed both of these cytokines (66).

In human bronchial epithelial cells, therapeutic doses of erythromycin and clarithromycin suppressed IL-6 release following stimulation with IL-1α. Additionally, erythromycin suppressed the constitutive release of IL-6 (64).

In the Fonseca-Aten et al. studies mentioned earlier, IL-1β, IL-10, and TNF-α concentrations in the nasal aspirates of clarithromycin-treated subjects were significantly reduced compared with placebo-treated subjects. In fact, the reduction in IL-1β, IL-10, and TNF-α persisted at the eight-week follow-up, suggesting that the five-day course of clarithromycin had long-term anti-inflammatory effects. Although the sample size of patients with atypical infections was too small to allow for statistically significant subanalysis, subjects with documented infection had a trend toward significance in the reduction of cytokine levels (28). Furthermore, IL-5 and TNF-α mRNA expression was significantly reduced in subjects receiving clarithromycin who were positive for *M. pneumoniae or C. pneumoniae* by PCR in the study by Kraft et al. mentioned previously (17).

Effects of Macrolides on Specific Cell Populations

The effects of macrolides on discrete cell types, ranging from leukocytes to epithelial cells, have been extensively reported. To expound on the mechanistic role that macrolide treatment has on neutrophil migration, neutrophil chemoattractant activity (NCA) was measured in 13 patients with DPB who were treated with erythromycin for 9 to 11 months. Improvement in FVC percent, FEV_1 percent predicted, and diffusion capacity of lung for carbon monoxide (DLCO) were also observed. Total neutrophil number and NCA were reduced (67). In a mouse model of bleomycin-induced pulmonary fibrosis, macrolide pretreatment inhibited neutrophil infiltration into the airspace following bleomycin treatment (68). Additionally, when treated with macrolides, alveolar macrophages have increased phagocytic activity for epithelial cells and neutrophils (69). As mentioned above, these findings implicate macrolide therapy in the downregulation of neutrophils and may offer an additional treatment modality in the NEA phenotype.

Macrolides potentially play a significant role in many other cells commonly associated with airway inflammatory responses. Eosinophil infiltration of the airway has been associated with hyperresponsiveness. In 17 mild to moderate atopic asthmatics on stable therapy and free of any active infection, clarithromycin treatment for eight weeks improved symptom scores, reduced both blood and sputum eosinophils and eosinophilic cationic protein levels, and decreased methacholine responsiveness (42). A similar effect was noted after treatment with sparfloxacin in the study by Horiguchi et al. mentioned earlier. As further evidence of immune-mediated cellular changes, T-cell proliferative response to mitogens and IL-2 production is suppressed after treatment with clarithromycin, josamycin, and midecamycin (70). The macrolides roxithromycin, clarithromycin, and azithromycin have direct effects on polymorphonuclear leukocyte function with inhibition of the oxidative burst and membrane protection against disruption by bioactive phospholipids (71,72).

Macrolide Effects on Cellular Interaction

In addition to having direct effects on individual cells and populations, macrolides effect the interaction between different cell types. Specifically, roxithromycin decreases intracellular adhesion molecule 1 (ICAM-1) expression in IFN-γ-treated bronchial epithelial cells (59). Roxithromycin also inhibits neutrophil adhesion in a concentration-dependent manner (59). Fourteen-member macrolides' inhibition of ICAM-1 and vascular cell adhesion molecule 1 (VCAM-1) causes a reduction in cellular adhesion between neutrophils and endothelial cells, thereby interrupting the inflammatory cascade (68).

Airway epithelial and goblet cell function is also altered by treatment with macrolides. Following methacholine challenge, nasal secretions were evaluated in ten subjects with purulent rhinitis before and after treatment with clarithromycin. After treatment, nasal secretions of rhinitis patients were similar to healthy controls in terms of hydration, cohesion, and transportability of secretions, and secretion volume was decreased (73). In in vitro studies of clarithromycin- and erythromycin-mediated effects on human nasal epithelial cells, both macrolides reduced mucin production in a dose-dependent manner, although only clarithromycin significantly reduced the TNF-α-mediated release of mucin (74).

Effects of Macrolides on Airway Smooth Muscle

As previously mentioned, erythromycin, roxithromycin, and clarithromycin have significant effects on airway hyperresponsiveness, as evidenced by significant reductions in

PC$_{20}$. The mechanism for this effect has not been completely elucidated. One explanation by Tamaoki et al. was a reduction in bronchial contractility. They noted that erythromycin, roxithromycin, and clarithromycin all significantly reduced the neurally mediated contractile response of human bronchial strips at all doses, suggesting that these medications effect the postganglionic prejunctional site in the cholinergic efferent pathway (75).

Endothelin-1 (ET-1) is a potent bronchoconstrictive peptide, which is increased in patients with asthma. ET-1 is constitutively expressed; increased production and release are observed when stimulated by the proinflammatory cytokines IL-1α, IL-1β, and TNF-α. Following treatment with erythromycin or clarithromycin, human bronchial epithelial cell expression and release of ET-1 were significantly reduced. This effect was also achieved by dexamethasone but not by theophylline, FK506, or salbutamol. Additionally, ET-1 release is significantly higher in culture of bronchial epithelial cells from asthmatics. Erythromycin, clarithromycin, and dexamethasone all induced suppression of ET-1 in this group of patients (76).

V. Conclusions

The antibacterial effects of macrolide antibiotics have been consistently demonstrated and well accepted by the scientific community. *C. pneumoniae* and *M. pneumoniae* are effectively treated with macrolides. While these atypical infections were not previously thought to impact asthma, studies reveal that *C. pneumoniae* and *M. pneumoniae* infections have important clinical relevance in acute exacerbations as well as disease severity and chronicity. Airway hyperresponsiveness, acute exacerbations, and disease chronicity are all impacted by the presence and subsequent elimination of *C. pneumoniae* and *M. pneumoniae* from the airway. Current studies clearly suggest the benefit of macrolide therapy in asthmatics. However, a Cochran review of the literature concluded at this time that there was insufficient evidence to advocate the use of macrolides as an add-on therapeutic option (77). Given the lack of conclusive evidence, further studies are needed to evaluate the effectiveness of macrolides in a large multicenter double-blind, placebo-controlled trial, as well as appropriate dosing and duration of therapy.

The immunomodulatory effects of macrolides extend beyond known antimicrobial effects. The expression and release of proinflammatory cytokines are likely modified by macrolides through the modification of transcription factors such as NF-κB. Cellular changes in the airway are also impacted by the administration of macrolides, specifically when mucous production and neurally mediated airway contraction are evaluated. Effects are noted even in the absence of atypical pathogens. Mounting clinical and scientific evidences suggest that macrolides may be beneficial in the treatment of acute and chronic asthma. However, characterization of the best candidates for macrolide therapy via evaluation of asthma phenotypes requires additional study.

References

1. Eder W, Ege MJ, and von Mutius E. The asthma epidemic. N Engl J Med 2006; 355(21): 2226–2235.
2. Johnston SL, Pattemore PK, Sanderson G, et al. The relationship between upper respiratory infections and hospital admissions for asthma: a time-trend analysis. Am J Respir Crit Care Med 1996; 154(3 pt 1):654–660.

3. Johnston, SL et al. Community study of role of viral infections in exacerbations of asthma in 9–11 year old children. BMJ 1995; 310(6989):1225–1229.
4. Nicholson KG, Kent J, and Ireland DC. Respiratory viruses and exacerbations of asthma in adults. BMJ 1993; 307(6910):982–986.
5. Johnston SL and Martin RJ. Chlamydophila pneumoniae and Mycoplasma pneumoniae: a role in asthma pathogenesis? Am J Respir Crit Care Med 2005; 172(9):1078–1089.
6. Blasi F and Johnston SL. The role of antibiotics in asthma. Int J Antimicrob Agents 2007; 29(5): 485–493.
7. Culic O, Erakovic V, and Parnham MJ. Anti-inflammatory effects of macrolide antibiotics. Eur J Pharmacol 2001; 429(1–3):209–229.
8. Shinkai M, Henke MO, and Rubin BK. Macrolide antibiotics as immunomodulatory medications: proposed mechanisms of action. Pharmacol Ther 2008; 117(3):393–405.
9. Szefler SJ. Anti-inflammatory drugs in the treatment of allergic disease. Med Clin North Am 1992; 76(4):953–975.
10. Saiman L et al. Azithromycin in patients with cystic fibrosis chronically infected with Pseudomonas aeruginosa: a randomized controlled trial. JAMA 2003; 290(13):1749–1756.
11. Kudoh S et al. Improvement of survival in patients with diffuse panbronchiolitis treated with low-dose erythromycin. Am J Respir Crit Care Med 1998; 157(6 pt 1):1829–1832.
12. Kudoh S et al. [Clinical effects of low-dose long-term erythromycin chemotherapy on diffuse panbronchiolitis]. Nihon Kyobu Shikkan Gakkai Zasshi 1987; 25(6):632–642.
13. Cunningham AF et al. Chronic Chlamydia pneumoniae infection and asthma exacerbations in children. Eur Respir J 1998; 11(2):345–349.
14. Freymuth F et al. Detection of viral, Chlamydia pneumoniae and Mycoplasma pneumoniae infections in exacerbations of asthma in children. J Clin Virol 1999; 13(3):131–139.
15. Graham VA et al. Routine antibiotics in hospital management of acute asthma. Lancet 1982; 1(8269):418–420.
16. Expert Panel Report 3 (EPR-3). Guidelines for the Diagnosis and Management of Asthma-Summary Report 2007. J Allergy Clin Immunol 2007; 120(5 suppl 1):S94–S138.
17. Biscione GL et al. Increased frequency of detection of Chlamydophila pneumoniae in asthma. Eur Respir J 2004; 24(5):745–749.
18. Hassan J, Irwin F, Dooley S, et al. Mycoplasma pneumoniae infection in a pediatric population: analysis of soluble immune markers as risk factors for asthma. Hum Immunol 2008; 69(12): 851–855.
19. Pietsch K, Ehlers S, and Jacobs E. Cytokine gene expression in the lungs of BALB/c mice during primary and secondary intranasal infection with Mycoplasma pneumoniae. Microbiology 1994; 140 (pt 8):2043–2048.
20. Zaitsu M. The development of asthma in wheezing infants with Chlamydia pneumoniae infection. J Asthma 2007; 44(7):565–568.
21. Pasternack R, Huhtala H, and Karjalainen J. Chlamydophila (Chlamydia) pneumoniae serology and asthma in adults: a longitudinal analysis. J Allergy Clin Immunol 2005; 116(5): 1123–1128.
22. Biscardi S et al. Mycoplasma pneumoniae and asthma in children (major article). Clin Infect Dis 2004; 38(10):1341(6).
23. Allegra L et al. Acute exacerbations of asthma in adults: role of Chlamydia pneumoniae infection. Eur Respir J 1994; 7(12):2165–2168.
24. Lieberman D et al. Atypical Pathogen Infection in Adults with Acute Exacerbation of Bronchial Asthma. Am J Respir Crit Care Med 2003; 167(3):406–410.
25. Miyashita N et al. Chlamydia pneumoniae and exacerbations of asthma in adults. Ann Allergy Asthma Immunol 1998; 80(5):405–409.
26. Johnston SL et al. The effect of telithromycin in acute exacerbations of asthma. N Engl J Med 2006; 354(15):1589–1600.

27. Kraft M et al. Mycoplasma pneumoniae and Chlamydia pneumoniae in asthma: effect of clarithromycin. Chest 2002; 121(6):1782–1788.
28. Fonseca-Aten M et al. Effect of clarithromycin on cytokines and chemokines in children with an acute exacerbation of recurrent wheezing: a double-blind, randomized, placebo-controlled trial. Ann Allergy Asthma Immunol 2006; 97(4):457–463.
29. Emre U et al. The association of Chlamydia pneumoniae infection and reactive airway disease in children. Arch Pediatr Adolesc Med 1994; 148(7):727–732.
30. Horiguchi T et al. Usefulness of sparfloxacin against Chlamydia pneumoniae infection in patients with bronchial asthma. J Int Med Res 2005; 33(6):668–676.
31. Hahn DL, Anttila T, and Saikku P. Association of Chlamydia pneumoniae IgA antibodies with recently symptomatic asthma. Epidemiol Infect 1996; 117(3):513–517.
32. Martin RJ et al. A link between chronic asthma and chronic infection. J Allergy Clin Immunol 2001; 107(4):595–601.
33. Black PN et al., Serological evidence of infection with Chlamydia pneumoniae is related to the severity of asthma. Eur Respir J 2000; 15(2):254–259.
34. Black PN et al. Trial of roxithromycin in subjects with asthma and serological evidence of infection with Chlamydia pneumoniae. Am J Respir Crit Care Med 2001; 164(4):536–541.
35. Garey KW et al. Long-term clarithromycin decreases prednisone requirements in elderly patients with prednisone-dependent asthma. Chest 2000; 118(6):1826–1827.
36. Hahn DL. Treatment of Chlamydia pneumoniae infection in adult asthma: a before-after trial. J Fam Pract 1995; 41(4):345–351.
37. Simpson JL et al. Clarithromycin targets neutrophilic airway inflammation in refractory asthma. Am J Respir Crit Care Med 2008; 177(2):148–155.
38. Miyatake H et al. Erythromycin reduces the severity of bronchial hyperresponsiveness in asthma. Chest 1991; 99(3):670–673.
39. Shimizu T et al. Roxithromycin reduces the degree of bronchial hyperresponsiveness in children with asthma. Chest 1994; 106(2):458–461.
40. Shimizu T et al. Roxithromycin attenuates acid-induced cough and water-induced bronchoconstriction in children with asthma. J Asthma 1997; 34(3):211–217.
41. Koh YY et al. Effect of roxithromycin on airway responsiveness in children with bronchiectasis: a double-blind, placebo-controlled study. Eur Respir J 1997; 10(5):994–999.
42. Amayasu H et al. Clarithromycin suppresses bronchial hyperresponsiveness associated with eosinophilic inflammation in patients with asthma. Ann Allergy Asthma Immunol 2000; 84(6):594–598.
43. Kostadima E et al. Clarithromycin reduces the severity of bronchial hyperresponsiveness in patients with asthma. Eur Respir J 2004; 23(5):714–717.
44. Ekici A, Ekici M, and Erdemoglu AK. Effect of azithromycin on the severity of bronchial hyperresponsiveness in patients with mild asthma. J Asthma 2002; 39(2):181–185.
45. Strunk RC et al. Azithromycin or montelukast as inhaled corticosteroid-sparing agents in moderate-to-severe childhood asthma study. J Allergy Clin Immunol 2008; 122(6):1138–1144.e4.
46. Itkin IH and Menzel ML. The use of macrolide antibiotic substances in the treatment of asthma. J Allergy 1970; 45(3):146–162.
47. Spector SL, Katz FH, and Farr RS. Troleandomycin: effectiveness in steroid-dependent asthma and bronchitis. J Allergy Clin Immunol 1974; 54(6):367–379.
48. Siracusa A et al. Troleandomycin in the treatment of difficult asthma. J Allergy Clin Immunol 1993; 92(5):677–682.
49. Zeiger RS et al. Efficacy of troleandomycin in outpatients with severe, corticosteroid-dependent asthma. J Allergy Clin Immunol 1980; 66(6):438–446.
50. Szefler SJ et al. The effect of troleandomycin on methylprednisolone elimination. J Allergy Clin Immunol 1980; 66(6):447–451.

51. Rosenberg SM et al. Use of TAO without methylprednisolone in the treatment of severe asthma. Chest 1991; 100(3):849–850.
52. Kamada AK et al. Efficacy and safety of low-dose troleandomycin therapy in children with severe, steroid-requiring asthma. J Allergy Clin Immunol 1993; 91(4):873–882.
53. Sher ER et al. Steroid-resistant asthma. Cellular mechanisms contributing to inadequate response to glucocorticoid therapy. J Clin Invest 1994; 93(1):33–39.
54. Spahn JD et al. Clarithromycin potentiates glucocorticoid responsiveness in patients with asthma: results of a pilot study. Ann Allergy Asthma Immunol 2001; 87(6):501–505.
55. Fost DA et al. Inhibition of methylprednisolone elimination in the presence of clarithromycin therapy. J Allergy Clin Immunol 1999; 103(6):1031–1035.
56. LaForce CF et al. Inhibition of methylprednisolone elimination in the presence of erythromycin therapy. J Allergy Clin Immunol 1983; 72(1):34–39.
57. Kohyama T et al. Fourteen-member macrolides inhibit interleukin-8 release by human eosinophils from atopic donors. Antimicrob Agents Chemother 1999; 43(4):907–911.
58. Takizawa H et al. Erythromycin modulates IL-8 expression in normal and inflamed human bronchial epithelial cells. Am J Respir Crit Care Med 1997; 156(1):266–271.
59. Kawasaki S et al. Roxithromycin inhibits cytokine production by and neutrophil attachment to human bronchial epithelial cells in vitro. Antimicrob Agents Chemother 1998; 42(6):1499–1502.
60. Tsuchihashi Y et al. Fourteen-member macrolides suppress interleukin-8 production but do not promote apoptosis of activated neutrophils. Antimicrob Agents Chemother 2002; 46(4):1101–1104.
61. Aoki Y and Kao PN. Erythromycin inhibits transcriptional activation of NF-kappa B, but not NFAT, through calcineurin-independent signaling in T cells. Antimicrob Agents Chemother 1999; 43(11):2678–2684.
62. Ichiyama T et al. Clarithromycin inhibits NF-{kappa}B activation in human peripheral blood mononuclear cells and pulmonary epithelial cells. Antimicrob Agents Chemother 2001; 45(1):44–47.
63. Khan AA et al. Effect of clarithromycin and azithromycin on production of cytokines by human monocytes. Int J Antimicrob Agents 1999; 11(2):121–132.
64. Takizawa H et al. Erythromycin suppresses interleukin 6 expression by human bronchial epithelial cells: a potential mechanism of its anti-inflammatory action. Biochem Biophys Res Commun 1995; 210(3):781–786.
65. Araujo FG, Slifer TL, and Remington JS. Inhibition of secretion of interleukin-1{alpha} and tumor necrosis factor alpha by the ketolide antibiotic telithromycin. Antimicrob Agents Chemother 2002; 46(10):3327–3330.
66. Morikawa K et al. Modulatory effect of antibiotics on cytokine production by human monocytes in vitro. Antimicrob Agents Chemother 1996; 40(6):1366–1370.
67. Oda H et al. Erythromycin inhibits neutrophil chemotaxis in bronchoalveoli of diffuse panbronchiolitis. Chest 1994; 106(4):1116–1123.
68. Li Y et al. Fourteen-membered ring macrolides inhibit vascular cell adhesion molecule 1 messenger RNA induction and leukocyte migration: role in preventing lung injury and fibrosis in bleomycin-challenged mice. Chest 2002; 122(6):2137–2145.
69. Yamaryo T et al. Fourteen-member macrolides promote the phosphatidylserine receptor-dependent phagocytosis of apoptotic neutrophils by alveolar macrophages. Antimicrob Agents Chemother 2003; 47(1):48–53.
70. Morikawa K et al. Immunomodulatory effects of three macrolides, midecamycin acetate, josamycin, and clarithromycin, on human T-lymphocyte function in vitro. Antimicrob Agents Chemother 1994; 38(11):2643–2647.
71. Feldman C et al. Roxithromycin, clarithromycin, and azithromycin attenuate the injurious effects of bioactive phospholipids on human respiratory epithelium in vitro. Inflammation 1997; 21(6):655–665.

72. Anderson R, Theron AJ, and Feldman C. Membrane-stabilizing, anti-inflammatory inter-actions of macrolides with human neutrophils. Inflammation 1996; 20(6):693–705.
73. Rubin BK et al. Effect of clarithromycin on nasal mucus properties in healthy subjects and in patients with purulent rhinitis. Am J Respir Crit Care Med 1997; 155(6):2018–2023.
74. Shimizu T et al. In vivo and in vitro effects of macrolide antibiotics on mucus secretion in airway epithelial cells. Am J Respir Crit Care Med 2003; 168(5):581–587.
75. Tamaoki J et al. Effects of macrolide antibiotics on neurally mediated contraction of human isolated bronchus. J Allergy Clin Immunol 1995; 95(4):853–859.
76. Takizawa H et al. Erythromycin and clarithromycin attenuate cytokine-induced endothelin-1 expression in human bronchial epithelial cells. Eur Respir J 1998; 12(1):57–63.
77. Richeldi L et al. Macrolides for chronic asthma. Cochrane Database Syst Rev 2005; (4): CD002997.

Index

Milton Keynes UK
Ingram Content Group UK Ltd.
UKHW020030071024
0327UK00032B/2997